DIABETES MELLITUS – INSIGHTS AND PERSPECTIVES

Edited by **Oluwafemi O. Oguntibeju**

Diabetes Mellitus – Insights and Perspectives
http://dx.doi.org/10.5772/3038
Edited by Oluwafemi O. Oguntibeju

Contributors

Alaa Badawi, Bibiana Garcia-Bailo, Paul Arora, Mohammed H. Al Thani, Eman Sadoun, Mamdouh Farid, Ahmed El-Sohemy, Changjin Zhu, Nienke M. Maas- van Schaaijk, Angelique B.C. Roeleveld-Versteegh, Roelof R.J. Odink, Anneloes L. van Baar, Xiaoyun Zhu, Wenglong Huang, Hai Qian, Olabiyi Folorunso, Oluwafemi O. Oguntibeju, Guillaume Aboua, Stefan S. du Plessis, E. J. Truter, A. J. Esterhuyse, Omiepirisa Yvonne Buowari, Yıldırım Çınar, Hakan Demirci, Ilhan Satman, Marco A. López Hernández, N.A. Odunaiya, Monica Daniela Dosa, Cecilia Ruxandra Adumitresi, Laurentiu Tony Hangan, Mihai Nechifor, A. Lukačínová, B. Hubková, O. Rácz, F. Ništiar, Hakan Demirci, Ilhan Satman, Yıldırım Çınar, Nazan Bilgel, Emilia Ciobotaru, Alireza Shahab Jahanlou, Masoud Lotfizade, Nader Alishan Karami

Published by InTech

Janeza Trdine 9, 51000 Rijeka, Croatia

Copyright © 2013 InTech

Notice

Publishing Process Manager Oliver Kurelic
Technical Editor InTech Prepress, Novi Sad
Cover InTech Design team

Additional hard copies can be obtained from orders@intechopen.com

Diabetes Mellitus – Insights and Perspectives, Edited by Oluwafemi O. Oguntibeju
p. cm.
ISBN 978-953-51-0939-6

For EU product safety concerns:
IN TECH d.o.o., Prolaz Marije Krucifikse Kozulić 3, 51000 Rijeka, Croatia,
info@intechopen.com or visit our website at intechopen.com.

Meet the editor

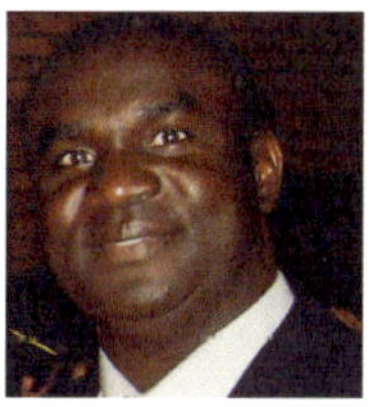

Prof Oluwafemi.O Oguntibeju is an Associate Professor and Group Leader (Nutrition and Chronic Disease Research Unit) at the Oxidative Stress Research Centre in the Department of Biomedical Sciences, Faculty of Health & Wellness, Cape Peninsula University of Technology Bellville, South Africa. He lectures and supervises postgraduate students and collaborates with national and international scientists. Over the years, he has been involved in the field of nutrition and HIV/AIDS and related-public health issues but more recently on diabetes. He has published over 90 scientific papers in peer-reviewed journals, presented over 30 papers at national and international conferences and reviewed manuscripts for over 30 international scientific journals. He has received various awards such as the Gold Research Excellence Award at his current university. Prof O.O Oguntibeju is a National Research Foundation (NRF) C-rated researcher and holds a master degree in Biochemistry from the University of Ibadan, Nigeria and a doctoral degree in Biomedical Science at the Central University of Technology, Bloemfontein, South Africa. He is a Chartered Scientist (CSci, UK) and Fellow of the Institute of Biomedical Science, London. He enjoys reading and music and he is married to Faustina and has four children.

Contents

Preface

The book "Diabetes Mellitus - Insights and Perspectives" is organized into 17 chapters and focused primarily on the management of diabetes mellitus from different perspectives. It also examines animal models in the study and potential management of diabetes mellitus. Each chapter is unique in content, style of writing and scientific and professional background and all these add flavour to the taste of the book. The book provides expert insights and perspectives in terms of scientific and professional knowledge on this important health issue-diabetes mellitus. I strongly believe that scientists, academics and different health professionals would find this book very useful. Students would equally find the scientific and professional insights and perspectives contained in the different chapters very helpful. It is my strong view that this book would add value to the pool of knowledge on the management of diabetes mellitus. The references cited in each chapter definitely acts as additional and important source of information for readers.

Oluwafem. O. Oguntibeju
Department of Biomedical Sciences,
Faculty of Health & Wellness Sciences, Cape Peninsula
University of Technology, Bellville,
South Africa

The Utility of Vitamins in the Prevention of Type 2 Diabetes Mellitus and Its Complications: A Public Health Perspective

Alaa Badawi, Bibiana Garcia-Bailo, Paul Arora, Mohammed H. Al Thani, Eman Sadoun, Mamdouh Farid and Ahmed El-Sohemy

Additional information is available at the end of the chapter

http://dx.doi.org/10.5772/47834

1. Introduction

Type 2 diabetes mellitus (T2DM) is currently considered as a global health problem where about six people die every minute from the disease worldwide. This rate will make T2DM one of the world's most prevalent causes of preventable mortality [1]. T2DM is caused by impaired glucose tolerance (IGT) as a result of insulin resistance and consequential islet β-cell exhaustion, with ensuing insulin deficiency [2]. In individuals with IGT, numerous genetic, host-related, and environmental factors contribute to the progression of insulin resistance to T2DM [3-7]. Obesity, however, is a major cause of insulin resistance [5] and can be complicated by metabolic dysregulation including hypertension and dyslipidemia [known collectively as the metabolic syndrome] which is a precursor of T2DM. The dyslipidemia involves high levels of triacylglycerides and circulating fatty acids originating from the diet or accelerated lipolysis in adipocytes. Direct exposure of muscle cells to these fatty acids impairs insulin-mediated glucose uptake and, therefore, may contribute to insulin resistance [8,9]. Within the last decade, a hypothesis was proposed to explain the pathogenesis of T2DM that connects the disease to a state of subclinical chronic inflammation [10,11]. Inflammation is a short-term adaptive response of the body elicited as a principle component of tissue repair to deal with injuries and microbial infections (e.g., cold, flu, etc.). It can be also elevated in chronic conditions such as peripheral neuropathy, chronic kidney disease and fatty liver. While the influence of fats is well known (see below), current thinking suggests that abnormal levels of chemokines released by the expanding adipose tissue in obesity activate monocytes and increase the secretion of pro-inflammatory adipokines. Such cytokines in turn enhance insulin resistance in adipose and other tissues, thereby increasing the risk for T2DM [12,13]. Together, lipid toxicity and low-grade inflammation appear to be major assaults on insulin sensitivity in insulin-responding tissues [9,14,15].

Activation of innate immunity promotes various inflammatory reactions that provide the first line of defense the body invokes against microbial, chemical, and physical injury, leading to repair of damage, isolation of microbial infectious threats and restoration of tissue homeostasis [16,17]. Inherited variations in the degree of innate immune response may determine the lifetime risk of diseases upon exposure to adverse environmental stimuli [18]. Therefore, innate immune responses can be viewed as the outcome of interaction between genetic endowment and the environment [19].

This article was undertaken in an attempt to evaluate the current knowledge linking vitamin intake to attenuating inflammation, and thereby reducing the risk of T2DM and its complications.

2. Micronutrients, T2DM and inflammation

Factors that attenuate inflammation could provide an important public health tool to reduce the burden of diseases related to this pathway, such as obesity, T2DM and cardiovascular diseases, in the general population. The feasibility of modulating innate immunity-related inflammation as an approach for the prevention of T2DM is based on reports that evaluated the efficacy of anti-inflammatory pharmaceutical agents on disease manifestation and outcome [12,20].

A therapeutic strategy for T2DM that would act primary on the inflammatory system has been proposed in the form of salicylates, an anti-inflammatory agent long known to have a hypoglycemic effect [21,22]. Nonsteroidal anti-inflammatory drugs (NSAIDs) and cyclooxygenase inhibitors are able to enhance glucose-induced insulin release, improve glucose tolerance, and increase the effect of insulin in patients with T2DM [15,23,24]. In humans, treatment with NSAIDs improved various biochemical indices associated with T2DM [25]. Although these observations support the notion that inflammation plays a pivotal role in T2DM, attenuating inflammation as a strategy for disease prevention in a public health setting will necessitate a substantially different perspective. In this case, a strategy that can be introduced into the general population with the least (if any) side effects and the maximal preventive outcome should be adopted. In this context, a nutritional intervention approach would be a desirable option.

Numerous nutritional factors can modify innate immune-related responses and, subsequently, modify the risk of a range of chronic conditions. With respect to T2DM, the consensus of available information suggests that micronutrient intake modulates the innate immune system [26] and can subsequently influence the predisposition to [and prevention of] disease [26-28]. By virtue of this observation, the hope is that the outcome of nutritional supplementation can be simply monitored via its modifying action on the levels of inflammatory biomarkers. Many micronutrients exhibit well-characterized anti-inflammatory or immunomodulatory functions [25]. Vitamins (e.g., D, E, and C), certain fatty acids (e.g., omega-3 fatty acid) and trace elements (e.g., selenium, zinc, copper and iron) are known to improve the overall function of the immune system, prevent excessive expression and synthesis of inflammatory cytokines, and increase the 'oxidative burst' potential of macrophages [25]. Vitamin C is the major water-soluble dietary antioxidant anti-inflammatory factor, exerting its actions in the aqueous phase. In contrast, vitamins E and D are lipid-soluble and protect against inflammation in the lipid phase, e.g., adipocytes. Although acting primarily in different phases, these micronutrients can function together by regenerating each other in the reduced form [29]. Indeed, exploring the possibility that supplementation with selected micronutrients can attenuate obesity-related inflammation in order to delay the development of T2DM should be considered alongside existing public health practices to reduce the disease rising rates.

3. Vitamin C

Vitamin C (ascorbic acid or ascorbate), an essential nutrient, is a 6-carbon lactone and the primary hydrophilic antioxidant found in human plasma [30]. Circulating concentrations of ascorbate in blood are considered adequate if at least 28 μM, but they are considerably higher in most cells due to active transport. The daily recommended dietary allowance for vitamin C is 75 mg for women and 90 mg for men, with an additional 35 mg for smokers due to the higher metabolic turnover of the vitamin in this group as compared to non-smokers [31]. Ascorbate appears in the urine at intakes of roughly 60 mg/day. However, the results of a depletion/repletion study in healthy young women showed that ascorbate plasma and white blood cell concentrations only saturate at intakes of 200 mg/day or higher [32]. These results suggest that the current dietary recommendations may not provide tissue-saturating ascorbate concentrations [33]. Indeed, epidemiologic findings suggest that serum ascorbic acid deficiency may be relatively common. For example, a recent cross-sectional survey of healthy young adults of the Toronto Nutrigenomics and Health (TNH) Study reported that 1 out 7 individuals is deficient in serum ascorbic acid [34].

Vitamin C has an important role in immune function and various oxidative and inflammatory processes, such as scavenging reactive oxygen species (ROS), preventing the initiation of chain reactions that lead to protein glycation [31;35] and protecting against lipid peroxidation [31, 36]. The oxidized products of vitamin C, ascorbyl radical and dehydroascorbic acid, are easily regenerated to ascorbic acid by glutathione, NADH or NADPH [31]. In addition, ascorbate can recycle vitamin E and glutathione back from their oxidized forms [31, 33]. For this reason, there has been interest in determining whether vitamin C might be used as a therapeutic agent against the oxidative stress and subsequent inflammation associated with T2DM.

A variety of epidemiologic studies have assessed the effect of vitamin C on biomarkers of oxidation, inflammation and/or T2DM risk [30, 37-42]. A large cross-sectional evaluation of healthy elderly men from the British Regional Heart Study reported that plasma vitamin C, dietary vitamin C and fruit intake were inversely correlated with serum CRP and tissue plasminogen activator [tPA], a biomarker of endothelial disfunction [134]. However, only plasma vitamin C was inversely associated with fibrinogen levels [30]. Another cross-sectional study of adolescents aged 13-17 found inverse associations between intakes of fruit, vegetables, legumes and vitamin C and urinary F_2-isoprostane, CRP, and IL-6 [43]. A recent cross-sectional evaluation of healthy young adults from the TNH Study demonstrated that serum ascorbic acid deficiency is associated with elevated CRP and other factors related to the metabolic syndrome such as waist circumference, BMI and high blood pressure [34]. Finally, the European Prospective Investigation of Cancer (EPIC)-Norfolk Prospective Study examined the link between fruit and vegetable intake and plasma levels of vitamin C and risk of T2DM. During 12-year follow-up, 735 incident cases of diabetes were identified among nearly 21,000 participants [44]. A significant inverse association was found between plasma levels of vitamin C and risk of diabetes (OR=0.38, 95% CI=0.28-0.52). In the same study, a similar association was observed between fruit and vegetable intake and T2DM risk (OR=0.78, 95% CI=0.60-1.00) [44].

Despite epidemiologic findings generally pointing towards an association between increased vitamin C and reduced oxidation and inflammation, intervention trials assessing the effect of vitamin C supplementation on various markers of T2DM have yielded inconsistent results. One randomized, cross-over, double-blind intervention trial reported no improvement in fasting plasma glucose and no significant differences in levels of CRP, IL-6, IL-1 receptor agonist or oxidized LDL after supplementation with 3000 mg/day of vitamin C for 2 weeks in a group of 20 T2DM patients, compared to baseline levels [45]. Chen and colleagues performed a randomized, controlled, double-blind intervention on a group of 32 diabetic subjects with inadequate levels of vitamin C and found no significant changes in either fasting glucose or fasting insulin after intake of 800 mg/day of vitamin C for 4 weeks [46].

On the other hand, Wang and colleagues showed that the red blood cell sorbitol/plasma glucose ratio was reduced after supplementation with 1000 mg/day vitamin C for 2 weeks in a group of eight diabetics, although no differences were found in fasting plasma glucose [47]. Since sorbitol is a product of the pro-oxidative polyol pathway, this observation may suggest an inhibition of the polyol pathway by vitamin C among subjects with diabetes. Another study has shown that daily intake of ascorbic acid at 2000 mg/day improved fasting plasma glucose, HbA1c, cholesterol levels and triglycerides in 56 diabetics [48]. In agreement, Paolisso *et. al.* found that 1000 mg/day of vitamin C for 4 months improved LDL and total cholesterol, fasting plasma insulin and free radicals, although it did not affect triglycerides or HDL levels in a group of 40 diabetics [49].

Overall, it remains unclear whether vitamin C intake has an effect on factors related to T2DM. Although the epidemiologic evidence suggests that vitamin C, whether as a supplement or as part of a diet rich in fruits and vegetables, beneficially affects inflammatory markers and disease risk, the results of intervention trials in T2DM are conflicting. Small sample sizes, genetic variation, short intervention duration, insufficient dosage and disease status of the assessed cohorts may account for the lack of effect and the inconsistent outcomes observed in intervention studies. However, it is possible also that the status of vitamin C deficiency is a result of the oxidative and pro-inflammatory challenges associated with T2DM rather than a determinant of disease pathogenesis. Therefore, further research and long-term prospective studies are needed to elucidate the role of vitamin C as a modulator of inflammation and T2DM risk, and to evaluate its potential role as a preventive agent at a population level.

4. Vitamin E

Vitamin E encompasses a group of 8 compounds, including α, β, γ, and δ tocopherols and α, β, γ, and δ tocotrienols, with differing biological activities. Each compound contains a hydroxyl-containing chromanol ring with a varying number and position of methyl groups between the α, β, γ, and δ forms [29]. It is known to have a significant impact on improving a variety of immune functions [50]. Supplementation with vitamin E increases the rate of lymphocyte proliferation by enhancing the ability of T cells to undergo cell division cycles [51]. The effective anti-inflammatory action of vitamin E was substantiated from observations such as the increased expression of the *IL-2* gene and IL-1 receptor antagonist and the decreased expression of IL 4 following vitamin E supplementation in animal models [50]. Furthermore, vitamin E reduced the serum levels of inflammatory factors such as IL-1β, IL-6, TNF-α , PAI-1, and CRP in T2DM patients [52, 53]. Furthermore, vitamin E downregulates NFκB [52], the principal mediator of inflammatory signaling cascade and its potent lipophilic antioxidant effect on internal and external cell membranes as well as plasma lipoproteins, notably LDL. Based on this latter characteristic, studies in both animal models and humans have demonstrated that vitamin E intake blocks LDL lipid peroxidation, prevents the oxidative stress linked to T2DM-associated abnormal metabolic patterns [hyperglycemia, dyslipidemia, and elevated levels of FFAs], and, subsequently, attenuates cytokine gene expression [50, 52, 56, 57]. Despite these findings, a recent study evaluated the effects of a combination of vitamin C (1000 mg/day) and vitamin E (400 IU/day) for four weeks on insulin sensitivity in untrained and trained healthy young men and concluded that such supplementation may preclude the exercise-induced amelioration of insulin resistance in humans [58]. This may relate to the source of vitamin E used, i.e., α-, β-, γ-, or δ-tocopherol [59].

Overall, the immunomodulatory, anti-inflammatory and anti-oxidative functions of vitamin E strongly support its possible application in designing effective prevention and/or treatment protocols for T2DM [25, 56]. Current practices for diabetes prevention in the general population include lifestyle change, dietary intervention and exercise. Vitamin E supplementation may further aid in T2DM prevention and control through its anti-oxidant, anti-inflammatory and immunomodulatory properties. It seems reasonable, therefore, to suggest supplementation with vitamin E together with lifestyle change may be combined into a single program to enhance the success and effectiveness of intervention. This strategy could be more efficient in reducing the low-grade inflammation associated with pre-clinical T2DM and, subsequently the disease burden, than when a single approach is considered. Moreover, such a combined strategy can be introduced in general practice settings and in a population-based fashion with low expenditure and minimal side effects.

5. Vitamin D

The role of vitamin D in calcium and phosphorus homeostasis and bone metabolism is well understood. However, more recently vitamin D and calcium homeostasis have also been linked to a number of conditions, such as neuromuscular function, cancer, and a wide range of chronic diseases, including autoimmune diseases, atherosclerosis, obesity, cardiovascular diseases, diabetes and associated conditions such as the metabolic syndrome and insulin resistance [25, 60-63]. In T2DM, the role of vitamin D was suggested from the presence of vitamin D receptors (VDR) in the pancreatic β-islet cells [63]. In these cells, the biologically active metabolite of vitamin D (*i.e.*, 1,25-dihydroxy-vitamin D; 1,25[OH]D) [64] enhances insulin production and secretion *via* its action on the VDR [63]. Indeed, the presence of vitamin D binding protein (DBP), a major predictor of serum levels of 25(OH)D and response to vitamin D supplementation [65, 66], and VDR initiated several studies demonstrating a relationship between single nucleotide polymorphisms (SNPs) in the genes regulating *VDR* and *DBP* and glucose intolerance and insulin secretion [67-69]. This further supports a role for vitamin D in T2DM and may explain the reduced overall risk of the disease in subjects who ingest >800 IU/d of vitamin D [61,70]. However, an alternative, and perhaps related, explanation was recently proposed for the role of vitamin D in T2DM prevention based on its potent immunomodulatory functions [71-73]. 1,25(OH)D modulates the production of the immunostimulatory IL-12 and the immunosuppressive IL-10 [74] and VDRs are present in most types of immune cells [75]. In this respect, supplementation with vitamin D [76] or its bioactive form, 1,25(OH)D [64], improved insulin sensitivity by preventing the excessive synthesis of inflammatory cytokines. This effect of vitamin D on cytokine synthesis is due to its interaction with vitamin D response elements (VDRE) present in the promoter region of cytokine-encoding genes. This interaction downregulates the transcriptional activities of cytokine genes and attenuates the synthesis of the corresponding proteins [76]. Vitamin D also deactivates NFκB, which transcriptionally upregulates the pro-inflammatory cytokine-encoding genes [77]. Downregulating the expression of NFκB and downstream cytokine genes inhibits β-cell apoptosis and promotes their survival [76].

As reviewed by Pittas et al [78], a number of cross-sectional studies in both healthy and diabetic cohorts have shown an inverse association between serum 25(OH)D and glycemic status measures such as fasting plasma glucose, oral glucose tolerance tests, hemoglobin A1c (HbA1c), and insulin resistance as measured by the homeostatic model assessment (HOMA-R), as well as the metabolic syndrome [79-84]. For example, data from the National Health and Nutrition Examination Survey (NHANES) showed an inverse, dose-dependent association between serum 25(OH)D and diabetes prevalence in non-Hispanic whites and Mexican Americans, but not in non-Hispanic blacks [81,84]. The same inverse trend was observed between serum 25(OH)D and insulin resistance as measured by HOMA-R, but there was no correlation between serum levels of vitamin D and β-cell function, as measured by HOMA-β [81,84]. Data from the same cohort also showed an inverse association between 25(OH)D and prevalence of the metabolic syndrome [81].

In prospective studies, dietary vitamin D intake has been associated with incidence of T2DM. For example, data from the Women's Health Study showed that, among middle-aged and older women, taking >511 IU/day of vitamin D reduced the risk of developing T2DM, as compared to ingesting 159 IU/day [85]. Furthermore, data from the Nurses Health Study also found a significant inverse correlation between total vitamin D intake and T2DM risk, even after adjusting for BMI, age, and non-dietary covariates [70]. Intervention studies have shown conflicting results about the effect of vitamin D on T2DM incidence. One study reported that supplementation with 1,25$[OH]_2D_3$ for 1 week did not affect fasting glucose or insulin sensitivity in 18 young healthy men [86]. Another study found that, among 14 T2DM patients, supplementing with 80 IU/day of 1 α-OHD_3 ameliorated insulin secretion but did not improve glucose tolerance after a 75 g oral load [87]. Yet another study showed that, among 65 middle-aged men who had IGT or mild T2DM and adequate serum vitamin D levels at baseline, supplementation with 30 IU/day of 1-α-OHD_3 for 3 months affected neither fasting nor stimulated glucose tolerance [88]. However, in a cross-over design, 20 diabetics with inadequate vitamin D serum levels who were given 40 IU/day of 1,25-OHD for 4 days had improved insulin secretion, but showed no changes in fasting or stimulated glucose or insulin concentrations [89]. Although the short duration of this cross-over trial may account for the lack of a significant overall effect, the results suggest that improving vitamin D status can modulate factors associated with the development and progression of T2DM.

The data from a 2-year-long trial designed to assess the effects of vitamin D_3 or 1-α-OHD_3 supplementation on bone health in non-diabetic postmenopausal women were analyzed *a posteriori* and found no significant effect on fasting glucose levels [90]. A *post-hoc* analysis of data from a 3-year trial for bone health showed that daily supplementation with 700 IU of vitamin D_3 and 500 mg of calcium citrate malate did not change blood glucose levels or insulin resistance in elderly adults with normal glucose tolerance. These measures, however, were significantly improved in subjects with IGT at baseline [91]. In this trial the effect of fasting glucose levels in the high-risk group (*i.e.*, IGT) was similar to that observed in the Diabetes Prevention Program after an intensive lifestyle intervention or metformin treatment [92]. Taken together, the available information warrants exploring the possibility that vitamin D (alone or in combination with calcium) can be employed in developing population-based strategies for T2DM prevention and control.

6. β-carotene and lycopene

As previously stated, oxidative stress is involved in the development and complications of T2DM [60]. Patients with T2DM exhibit a reduced antioxidative defence, which negatively correlates with glucose levels and duration of the disease [93]. In diabetic subjects, the lack of metabolic homeostasis, the increased plasma ROS generation and the decreased efficiency of inhibitory and scavenger systems [60], all can that result in a status of oxidative stress that can have an etiological role in T2DM complications, e.g., retinopathy, chronic kidney disease, and cardiovascular diseases [94]. The synthesis of ROS was proposed to be primarily due to hyperglycaemia [95] resulting in stimulation of the polyol pathway, formation of advanced glycosylation endproducts, and subsequent formation of ROS. Hyperinsulinaemia, insulin resistance and inflammation, may all play a role in the synthesis of ROS in pre-diabetic and diabetic patients [60].

As we reviewed recently, the risk of T2DM can be mitigated by increased antioxidants intake [60]. Intake of α- and β-carotene and lycopene has been shown to improve glucose metabolism in subjects at high risk of T2DM [96], and glucose metabolism has been associated with oxidative stress [95]. Indeed, diabetic patients have shown a predominantly elevated levels of lipid peroxidation (F_2-isoprostanes) [97]. *In vivo* lipid peroxidation, measured as F_2-isoprostanes, apprears to be influenced by the consumption of dietary components such as antioxidants. It is therefore critical to examine the dietary effects of α- and β-carotene and lycopeneon lipid peroxidation in patients with T2DM. The relationship between plasma levels of antioxidants and markers of oxidative stress and inflammation have been described in healthy population [58,98] and is yet to be identified in diabetic subjects. This will allow us to better define the role of α- and β-carotene and lycopene in attenuating inflammation and modulating the oxidative stress during the course of T2DM development and progression.

7. T2DM complications: Cardiometabolic disease

It is well-established that T2DM is a risk factor for cardiometabolic diseases. Studies from our group demonstrated a relationship between T2DM and its risk factors and cardiometabolic disease markers [98,99]. We observed an apparent profile of metabolic phenotypes and inflammatory biomarkers, known to be related to the cardiometabolic disease risk, that emerges with the susceptibility to T2DM. These findings allowed us to establish a composite metabolic trait that lead to the development of improved strategies for early risk prediction and intervention.

In the same study population, we further demonstrated an association between plasma vitamin D level and T2DM risk, e.g., insulin resistance [100]. We found that the likelihood that T2DM develops and results in related complications is further increased as plasma vitamin D levels decrease. These studies highlights the possibility that micronutrient supplementation can be employed in the prevention of various T2Dm complications including cardimetabolic diseases. Moreover, there is a need to develop adequately powered randomized controlled clinical trials to evaluate the value of replenishment of vitamin D on T2DM and the related conditions, e.g., obesity, insulin resistance and cardiovascular diseases, as an approach for an effective population based strategy for disease prevention.

8. Public health prespectives

Introducing novel and effective prevention strategies in a public health setting necessitates considering approaches with the least [if any] side effects and the maximal preventive efficacy and outcome. Furthermore, the heterogeneity of the general Western population in terms of culture, location and resources renders creating a unified intervention program a formidable endeavour. In this context, applying nutritional intervention as an approach to attenuate inflammation and oxidative stress would be a feasible public health strategy for the T2DM. A conceptual model need to be implemented to improve the availability and accessibility of nutritious food as a factor that can be integrated into a comprehensive public health intervention strategy aimed at T2DM prevention.

Combining micronutrients supplementation or encouraging the consumption of nutritious diet should be explored in pre-diabetic subjects and the outcome should be compared to the effect(s) of changing current practices, such as lifestyle change, dietary intervention and exercise. The effectiveness of lifestyle-change intervention programmes for pre-diabetes also shows a promising effect on the reduction of overall incidence of T2DM or its complications, and it can be implemented in general clinical practice [95]. A lifestyle-change programme including increased exercise and diet change (either by reduction in glycemic load or reduced-fat diet) demonstrated a significant difference between control and intervention groups in markers for risk of progression to T2DM including weight, BMI, and waist circumference [101]. In general, current approaches for the prevention of T2DM have been shown to be effective in delaying or preventing the progression from pre-diabetes to diabetes [102]. In patients with insulin resistance, these practices are known to improve insulin sensitivity and the overall predisposition to T2DM [103]. On the other hand, increasing intake of vitamin D to greater than 800 IU daily along with 1200 mg of calcium was reported to reduce the risk of developing T2DM by 33% [78]. In agreement, healthy older adults with impaired fasting glucose showed significant improvement in attenuating the glycemic response and insulin resistance when they increased the vitamin D to 700 IU/d and calcium to 500 mg/d for 3 yrs [70]. It seems reasonable, therefore, to suggest that the two preventive approaches for T2DM, *i.e.*, micronutrient supplementation and lifestyle change, may be combined into a single successful intervention programme. This strategy may be more efficient in reducing the burden of the disease in the general population and in vulnerable subpopulations than when a single approach is proposed. Moreover, such a combined approach may be introduced into the general practice setting and to the general population with low expenditure and minimal side effects [25,60].

Overall, the current state of knowledge warrants further study into the extent to which micronutrients can modify the association between markers of inflammation and oxidative stress and early stages of T2DM. There is evidence supporting the idea that vitamin supplementation can modify the genotype-phenotype association within the innate immune response (*i.e.*, the pro-inflammatory and inflammatory markers), and that it has an ameliorating effect on oxidative stress and the subsequent inflammatory signalling. This proposition may provide the mechanism by which nutritional factors prevent or delay disease development and can be introduced into the general population, as well as susceptible subpopulations. In relation to the current preventive approaches for T2DM, *e.g.*, lifestyle changes, exercise, and dietary intervention, exploring the efficacy of micronutrient supplementation on attenuating oxidative stress, the innate immune response and the ensuing inflammation and evaluating the outcome of this strategy on T2DM incidence may be assessed through a series of prospective population-based studies, first, to determine the feasibility and effectiveness of this protocol; second, to validate and evaluate this strategy and ensure replication of results; and, third, to monitor the outcome to quantify the overall preventive response in comparison with the current approaches.

Author details

Alaa Badawi*

Office for Biotechnology, Genomics and Population Health, Public Health Agency of Canada, Toronto, ON, Canada

---

* Corresponding Author

Bibiana Garcia-Bailo
Office for Biotechnology, Genomics and Population Health, Public Health Agency of Canada, Toronto, ON, Canada
Department of Nutritional Sciences, Faculty of Medicine, University of Toronto, ON, Canada

Paul Arora
Office for Biotechnology, Genomics and Population Health, Public Health Agency of Canada, Toronto, ON, Canada
Dalla Lana School of Public Health, University of Toronto, Toronto, ON, Canada

Mohammed H. Al Thani and Eman Sadoun
Supreme Council of Health, Doha, Qatar

Mamdouh Farid
Queen Medical research Office, Doha, Qatar

Ahmed El-Sohemy
Department of Nutritional Sciences, Faculty of Medicine, University of Toronto, ON, Canada

Acknowledgement

This work is supported by the Public Health Agency of Canada.

9. References

[1] Wild S, Rolic C, Green A. Global prevalence of diabetes: Estimates for the year 2000 and projection for 2030. Diabetes Care. 2004;37:1047–1053.
[2] Stumvoll M, Goldstein B, van Haeften T. Type 2 diabetes: principles of pathogenesis and therapy. Lancet. 2005;365:1333–1346.
[3] Zimmet P, Alberti KG, Shaw J. Global and societal implications of the diabetes epidemic. Nature. 2001;414:782–787.
[4] Alberti KG. Treating type 2 diabetes–today's targets, tomorrow's goals. Diabetes Obesity Metabolism. 2001;3(Suppl 1):S3–S10.
[5] Dandona P, Aljada A, Bandyopadhyay A. Inflammation: the link between insulin resistance, obesity and diabetes. Trends Immunology. 2004;25:4–7.
[6] Dandona P, Aljada A. A rational approach to pathogenesis and treatment of type 2 diabetes mellitus, insulin resistance, inflammation, and atherosclerosis. American Journal Cardiology. 2002;90:27G–33G.
[7] Dandona P, Aljada A, Chaudhuri A, Bandyopadhyay A. The potential influence of inflammation and insulin resistance on the pathogenesis and treatment of atherosclerosis-related complications in type 2 diabetes. Journal Clinical Endocrinology Metabolism. 2003;88:2422–2429.
[8] Dimopoulos N, Watson M, Sakamoto K, Hundal HS. Differential effects of palmitate and palmitoleate on insulin action and glucose utilization in raty L6 skeletal muscle cells. Biochemistry Journal. 2006;399:473–481.

[9] Bilan PJ, Samokhvalov V, Koshkina A, Schertzer JD, Samaan MC, Klip A. Direct and macrophage-mediated actions of fatty acids causing insulin resistance in muscle cells. Archive Physiology Biochemistry. 2009;115:176–190.
[10] Pickup JC, Crook MA. Is type II diabetes mellitus a disease of the innate immune system? Diabetologia. 1998;41:1241–1248.
[11] Pickup JC, Matttock MB, Chusney GD, Burt D. NIDDM as a disease of the innate immune system: association of acute phase reactants and interleukin-6 with metabolic syndrome X. Diabetologia. 1997;40:1286–1292.
[12] King GL. The role of inflammatory cytokines in diabetes and its complications. Journal Periodontology. 2008;79:1527–1534.
[13] Larsen GL, Henson PM. Mediators of inflammation. Annals Review Immunology. 1983;1:335–359.
[14] Hotamisligil GS, Shargill NS, Spiegelman BM. Adipose expression of tumor necrosis factor-alpha: direct role in obesity-linked insulin resistance. Science. 1993;259:87–91.
[15] Hotamisligil GS. Inflammation and metabolic disorders. Nature. 2006;444:860–867.
[16] Beutler B. Innate immunity: an overview. Molecular Immunology. 2004;40:845–859.
[17] Takeda K, Akira S. TLR signaling pathways. Seminars Immunology. 2004;16:3–9.
[18] Le Souëf PN. Gene-environmental interaction in the development of atopic asthma: new developments. Current Opinion Allergy Clinical Immunology. 2009;9:123–127.
[19] Fernandez-Real JM, Pickup JC. Innate immunity, insulin resistance and type 2 diabetes. Trends Endocrinology Metabolism. 2007; 19:10–16.
[20] Liu G, Rondinone CM. JNK: bridging the insulin signaling and inflammatory pathway. Curr Opin Investig Drugs. 2005; 6:979–987.
[21] Robertson RP. Prostaglandins as modulators of pancreatic islet function. Diabetes. 1979;28:942–948.
[22] Robertson RP. Arachidonic acid metabolism, the endocrine pancreas, and diabetes mellitus. Pharmacology Therapy. 1984;24:91–106.
[23] Wellen KE, Hotamisligil GS. Inflammation, stress, and diabetes. Journal Clinical Investigation. 2005;115:1111–1119.
[24] Hundal RS, Peterson KF, Mayerson AB, et al. Mechanism by which high-dose aspirin improves glucose metabolism in type 2 diabetes. Journal Clinical Investigation. 2002;109:1321–1326.
[25] Badawi, A., Klip, A., Haddad, P., Cole, D.E.C., Bailo, B.G., El-Sohemy, A., and Karmali, M. Type 2 diabetes mellitus and inflammation: Prospects for biomarkers of risk and nutritional intervention. Diabetes Metabolic Syndrome Obesity. 2010;3:173-186.
[26] Maggini S, Wintergerst ES, Beveridge S, Hornig DH. Selected vitamins and trace elements support immune function by strengthening epithelial barriers and cellular and humoral immune responses. British Journal Nutrition 2007;98(Suppl 1):S29–S35.
[27] Pittas AG, Lau J, Hu FB, Dawson-Hughes B. Review: The role of vitamin D and calcium in type 2 diabetes. A systematic review and meta-analysis. Journal Clinical Endocrinology Metabolism. 2007;92:2017–2029.
[28] Pittas AG, Dawson-Hughes B, Li T, et al. Vitamin D and calcium intake in relation to type 2 diabetes in women. Diabetes Care. 2006;29:650–656.

[29] Da Costa, L.A., García-Bailo, B., Badawi, A., and El-Sohemy, A. Genetic determinants of dietary antioxidant status. In: Bouchard, C. and Ordovas, J.M. [eds.]. Recent Advances in Nutrigenetics and Nutrigenomics. Elsevier, New York, NY. 2012, in press.

[30] Wannamethee SG, Lowe GD, Rumley A, Bruckdorfer KR, Whincup PH. Associations of vitamin C status, fruit and vegetable intakes, and markers of inflammation and hemostasis. American Journal Clinical Nutrition 2006;83:567-574.

[31] Calder PC, Albers R, Antoine JM, Blum S, Bourdet-Sicard R, Ferns GA, Folkerts G, Friedmann PS, Frost GS, Guarner F, Lovik M, Macfarlane S, Meyer PD, M'Rabet L, Serafini M, et al. Inflammatory disease processes and interactions with nutrition. British Journal Nutrition 2009;101 (Suppl 1):S1-S45.

[32] Levine M, Wang Y, Padayatty SJ, Morrow J. A new recommended dietary allowance of vitamin C for healthy young women. Proceedings National Acadamy Science USA. 2001; 98:9842-9846.

[33] Aguirre R, May JM. Inflammation in the vascular bed: importance of vitamin C. Pharmacolocial Therapy. 2008;119:96-103.

[34] Cahill L, Corey PN, El-Sohemy A. Vitamin C deficiency in a population of young Canadian adults. American Journal Epidemiology. 2009;170:464-471.

[35] Bartlett HE, Eperjesi F. Nutritional supplementation for type 2 diabetes: a systematic review. Ophthalmic Physiology Opt. 2008; 28:503-523.

[36] Young IS, Tate S, Lightbody JH, McMaster D, Trimble ER. The effects of desferrioxamine and ascorbate on oxidative stress in the streptozotocin diabetic rat. Free Radical Biology Medicine 1995;18:833-840.

[37] Ford ES, Liu S, Mannino DM, Giles WH, Smith SJ. C-reactive protein concentration and concentrations of blood vitamins, carotenoids, and selenium among United States adults. European Journal Clinical Nutrition 2003; 57:1157-1163.

[38] Hamer M, Chida Y. Intake of fruit, vegetables, and antioxidants and risk of type 2 diabetes: systematic review and meta-analysis. Journal Hypertension 2007;25:2361-2369.

[39] Woodward M, Lowe GD, Rumley A, Tunstall-Pedoe H, Philippou H, Lane DA, Morrison CE. Epidemiology of coagulation factors, inhibitors and activation markers: The Third Glasgow MONICA Survey. II. Relationships to cardiovascular risk factors and prevalent cardiovascular disease. British Journal Haematology. 1997;97:785-797.

[40] Woodward M, Rumley A, Tunstall-Pedoe H, Lowe GD. Associations of blood rheology and interleukin-6 with cardiovascular risk factors and prevalent cardiovascular disease. British Journal Haematology. 1999; 104:246-257.

[41] Woodward M, Rumley A, Lowe GD, Tunstall-Pedoe H. C-reactive protein: associations with haematological variables, cardiovascular risk factors and prevalent cardiovascular disease. British Journal Haematology 2003;122:135-141.

[42] Gao X, Bermudez OI, Tucker KL. Plasma C-reactive protein and homocysteine concentrations are related to frequent fruit and vegetable intake in Hispanic and non-Hispanic white elders. Journal Nutrition. 2004;134:913-918.

[43] Holt EM, Steffen LM, Moran A, Basu S, Steinberger J, Ross JA, Hong CP, Sinaiko AR. Fruit and vegetable consumption and its relation to markers of inflammation and

oxidative stress in adolescents. Journal American Dietetics Association 2009;109:414-421.

[44] Harding AH, Wareham NJ, Bingham SA, Khaw K, Luben R, Welch A, Forouhi NG. Plasma vitamin C level, fruit and vegetable consumption, and the risk of new-onset type 2 diabetes mellitus: the European prospective investigation of cancer--Norfolk prospective study. Archives Internal Medicine. 2008; 168:1493-1499.

[45] Lu, Q, Bjorkhem,I, Wretlind,B, Diczfalusy,U, Henriksson,P, Freyschuss,A: Effect of ascorbic acid on microcirculation in patients with Type II diabetes: a randomized placebo-controlled cross-over study. Clinical Science. 2005;108:507-513.

[46] Chen H, Karne RJ, Hall G, Campia U, Panza JA, Cannon RO, III, Wang Y, Katz A, Levine M, Quon MJ. High-dose oral vitamin C partially replenishes vitamin C levels in patients with Type 2 diabetes and low vitamin C levels but does not improve endothelial dysfunction or insulin resistance. American Journal Physiology Heart Circulation Physiology. 2006; 290:H137-H145.

[47] Wang H, Zhang ZB, Wen RR, Chen JW. Experimental and clinical studies on the reduction of erythrocyte sorbitol-glucose ratios by ascorbic acid in diabetes mellitus. Diabetes Research Clinical Practice 1995; 28:1-8.

[48] Eriksson J, Kohvakka A. Magnesium and ascorbic acid supplementation in diabetes mellitus. Annals Nutrition Metabolism. 1995;39:217-223.

[49] Paolisso G, Balbi V, Volpe C, Varricchio G, Gambardella A, Saccomanno F, Ammendola S, Varricchio M, D'Onofrio F. Metabolic benefits deriving from chronic vitamin C supplementation in aged non-insulin dependent diabetics. Journal American College Nutrition. 1995;14:387-392.

[50] Han SN, Adolfsson O, Lee CK, Prolla TA, Ordovas J, Meydani SN. Vitamin E and gene expression in immune cells. Annals NY Academy Science. 2004;1031:96–101.

[51] Adolfsson O, Huber BT, Meydani SN. Vitamin E-enhanced IL-2 production in old mice: naive but not memory T cells show increased cell division cycling and IL-2 -producing capacity. Journal Immunology. 2001;167:3809–3817.

[52] Singh U, Jialal I. Anti-inflammatory effects of α-tocopherol. Annals NY Academy Science. 2004;1031:195–203.

[53] Devaraj JS, Jialal I. Alpha-tocopherol decreases interleukin-1 beta release from activated human monocytes by inhibition of 5-lipoxygenase. Arteriosclerosis Thrombosis Vascular Biology. 1999;19:1125–1133.

[54] Scott JA, King GL. Oxidative stress and antioxidant treatment in diabetes. Annals NY Academy Science. 2004;1031:204–213.

[55] Thomas SR, Stocker R. Molecular action of vitamin E in lipoprotein oxidation: Implications for athrosclerosis. Free Radical Biology Medicine. 2000;28:1795–1805.

[56] Ristow M, Zarse K, Oberbach A, et al. Antioxidants prevent healthpromoting effects of physical exercise in humans. Proceeding National Academy Science USA. 2009;106:8665–8670.

[57] Buijsee B, Feskens EJM, Kwape L, Kok FJ, Kormhout D. Both alphaand beta-carotene, but not tocopherols and vitamin C, are inversely related to 15-year cardiovascular mortality in Dutch elderly men. Journal Nutrition. 2008;138:344–350.

[58] Garcia-Bailo, B., El-Sohemy, A., Haddad, P., Arora, P., BenZaied, F., Karmali, M. and Badawi, A. Vitamins D, C and E in the prevention of type II diabetes mellitus: modulation of inflammation and oxidative stress. Biologics, 2011;5:7-19.
[59] Pittas AG, Lau J, Hu FB, Dawson-Hughes B. Review: The role of vitamin D and calcium in type 2 diabetes. A systematic review and meta-analysis. Journal Clinical Endocriology Metabolism 2007; 92:2017-2029.
[60] Botella-Carretero JI, Alvarez-Blasco F, Villafruela JJ, Balsa JA, Vazquez C, Escobar-Morreale HF. Vitamin D deficiency is associated with the metabolic syndrome in morbid obesity. Clinical Nutrition. 2004;26:573-580.
[61] Teegarden D, Donkin SS. Vitamin D: emerging new roles in insulin sensitivity. Nutrition Research Reviews, 2009; 22:82-92.
[62] Holick MF. Diabetes and the vitamin D connection. Current Diabetes Reports 2008; 8:393-398.
[63] Maggini S, Wintergerst ES, Beveridge S, Hornig DH. Selected vitamins and trace elements support immune function by strengthening epithelial barriers and cellular and humoral immune responses. British Journal Nutrition. 2007;98(Suppl 1):S29-S35.
[64] Anan F, Takahashi N, Nakagawa M, Ooie T, Saikawa T, Yoshimatsu H. High-sensitivity C-reactive protein is associated with insulin resistance and cardiovascular autonomic dysfunction in type 2 diabetic patients. Metabolism 2005;54:552-558.
[65] Fu L, Yun F, Oczak M, Wong BY, Vieth R, Cole DE. Common genetic variants of the vitamin D binding protein (DBP) predict differences in response of serum 25-hydroxyvitamin D (25(OH)D) to vitamin D supplementation. Clinical Biochemistry. 2009;42:1174-1177.
[66] Szathmary EJ. The effect of Gc genotype on fasting insulin level in Dogrib Indians. Human Genetics. 1987;75:368-372.
[67] Hirai M, Suzuki S, Hinokio Y, Hirai A, Chiba M, Akai H, Suzuki C, Toyota T. Variations in vitamin D-binding protein (group-specific component protein) are associated with fasting plasma insulin levels in Japanese with normal glucose tolerance. Journal Clinical Endocrinology Metabolism. 2000;85:1951-1953.
[68] Baier LJ, Dobberfuhl AM, Pratley RE, Hanson RL, Bogardus C. Variations in the vitamin D-binding protein (Gc locus) are associated with oral glucose tolerance in nondiabetic Pima Indians. Journal Clinical Endocrinology Metabolism. 1998;83:2993-2996.
[69] Pittas AG, Dawson-Hughes B, Li T, Van Dam RM, Willett WC, Manson JE, Hu FB. Vitamin D and calcium intake in relation to type 2 diabetes in women. Diabetes Care. 2006;29:650-656.
[70] Hayes CE, Nashold FE, Spach KM, Pedersen LB. The immunological functions of the vitamin D endocrine system. Cellular Molecular Biology. 2003; 49:277-300.
[71] Griffin MD, Xing N, Kumar R. Vitamin D and its analogs as regulators of immune activities and antigen presentation. Annual Reviews Nutrition. 2003;23:117-145.
[72] Cantorna MT, Zhu Y, Froicu M, Wittke A. Vitamin D status, 1,25-dihydroxy- vitamin D3, and the immune system. American Journal Clinical Nutrition. 2004;80:1717S-1720S.

[73] DeLuca HF, Cantorna MT. Vitamin D: its role and uses in immunology. FASEB Journal. 2001;15:2579-2585.

[74] Veldman CM, Cantorna MT, DeLuca HF. Expression of 1,25-dihydroxyvitamin D3 receptor in the immune system. Archive Biochemistry Biophysics. 2000;374:338.

[75] Riachy R, Vandewalle B, Kerr CJ, Moerman E, Sacchetti P, Lukowiak B, Gmyr V, Bouckenooghe T, Dubois M, Pattou F. 1,25-dihydroxyvitamin D3 protects RINm5F and human islet cells against cytokine-induced apoptosis: implication of the antiapoptotic protein A20. Endocrinology. 2002;143:4809-4819.

[76] van Etten E, Mathieu C. Immunoregulation by 1,25-dihydroxyvitamin D3: basic concepts. Journal Steroides Biochemistry Molecular Biology. 2005;97:93-101.

[77] Pittas AG, Lau J, Hu FB, Dawson-Hughes B. Review: The role of vitamin D and calcium in type 2 diabetes. A systematic review and meta-analysis. Journal Clinical Endocriology Metabolism. 2007;92:2017-2029.

[78] Mokdad AH, Bowman BA, Ford ES, Vinicoor F, Marks JS, Koplan JP. The continuing epidemics of obesity and diabetes in the United States. Journal American Medical Association. 2001;286:1195-1200.

[79] Chiu KC, Chu A, Go VL, Saad MF. Hypovitaminosis D is associated with insulin resistance and beta cell dysfunction. American Journal Clinical Nutrition. 2004;79:820-825.

[80] Ford ES, Ajani UA, McGuire LC, Liu S. Concentrations of serum vitamin D and the metabolic syndrome among U.S. adults. Diabetes Care. 2005;28:1228-1230.

[81] Hypponen E, Power C. Vitamin D status and glucose homeostasis in the 1958 British birth cohort: the role of obesity. Diabetes Care. 2006;29:2244-2246.

[82] Need AG, O'Loughlin PD, Horowitz M, Nordin BE. Relationship between fasting serum glucose, age, body mass index and serum 25 hydroxyvitamin D in postmenopausal women. Clinical Endocrinology. 2005;62:738-741.

[83] Scragg R, Sowers M, Bell C. Serum 25-hydroxyvitamin D, diabetes, and ethnicity in the Third National Health and Nutrition Examination Survey. Diabetes Care. 2004;27:2813-2818.

[84] Liu S, Song Y, Ford ES, Manson JE, Buring JE, Ridker PM. Dietary calcium, vitamin D, and the prevalence of metabolic syndrome in middle-aged and older U.S. women. Diabetes Care, 2005;28:2926-2932.

[85] Fliser D, Stefanski A, Franek E, Fode P, Gudarzi A, Ritz E. No effect of calcitriol on insulin-mediated glucose uptake in healthy subjects. European Journal Clinical Investigation. 1997;27:629-633.

[86] Inomata S, Kadowaki S, Yamatani T, Fukase M, Fujita T. Effect of 1 alpha (OH)-vitamin D3 on insulin secretion in diabetes mellitus. Bone Mineral 1986;1:187-192.

[87] Ljunghall S, Lind L, Lithell H, Skarfors E, Selinus I, Sorensen OH, Wide L. Treatment with one-alpha-hydroxycholecalciferol in middle-aged men with impaired glucose tolerance--a prospective randomized double-blind study. Acta Medica Scandnavia. 1987;222:361-367.

[88] Orwoll E, Riddle M, Prince M. Effects of vitamin D on insulin and glucagon secretion in non-insulin-dependent diabetes mellitus. American Journal Clinical Nutrition. 1994;59:1083-1087.

[89] Nilas L, Christiansen C. Treatment with vitamin D or its analogues does not change body weight or blood glucose level in postmenopausal women. Intnational Journal Obesity. 1984;8:407-411.

[90] Pittas AG, Harris SS, Stark PC, Dawson-Hughes B. The effects of calcium and vitamin D supplementation on blood glucose and markers of inflammation in nondiabetic adults. Diabetes Care 2007; 30:980-986.

[91] Knowler WC, Barrett-Connor E, Fowler SE, Hamman RF, Lachin JM, Walker EA, Nathan DM. Reduction in the incidence of type 2 diabetes with lifestyle intervention or metformin. New England Journal Medicine. 2002;346:393-403.

[92] Colak E, Majkic-Singh N, Stankovic S, Sreckovic-Dimitrijevic V, Djordjevic PB, Lalic K, Lalic N. Parameters of antioxidative defense in type 2 diabetic patients with cardiovascular complications. Annals Medicine. 2005;37:613–620.

[93] Baynes JW. Role of oxidative stress in development of complications in diabetes. Diabetes. 1991;40:405–412.

[94] Ceriello A. Acute hyperglycaemia and oxidative stress generation. Diabet Med. 1997;14:45–49.

[95] Ylönen K, Alfthan G, Groop L, Saloranta C, Aro A, Virtanen SM. Dietary intakes and plasma concentrations of carotenoids and tocopherols in relation to glucose metabolism in subjects at high risk of type 2 diabetes: the Botnia Dietary Study. American Journal Clinical Nutrition. 2003;77:1434–1441.

[96] Helmersson J, Vessby B, Larsson A, Basu S. Association of type 2 diabetes with cyclooxygenase-mediated inflammation and oxidative stress in an elderly population. Circulation. 2004;109:1729–1734.

[97] Block G, Dietrich M, Norkus E, Jensen C, Benowitz NL, Packer L, et al. Intraindividual variability of plasma antioxidants, markers of oxidative stress, C-reactive protein, cotinine, and other biomarkers. Epidemiology. 2006;17:404–412.

[98] Brenner DR, Arora P, Garcia-Bailo B, El-Sohemy A, Karmali M and Badawi A. The relationship between metabolic syndrome components and inflammatory markers among non-diabetic Canadian adults. Journal Diabetes Metabolism. 2012; doi:10.4172/2155-6156.S2-003.

[99] Brenner DR, Arora P, Garcia-Bailo B, Wolever TMS, Morrison H, El-Sohemy A, Karmali M, and Badawi A. Plasma vitamin D and risk of the metabolic syndrome in Canadians. Clinical Investigative Medicine. 2011;34: E377-E384.

[100] Barclay C, Procter KL, Glendenning R, Marsh P, Freeman J, Mathers N. Can type 2 diabetes be prevented in UK general practice? A lifestyle-change feasibility study [ISAIAH]. British Journal General Practice. 2008;58:541-547.

[101] Norris SL, Zhang X, Avenell A, Gregg E, Bowman B, Schmid CH, Lau J. Long-term effectiveness of weight-loss interventions in adults with pre-diabetes: a review. American Journal Preventive Medicine. 2005;28:126-139.

[102] Frost G, Leeds A, Trew G, Margara R, Dornhorst A. Insulin sensitivity in women at risk of coronary heart disease and the effect of a low glycemic diet. Metabolism 1998;47:1245-1251.

Chapter 2

Aldose Reductase Inhibitors as Potential Therapeutic Drugs of Diabetic Complications

Changjin Zhu

Additional information is available at the end of the chapter

http://dx.doi.org/10.5772/54642

1. Introduction

Diabetes mellitus has become a major health threat as a global rise in it has been seen. The chronic disease has afflicted over 171 million people worldwide in 2000 and the incidence is expected to grow steadily to 366 million by 2030. As of May 2008, an estimated 92 million adults in China of the most populous country were living with diabetes and 148 million adults with prediabetes [1]. Diabetes mellitus is one of the leading causes of death across the globe particularly in the developing world. Most diabetic patients suffer from so-called long-term complications such as neuropathy, nephropathy, retinopathy, cataracts and even stroke. These complications arise from chronic hyperglycemia, which causes damage to blood vessels and peripheral nerves, greatly increasing the risk of heart attack. A number of mechanistic explanations for the complications have been proposed (for the reviews, see Refs. [2-5]). First, they include hyperactivity of polyol metabolic pathway that produces elevated accumulation of cellular sorbitol leading to osmotic stresses on cells, and is then implicated mainly in microvascular damage to retina, kidney, and nerve systems. As the second mechanism, increased formation of advanced glycation end products (AGEs) activates nonenzymatic glycosylation of proteins and lipids, and in turn leads to dysfunctional behaviors of related enzymes and receptors. The third of them is hyperglycemia-induced activation of protein kinase C (PKC) isoforms which evokes pathological changes in growth factor expression. The fourth is diverting of excess intracellular glucose into the hexosamine pathway and consequent overmodification of enzymatic proteins by N-acetylglucosamine along with abnormal enzyme behaviors. Finally, the fifth mechanism is recently proposed in which an hyperglycemia-induced impairment of antioxidant defense such as the overproduction of reactive oxygen species (ROS) readily initiates inflammation responses.

Among these mechanisms, the polyol pathway was first discovered and in fact is generally accepted to be the mechanism of prime importance in the pathogenesis of diabetic complications. Aldose reductase (AR, EC 1.1.1.21) that is the first and rate-controlling enzyme in the polyol pathway is of importance for the pathway and in turn has been a potential target for drug design, therefore, the inhibition of aldose reductase has been an attractive approach to the prevention and treatment of diabetic complications. In line with the focus of this chapter, ARIs and their therapeutic functions will be discussed in the following sections.

2. Aldose reductase and the polyol metabolic pathway of glucose

2.1. The polyol pathway

Aldose reductase together with sorbitol dehydrogenase (SDH) forms the polyol pathway as shown in Figure 1. In the polyol pathway, AR initially catalyzes the NADPH-dependent reduction of the aldehyde form of glucose to form sorbitol. Sorbitol dehydrogenase then utilizing NAD oxidizes the intermediate sorbitol to fructose. The conversion of glucose to sorbitol catalyzed by AR was first identified in 1956 by Hers in the seminal vesicles where glucose is converted into fructose to provide an energy source for sperm [6]. Soon after, the polyol pathway sorbitol was found in diabetic rat lens by Van Heyningen [7]. In 1965, pathogenic effects of AR and its associated polyol pathway were first identified in the lens by Kinoshita, and these works formed the basis for the osmotic stress hypothesis of sugar cataract formation [8]. It proposes that intracellular excess sorbitol produced by AR accumulates in cells and is difficult to diffuse across the cell membranes, and consequently the osmotic damage to cells occurs which eventually leads to diabetic cataract complication [9]. These discoveries taken together led to the opening for studies on the pathogenic role of AR and the polyol pathway in the development of diabetic complications, and also made the beginning of research for the mechanism of diabetic complications. AR is now known to be present in most of the mammalian cells. Normally, the cellular glucose is oxidatively metabolized through the glycolysis pathway and then the Krebs cycle to produce the building blocks and energy for cells. Under hyperglycemic conditions, however, the increased amount of glucose activates AR and is metabolized by the activated polyol pathway.

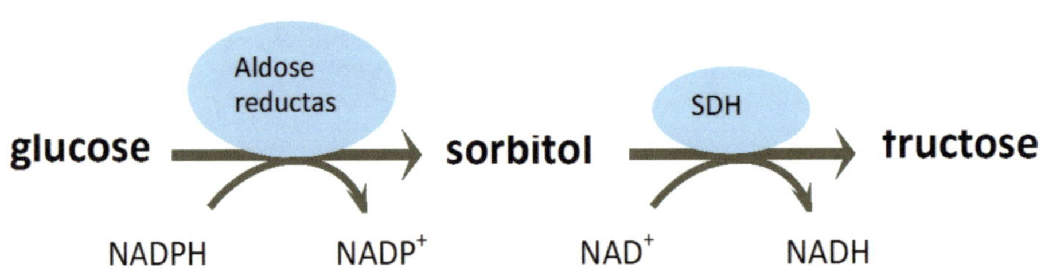

Figure 1. Polyol metabolic pathway of glucose

After finding the AR-mediated glucose metabolism, several mechanisms other than the AR-initiated polyol pathway for diabetic complications were successively proposed. Nevertheless, the polyol pathway appears still to be a compelling mechanism of diabetic complications because growing evidences have been shown for an involvement of the abnormally activated polyol pathway in the pathogenesis of diabetic complications.

Biomolecular evidences for the role of the polyol pathway are recently provided by cellular experiments and regulations of AR gene expression in the presence of high glucose induction. The protein expression of AR, and the intracellular sorbitol and fructose contents appeared to be up-regulated in mouse Schwann cells under high glucose conditions [10, 11]. In transgenic mice with AR overexpression, an elevated accumulation of sorbitol and fructose along with a simulteneous decrease in tibial motor nerve conduction velocity were found [12]. In peripheral blood mononuclear cells from nephropathy, high glucose increased NF-kB binding activities, which in turn induced an expression of AR protein [13]. Observations in high glucose-induced rat mesangial cells suggested that altered protein kinase C activity mediated through activation of the polyol-pathway contributes to a loss of mesangial cell contractile responsiveness [14]. A particular convincing finding is that these detrimental alterations could be prevented or reversed by the treatment with AR inhibitors (ARIs).

Consistent findings can be also traced in the animals with a deficient AR gene expression. In db/db mice with an AR null mutation, diabetes-induced reduction of platelet/endothelial cell adhesion molecule-1 expression and increased expression of vascular endothelial growth factor were prevented which may have contributed to blood-retinal barrier breakdown. As a result, long-term diabetes-induced neuro-retinal stress and apoptosis and proliferation of blood vessels were less present [15]. This suggests that AR is responsible for the early events in the pathogenesis of diabetic retinopathy, leading to a cascade of retinal lesions. Also, AR-deficient mice were protected from delayed motor nerve conduction velocity, increased c-Jun NH2-terminal kinase activation, depletion of reduced glutathione, increased superoxide accumulation, and DNA damage [16]. AR-deficient or ARI-treated mice were protected from severe ischaemic limb injury and renal failure, showing only modest muscle necrosis and significant suppression of serum markers of renal failure and inflammation [17]. In addition, AR inhibition counteracted diabetes-induced oxidative-nitrosative stress and poly(ADP-ribose) polymerase activation in sciatic nerve and retina [18]. Very recently in human mesangial cells in culture, exposure to high glucose and overexpression AR increased the expression of fibronectin. This increase was prevented by the AR inhibitors sorbinil and zopolrestat. Treatment with high glucose and transfected with plasmid PcDNA3.0-AR, resulted in phosphorylation and activation of ERK, JNK and AKT signaling pathway, and an increase in the expression of fibronectin. Treatment with inhibitor of JNK and AKT signaling pathway decreased the expression of fibronectin. Obviously, AR may be linked to extracellular matrix deposition in diabetic nephropathy, which is regulated by JNK and AKT [19].

On the other hand, in streptozotocin-diabetic rats, significantly delayed motor nerve conduction velocity, decreased R-R interval variation, reduced sciatic nerve blood flow and decreased erythrocyte 2,3-diphosphoglycerate concentrations were all ameliorated by treatment with ARI [5-(3-thienyl) tetrazol-1-yl]acetic acid. The inhibitor also reduced platelet hyperaggregation activity, decreased sorbitol accumulation and prevented not only myo-inositol depletion but also free-carnitine deficiency in diabetic nerves. Therefore, there is a close relationship between increased polyol pathway activity and carnitine deficiency in the development of diabetic neuropathy [20].

Similar to the results from cellular experiments and gene expression regulations, the role of the polyol pathway has been confirmed by animal models. Marked muscle necrosis and renal failure with accumulation of sorbitol and fructose were identified in ischaemic muscles of mice [17], and the disturbance in the renal medulla including oxygen tension, oxygen consumption, lactate/pyruvate ratio and pH were observed in diabetic rats [21]. Notably, these alterations were preventable by either ARI treatment or AR-deficient suggesting the involvement of the polyol pathway in the acute kidney injury.

Besides, the pathways of AGEs, PKC, hexosamine, and ROS can be causally linked to downstream events of the increased polyol pathway flux including alterations in cellular redox balance and fructose concentration [2, 5, 22, 23]. As described above, for example, the loss of mesangial cell contractile responsiveness in high glucose-induced rat mesangial cells resulted from the activation of the polyol-pathway could be mediated by altered PKC activity [14]. In vitro studies on cultured human mesangial cells and in vivo studies in the diabetic renal cortex of streptozotocin-diabetic rats have indicated the presence of both increased AR activity and oxidative/nitrosative stress in the pathogenesis of diabetic nephropathy, and the nitrosative stress and polymerase activation could be counteracted by AR inhibition [24]. Moreover, the increased kinase activation, depletion of reduced glutathione, increased superoxide accumulation, and DNA damage could be prevented by AR-deficiency in the amelioration of motor nerve conduction velocity [16]. Recently, osmotic stress resulting from the accumulation of sugar alcohols in lens epithelial cells which contain mitochondria, has been shown to induce endoplasmic reticulum stress that leads to the generation of reactive ROS and apoptotic signaling [25].

The polyol pathway is in fact supported by successfully therapeutic applications of ARI drugs epalrestat and tolrestat in diabetic complications such as neuropathy. Epalrestat is now on the markets in Japan, China, and India while tolrestat was marketed in several countries although it was withdrawn. Also, a few of other ARIs involving fidalrestat and ranirestat have been advanced to late stage of clinical trials.

2.2. Properties of AR

AR belongs to the aldo-keto reductase enzyme superfamily. Crystallized complexes of AR with ligands and site directed mutagenesis allowed the enzyme structure to be identified. The enzyme is a single polypeptide domain composed of 315 amino acid residues [26]. The peptide chain blocked at the amino terminus folds into a β/α-barrel structural motif containing eight parallel β strands which are connected to each other by eight peripheral α-helical segments running anti-parallel to the β sheet. The active site is located in a large and deep crevice in the C-terminal end of the β barrel, and the NADPH cofactor binds in an extended conformation to the bottom of the active site [27, 28]. However, it is likely that the active site often changes its conformational shape because a variety of binding conformations bound by ARIs, represented by the complexes with ligands sorbinil (PDB entry code 1AH051), tolrestat (PDB entry code 2FDZ52), and IDD594 (PDB entry code 1US053), have been reported [29-32]. These ligand-dependent conformations indicate a remarkable induced fit or flexibility of the active site. Nevertheless, at least three distinct binding pockets in the active site can be proposed as shown in Figure 2 according to a number of studies on crystal structures of AR by X-ray crystallography and mutagenesis [30, 33-38]. The first is usually occupied by the anion head of ligand and thus named "anion binding pocket". It is made up of Tyr48, His110, Trp20, and Trp111 side chains and the positively charged nicotinamide moiety of the cofactor NADP+. The second is a hydrophobic pocket, known as specificity pocket, and lined by the residues Leu300, Cys298, Cys303, Trp111, Cys303, and Phe122 [30]. The specificity pocket displays a high degree of flexibility and the residues lining this pocket are not conserved in other aldo-keto reductases such as aldehyde reductase, The third is another hydrophobic pocket formed by the residues Trp20, Trp111, Phe122, and Trp219 [34].

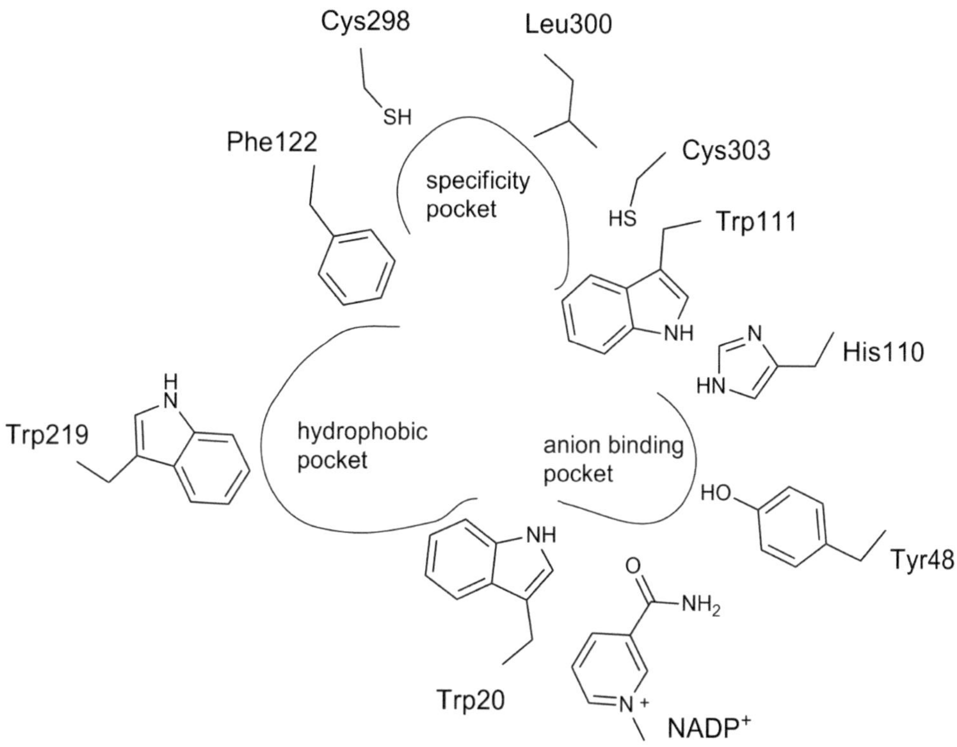

Figure 2. Proposed binding pockets in the active site of AR

Aldehyde reductase (EC 1.1.1.2) , another member of the aldo-keto reductase superfamily, is mentioned here because of its close similarities to AR which may be associated with the specificity of ARIs. The two closely related enzymes share a high degree of sequence (~65%) and three dimensional structure homology with the majority of the differences present at the C-terminal end of the enzyme proteins, where is the region containing the least conserved residues and lining the hydrophobic pocket of the active site called the specificity pocket [30, 39-42]. The specificity pocket is responsible for substrate and inhibitor specificity in the aldo-keto reductases.

Aldehyde reductase plays a detoxification role, as it specifically metabolizes toxic aldehydes such as hydroxynonenal (HNE), 3-deoxyglucosone, and methylglyoxal, which arise in large quantities from pathological conditions connected with oxidative stress, as in hyperglycemia, and are intermediates for the formation of AGEs [43-45]. Thus, aldehyde reductase inhibition may account for some of the undesirable toxicities associated with the present ARIs. It is believable that the development of more structurally diverse ARIs and in turn the identification of molecularly targeted candidates that specifically block AR are important approaches in the search of new drugs.

3. AR inhibitors

In spite of a range of structurally varied ARIs developed up to date [46, 47], carboxylic acids have been the most important and largest class of ARIs. This class readily shows activity in the AR inhibition because of the structural feature of carboxylate anion head group which may fit well in the so-called anion binding pocket of AR as described above (Figure. 2). At the beginning of research on AR properties, it was found that the enzyme is sensitive to organic anions, particularly to long-chain fatty acids [48], leading to the identification of tetramethyleneglutaric acid (TMG) as the first decent ARI in the 1960s. Since then, the more

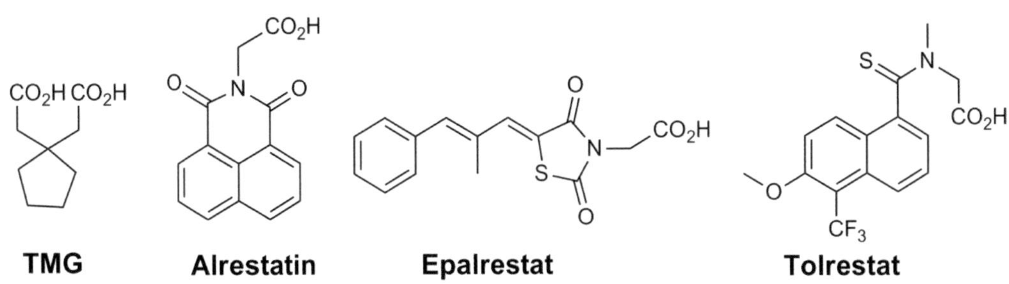

potent and early inhibitor alrestatin (AY-22,284) was developed [46]. Now the number of carboxylic acid ARIs is still growing. Among them is epalrestat, the only ARI given marketing approval as a therapeutic drug applied in the clinical treatment of diabetic neuropathy. Epalrestat was developed in 1983 [49] and has been marketed in Japan, and recently in China and India. Tolrestat, a strong ARI and potential drug for the treatment of diabetic complications [50], was approved to several markets, but withdrawn for the reason of risk of severe liver toxicity and death.The typical carboxylic acid ARIs also include zenarestat [51], zopolrestat [52], and ponalrestat [53]. Zenarestat is a potential drug for the treatment of diabetic neuropathy, retinopathy and cataracts. Both zenarestat and zopolrestat proceeded into late phase research of clinical trials. However, research results from Phase III trials showed zenarestat therapy in the dose level of 1200 mg/day to be linked with renal toxicity in a small number of patients [54]. Ponalrestat was withdrawn from clinical trials

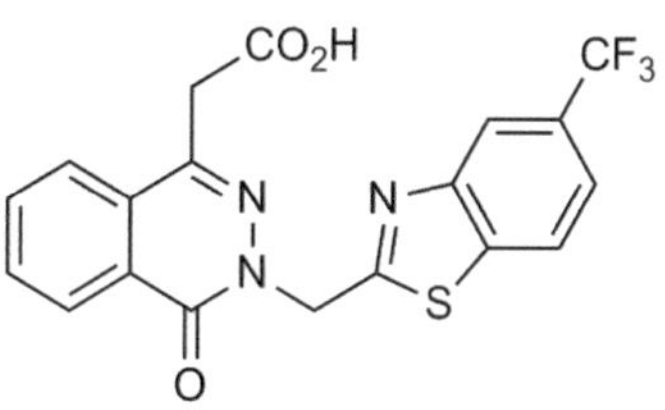

Zopolrestat

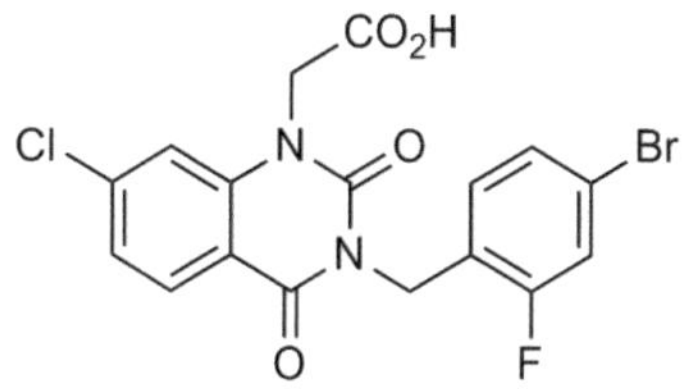

Zenarestat

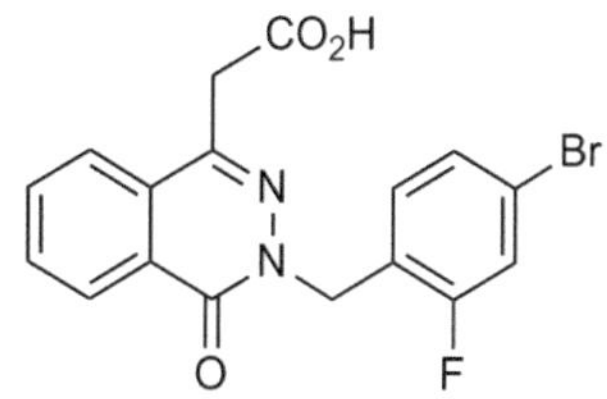

Ponalrestat

due to lack of efficacy. Besides, a number of potent ARIs were recently designed and synthesized based on various chemical core structures including (benzothiazol-2-yl)methyl-indole (lidorestat) [36], naphtho[1,2-d]isothiazole [55], oxadiazole [56], aromatic thiadiazine-1,1-dioxide [57, 58], and quinoxalinone [59]. All of them bear a chemical group of acetic acid on the core. However, poor tissue penetration has been observed as the major shortcoming for some individual inhibitors of the carboxylic acid ARI class [60, 61].

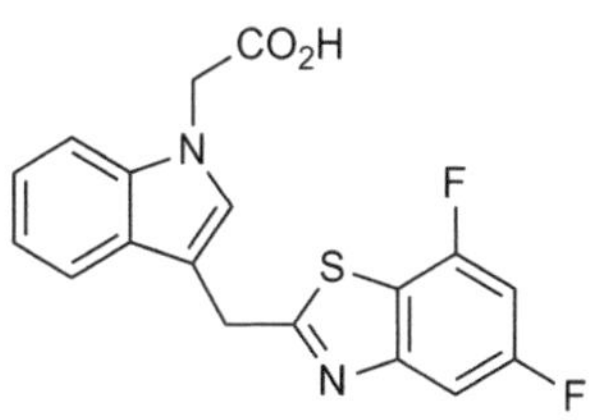

Lidorestat

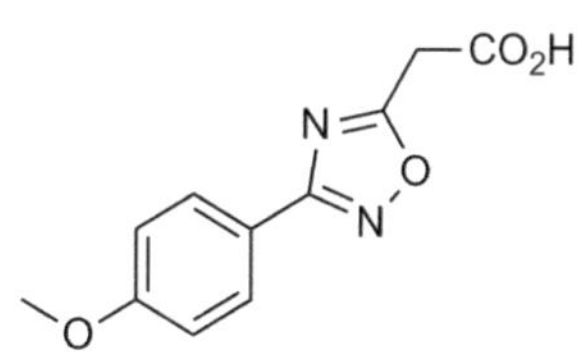

Acetic acid derivative of oxadiazole

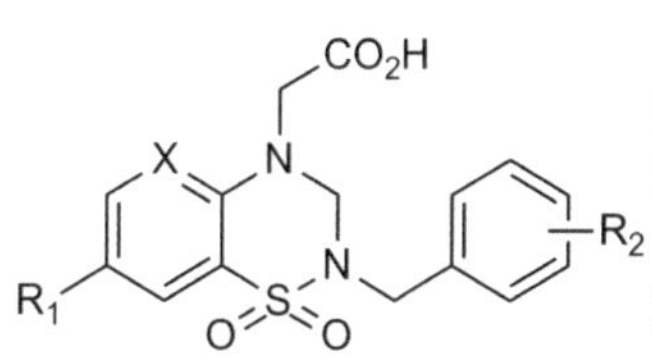

R_1 = halogens
R_2 = 2-F,4-Br
2,4,5-F_3
X = CH, N

Aromatic thiadiazine 1,1-dioxides

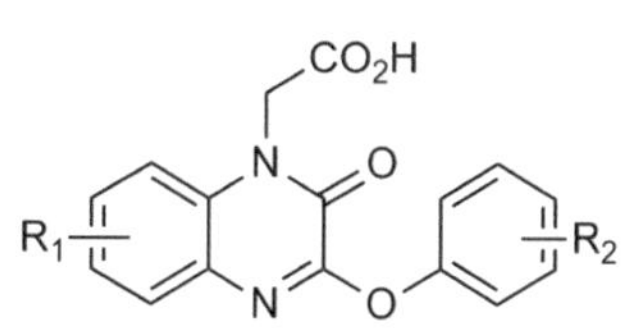

R_1 = halogens
R_2 = 2-F,4-Br
4-F
4-Br

Quinoxalinones

The second chemical class of ARIs includes spirohydantoin derivatives and their analogs. In this class, sorbinil was the first ARI capable of preventing the entire cataractogenic process in diabetic rats [62, 63]. The exquisite spiro system is well formed based on the combination of structures chroman and hydantoin. The hydantoin and the spiro in sorbinil may be key structures responsible for the strong inhibition against AR. In the binding interaction in the active site of AR, the hydantoin ring occupies the anion pocket as does the anion head group of carboxylate ARIs. Carbonyl oxygens and amino nitrogens in the hydantoin could make a

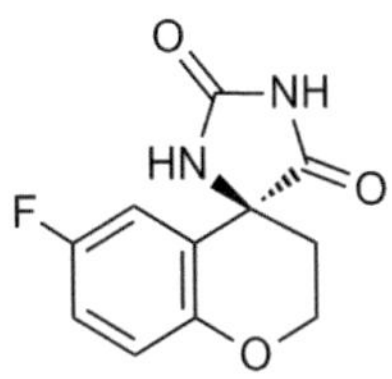

Sorbinil

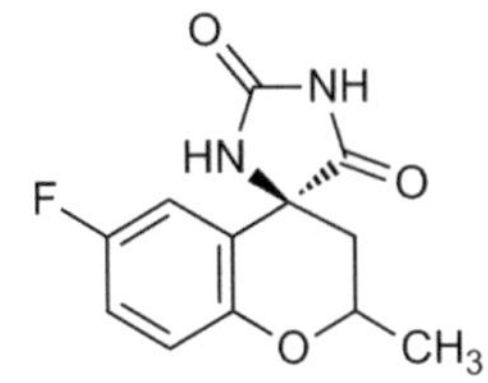

M79175

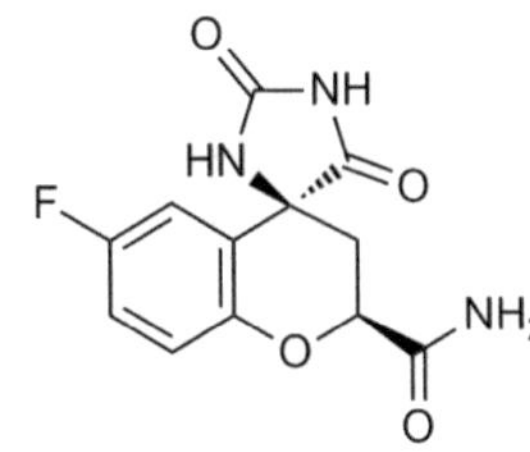

Fidarestat

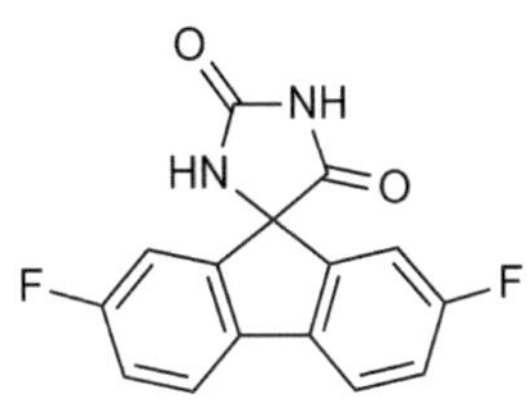

Imirestat

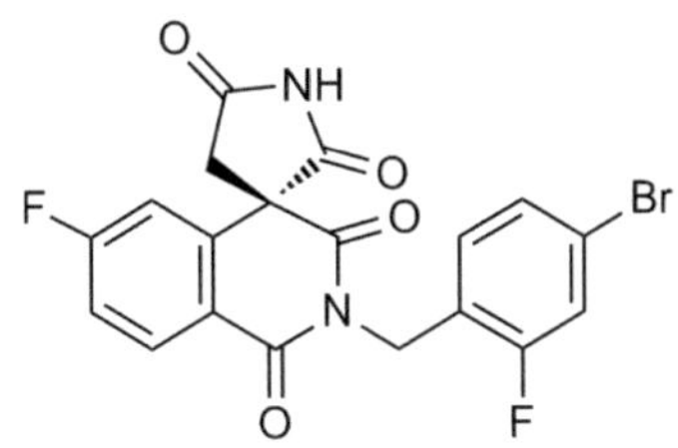

Minalrestat

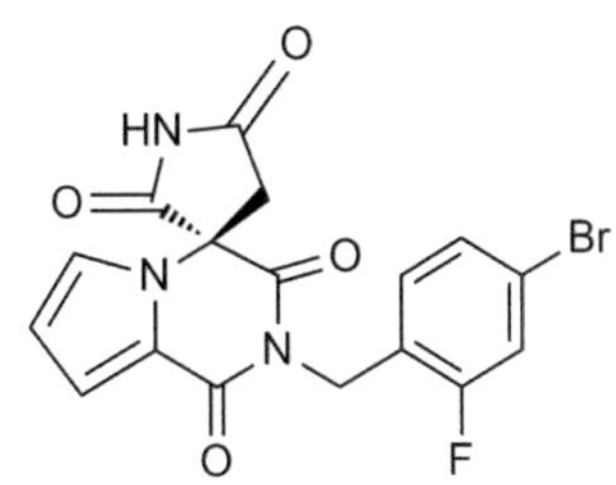

Ranirestat

tight hydrogen-bonding network with residues Tyr48, His110 and Trp111 of AR [30]. The conformationally constrained spiro system made the ring planes of the hydantoin and chroman perpendicular to each other which may be the conformational shape of the inhibitor favored for the binding to AR. Sorbinil has proved an excellent ARI both in vitro and in vivo. However, in the research of clinical trials it was found that as many as 10% of patients receiving sorbinil may be at increased risk for developing hypersensitivity reactions characterized by fever, skin rash, and myalgia due to a potentially toxic intermediate oxidatively metabolized from sorbinil [64, 65]. The adverse reaction may also be attributed to the poor selectivity of sorbinil for AR versus aldehyde reductase [42].

While development of this important drug was hampered by potentially severe reactions, sorbinil has been a distinguish leading inhibitor or a reference widely used in the development of new ARIs and in the research of AR and the polyol pathway.

Based on the structure of sorbinil, several other spirohydantoins and related cyclic amides were developed. Addition of a methyl or a carbamoyl substituent at the 2-position of sorbinil resulted in the formation of M79175 and fidarestat, respectively. Replacement of the chroman ring system with a planar fluorene ring produced imirestat. Then, the spirohydantoin-like spiroimide minalrestat was formed by the replacements of both the chroman and hydantoin with isoquinoline-1,3(2H,4H)-dione ring and succinimide ring, respectively, and the addition of benzyl side chain at the 2-position. Further replacement of the isoquinoline-1,3(2H,4H)-dione ring of minalrestat with pyrrolo[1,2-a]pyrazine-1,3(2H,4H)-dione led to ranirestat (AS-3201) [66]. Imirestat was withdrawn from clinical trials due to toxicity. However, fidarestat and ranirestat have been identified as powerful ARIs with beneficial efficacy in diabetic complications [67-69]. There are no adverse effects reported to the two agents.

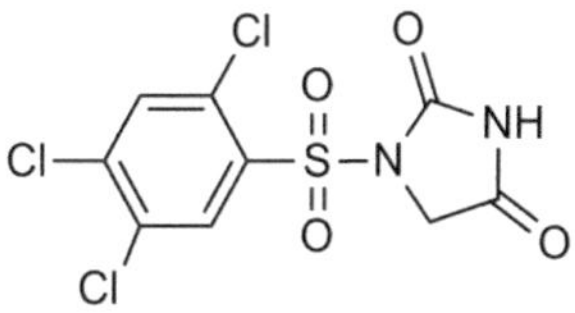

Tri-Cl-PSH

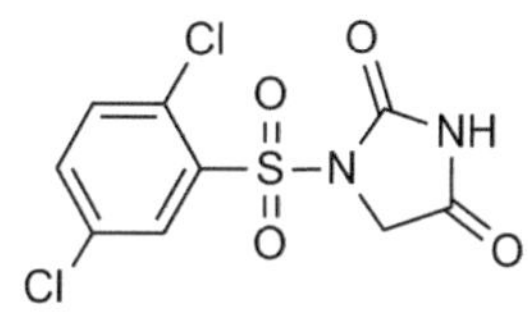

Di-Cl-PSH

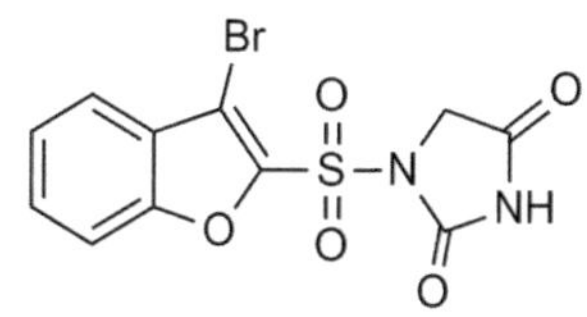

M16209

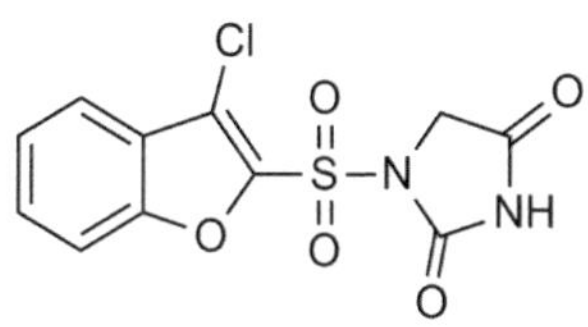

M16287

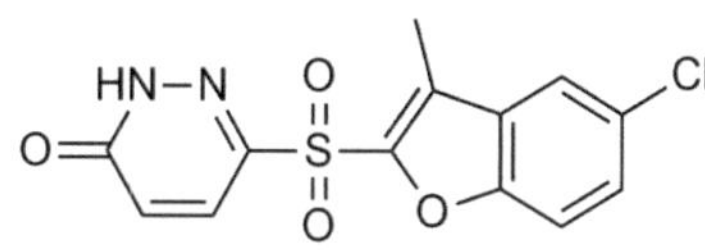

ARI-809

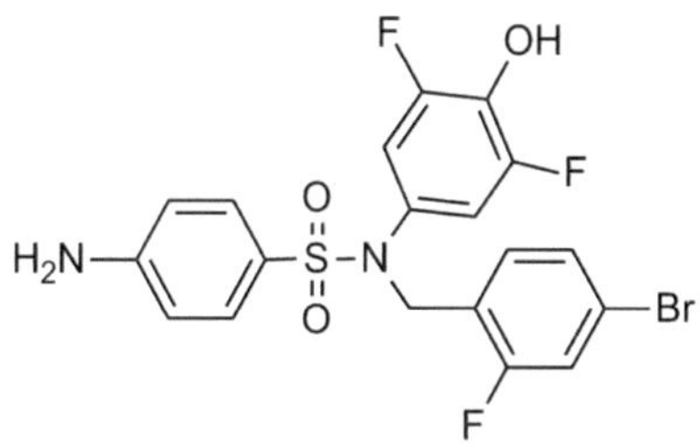

Benzenesulfonamide

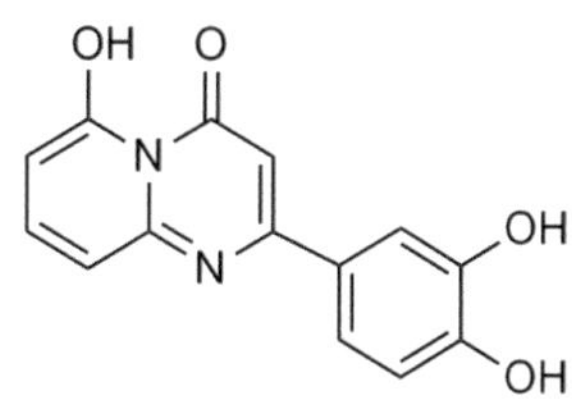

ppp

In another design, the orthogonal spirohydantoin moiety of the above ARIs was changed into a more flexible structure, which is bridged by sulfonyl group leading to Tri-CI-PSH and Di-CI-PSH with IC_{50} values of 0.28 μM and 0.36 μM, respectively [70, 71]. They were found to inhibit sorbitol accumulation in the sciatic nerve completely and in the lens by up to 92%. Modification of aryl moieties of the arylsulfonylhydantoins has generated a group of benzofuransulfonylhydantoins. Of these, two compounds M16209 and M16287 indicated potent AR inhibition [72]. Recently, more modifications of the arylsulfonylhydantoins resulted in a new series of ARIs that are designed based on SO_2 linker-bearing sulfonylpyridazinone. Among them, the most potent and selective compound was profiled to be 6-(5-chloro-3-methylbenzofuran-2-sulfonyl)-2H-pyridazin-3-one (ARI-809) with IC_{50} value of 1 nM in vitro and ED_{50} of 0.8 mg/kg in vivo. ARI-809 is a highly selective (1:930) inhibitor of AR relative to aldehyde reductase, and such selectivity distinguishes it from sorbinil, which inhibits AR and aldehyde reductase to a comparable extent [73, 74]. In addition, introduction of phenol moiety into the sulfonyl-bridged system has provided benzenesulfonamide ARIs, which could not only inhibit AR but also exhibit potent antioxidant activity [75]. Moreover, phenylpyridopyrimidinone (PPP) was developed as a flavinoid bioisoster, and exhibited AR inhibition activity level in the submicromolar range and significant antioxidant properties [76].

4. Therapeutic properties of ARIs in the diabetic complications

The diabetic complications include typically neuropathy, nephropathy, and retinopathy and cataract although a substantial increase of atherosclerotic disease of large vessels, including cardiac and cerebral diseases, has been seen in the complications. ARIs appear to be a specific option for the improvement of the diabetic abnormalities according to the study results from experiments in vitro, in animal models, and clinical trials.

4.1. Retinopathy and cataract

Diabetic eye damages including retinopathy and cataract are characteristic of diabetes. ARIs sorbinil, ARI-809, ranirestat, fidarestat, zenarestat, M79175, and Kinostat™ have shown an activity for the treatment of the diabetic retinopathy and cataract. Kinostat™ is a new ARI developed by Kador [77].

It was found early that potent ARI sorbinil was effective in preventing cataractous changes in diabetic rats. Diabetic rats treated with sorbinil showed no lens changes during the 5-month period of the experiment. In contrast, untreated diabetic rats developed early lens changes by 3 weeks and dense nuclear opacities by 6 to 9 weeks [62]. It was evident by later independent studies in which sorbinil prevented the galactose-induced retinal microangiopathies and was also effective in preventing cataractous changes in diabetic rats [63]. In recent studies, treatment of diabetic Sprague Dawley rats with oral ARI imirestat prevented cataract by inhibiting sorbitol formation in the lens [78]. In insulinized streptozotocin-induced diabetic rats, ARI-809 improved survival, inhibited cataract development, normalized retinal sorbitol and fructose, and protected the retina from abnormalities that also occur in human diabetes: neuronal apoptosis, glial reactivity, and complement deposition [74]. Streptozotocin-diabetic rats could developed early lens opacities 8 weeks after streptozotocin injection and could have cataract. These alterations were prevented by the ranirestat treatment [69].

From several investigations performed recently with rat models, it appears that ARI fidarestat is active in the treatment of diabetic retinopathy. In streptozotocin-diabetic rats, fidarestat treatment reduced diabetes-associated cataract formation, and retinal oxidative-nitrosative stress, glial activation, and apoptosis [79]. Similar results were obtained in the rat model with retinal ischemia-reperfusion injury. The retinal injury-associated dramatic increase in cell death, elevated AR expression, and sorbitol pathway intermediate accumulation were prevented or alleviated by fidarestat treatment [80]. Also in the streptozotocin-diabetic rats, fidarestat treatment significantly decreased concentrations of sorbitol and fructose in the rat retinas. The expression of ICAM-1 mRNA and eukocyte accumulation in the retinas were significantly reduced. Immunohistochemical study also revealed the suppressive effect of fidarestat on the expression of ICAM-1 [81].

In addition, the study using Zucker diabetic fatty rats, an animal model of type 2 diabetes, showed that the administration of a combination of four plant extracts inhibited the development of diabetic cataract through the inhibition of AR activity and protein expression in diabetic lenses [82].

In galactose-fed dogs, cataract formation was delayed or prevented either by oral administration of the ARI M79175 [83, 84], or topical administration of the formulation Kinostat™ [77]. This has been further confirmed by the more recent experiment in a similar dog model. In a randomized, prospective, double-masked placebo control pilot study conducted with 40 dogs diagnosed with diabetes mellitus by topical administration of the ARI Kinostat™ for 12 months, the cataract score was significantly less with seven developing anterior equatorial vacuoles, two developing incipient anterior cortical cataracts, and four developing mature cataracts. It was noted that the cataract scores of the Kinostat™ group at 12 months did not in fact significantly increase from the score at the time of enrollment [85].

According to the results from phase III trial research in Japan, zenarestat developed as an eyedrop formulation was specifically effective for the treatment of diabetic retinopathy [54].

The beneficial effects of these different types of ARIs on the diabetic cataract and retinopathy support the notion that AR is the key relay that converts hyperglycemia into glucose toxicity in neural and glial cell types in the retina [74]. This provides a rationale for the development of ARIs, and in particular for the prevention and treatment of diabetic ocular complications [79].

4.2. Neuropathy

Nerve injuries of the respective organs are thought to be the root cause of diabetes complications. Pharmaceutical options in the treatment of diabetic neuropathy include antidepressants, anticonvulsants, tramadol, serotonin–norepinephrine reuptake inhibitors, and capsaicin [86]. These agents are modestly effective for symptomatic relief, but they do not affect the underlying pathology nor do they slow progression of the disease. In addition, they carry a risk of side effects. Therefore, the application of ARIs are expected to address this issue. Epalrestat, fidarestat, ranirestat (AS-3201), zenalrestat, sorbinil, and tolrestat will be described in this section.

4.2.1. Epalrestat

Epalrestat is undoubtedly the first agent for the treatment of diabetic neuropathy because of its effectiveness and safety. It is approved in Japan, China and India for the improvement of subjective neuropathy symptoms, abnormality of vibration sense and abnormal changes in heart beat associated with diabetic peripheral neuropathy. Long-term treatment with epalrestat in a clinic trial was well tolerated and could effectively delay the progression of diabetic neuropathy and ameliorate the associated symptoms of the disease, particularly in subjects with good glycemic control and limited microangiopathy [87]. Epalrestat is easily absorbed into neural tissue and potently inhibits AR with minimum adverse effects. Unlike the current pharmaceutical options for diabetic neuropathy, epalrestat may affect or delay progression of the underlying disease process. Data from experimental studies indicate that epalrestat reduces sorbitol accumulation in the sciatic nerve, erythrocytes, and ocular tissues in animals, and in erythrocytes in humans. On the bases of several clinical trials, treatment with epalrestat in a dose of 50 mg 3 times/day may improve motor and sensory nerve conduction velocity and subjective neuropathy symptoms. The most frequently reported adverse effects for epalrestat include elevations in liver enzyme levels and gastrointestinal-related events such as nausea and vomiting [88].

The diabetic patients treated with epalrestat for 2 years showed a significant suppression of deterioration of motor nerve conduction velocity and minimum F-wave latency in the tibial nerve, and sensory nerve conduction velocity in the sural nerve. In fact, there was a significant difference in change in the level of serum N(ε)-carboxymethyl lysine after 1 year treatment. Therefore, it is suggested that epalrestat suppressed the deterioration of diabetic peripheral neuropathy, especially in the lower extremity, and the effects might be mediated by improvement of the polyol pathway and suppression of production of AGEs [89]. In a clinical trial in India, more than 2000 patients with diabetic neuropathy were treated with epalrestat for 3-12 months, the results showed that the improvement rate of the subjective symptoms was 75% and that of the nerve function tests 36%. Adverse drug reactions were encountered in 52 (2.5%) of the 2190 patients, none of which was severe [90]. Although data are limited, it is strongly suggested that epalrestat is a highly effective and safe agent for the treatment of diabetic neuropathy.

Clinical efficacy of epalrestat for diabetic peripheral neuropathy has been well documented by Hotta and coworkers [87, 91]. When patients with diabetic peripheral neuropathy were treated with epalrestat for period of 3 years, significantly better efficacy was found in patients with good glycaemic control and less severe diabetic complications. Nerve function deteriorated less or improved in patients whose symptoms improved. The odds ratio of the efficacy of epalrestat versus control subjects was approximately 2:1 [91].

In diabetic nerves, activation of the polyol pathway via AR and the resulting impairment of the Na(+)-K(+) pump would lead to a decreased transaxonal Na+ gradient, and thereby reduced nodal Na+ currents. In a 6-month, open clinical trial with epalrestat in 30 patients with mild-to-moderate diabetic neuropathy, results from excitability testing and extensive nerve conduction studies including F-wave analyses displayed that within a month of the start of treatment, there was a significant improvement in nerve conduction, particularly in conduction times across the carpal tunnel and F-wave latencies. It suggested an increased nodal persistent Na+ currents. At 6 months, nerve conduction continued to improve. Therefore, AR pathway inhibition could rapidly increase nodal Na+ currents and thereby improve the slowing of nerve conduction, presumably because of a restoration of the membranous Na+ gradient [92].

Earlier investigation on streptozotocin-induced diabetic neuropathy in rats showed that the treatment with epalrestat resulted in a significant improvement of nerve growth factor content and faster H-wave-related sensory nerve conduction velocity. At the same time, epalrestat treatment showed the stimulating effect on nerve growth factor synthesis/secretion in rat Schwann cell culture in vitro. Consequently, these results suggest that decreased levels of nerve growth factor in diabetic sciatic nerves may be involved in the pathogenesis of diabetic neuropathy in these rats and indicated that epalrestat can be useful for the treatment of diabetic neuropathy through nerve growth factor-induction and inhibition of the polyol pathway [93].

Therefore, epalrestat may serve as a new therapeutic option to prevent or slow the progression of diabetic neuropathy. However, long-term, comparative studies in diverse patient populations are needed for clinical application.

4.2.2. *Fidarestat*

In a 52-week multicenter placebo-controlled double-blind parallel group study in 279 patients with diabetes and associated peripheral neuropathy, the group of fidarestat-treated at a daily dose of 1 mg was significantly improved compared with the placebo group in two electro physiological measures (i.e., median nerve F-wave conduction velocity and minimal latency). Subjective symptoms (including numbness, spontaneous pain, sensation of rigidity, paresthesia in the sole upon walking, heaviness in the foot, and hypesthesia) benefited from fidarestat treatment, and all were significantly improved in the treated versus placebo group. At the dose used, fidarestat was well tolerated, with an adverse event profile that did not significantly differ from that seen in the placebo group [94].

In experimental rats with diabetic neuropathy, oral administration of fidarestat at a dose of 1 or 4 mg/kg for 10 weeks significantly improved nerve blood flow, compound muscle action potential, and amplitude of C-potential. Fidarestat suppressed the increase in sorbitol and fructose, normalised reduced glutathione in sciatic nerve, and reduced the number of 8-hydroxy-2'-deoxyguanosine-positive cells in dorsal root ganglion neurons. This indicates that the fidarestat-improved neuropathy may be via an improvement in oxidative stress and supports a role for fidarestat in the treatment of diabetic neuropathy [95].

4.2.3. *Ranirestat (AS-3201)*

Ranirestat is an orally available ARI under development for the potential treatment of diabetic complications, such as neuropathy, cataracts, retinopathy and nephropathy [96]. It appears to be in late phase of clinical trials.

In the sciatic nerve and lens of streptozotocin-diabetic rats, ranirestat treatment reduced sorbitol accumulation in the sciatic nerve and improved the decrease in motor nerve conduction velocity. Morphological and morphometric examination of changes in sural nerve revealed that the treatment with ranirestat prevented both the deformity of myelinated fibers and the decrease in their axonal and myelin areas (atrophy). Ranirestat also averted the changes in the size frequency histogram of myelinated fibers. The studies showed that ranirestat is an agent for the management of diabetic sensorimotor polyneuropathy [69, 97].

Ranirestat has been well studied by Bril and coworkers [98, 99]. In a double-blind, placebo-controlled nerve biopsy trial study, 12-week-treatment with ranirestat at a dose of 5 or 20 mg/day improved nerve function in patients with diabetic sensorimotor polyneuropathy, and the improvement could be maintained. When patients completing this biopsy study were offered a 48-week extension at the same ranirestat dose or at 5 mg/day ranirestat if they were originally treated with placebo, it was found that nerve conduction velocity of peroneal motor improved in the 20 mg/day group following 60 weeks of treatment while those of sural and median sensory improved after both 12 and 60 weeks of treatment with 20 mg/day. Vibration perception threshold improved after 60 weeks of treatment with 20 mg/day. The improved sensory nerve function observed after 12 weeks of therapy was maintained at 60 weeks, and improved motor nerve function was observed at 60 weeks. Ranirestat was found to be well tolerated with no difference in adverse events between the 5- and 20-mg/day groups [98]. In a further multicenter, double-blind study, patients with diabetic sensorimotor polyneuropathy were treated with 10, 20, or 40 mg/day ranirestat for 52 weeks. At week 52, the summed sensory (bilateral sural plus proximal median sensory) nerve conduction velocity did not show significant changes from baseline. However, significant improvement in the summed motor (peroneal, tibial, and median) nerve conduction velocity was observed with 20 and 40 mg/day ranirestat treatment at week 12 and at weeks 24 and 36. The peroneal motor nerve conduction velocity was improved at weeks 36 and 52 for the 20 mg/day ranirestat group. Therefore, the treatment with ranirestat might have an effect on motor nerve function in mild to moderate diabetic sensorimotor polyneuropathy. However, it failed to show a statistically significant difference in sensory nerve function relative to placebo. Ranirestat was well tolerated with no pertinent differences in drug-related adverse events or in effects on clinical laboratory parameters, vital signs, or electrocardiograms among the four groups [99].

4.2.4. Zenarestat

Zenarestat has proved to affect peripheral neuropathy in Zucker diabetic fatty rats, an animal model of type 2 diabetes. In the control group of Zucker diabetic fatty rats, a remarkable accumulation of sorbitol, a delay in F-wave minimal latency, and a slowing of motor nerve conduction velocity were observed compared with lean rat counterparts. Zenarestat, orally administrated at a dose of 3.2 mg/kg/day for 8 weeks, had no significant effect on the delay in F-wave minimal latency and the slowing of motor nerve conduction velocity, although the sorbitol accumulation in the sciatic nerve was partially inhibited. On the other hand, 32 mg/kg zenarestat treatment improved these nerve dysfunctions, along with a reduction of nerve sorbitol accumulation almost to the normal level [100]. Obviously, zenarestat could improve diabetic peripheral neuropathy in Zucker diabetic fatty rats. Also, the effects of zenarestat on nerves were confirmed in streptozotocin-induced diabetic rat model. When the diabetic model rats were maintained on a diet of containing 0.09% zenarestat for 8 weeks, endoneurial blood flow was significantly reduced by the application of nitric oxide synthase inhibitor, NG-nitro-L-arginine, whereas that in diabetic control rats was not affected by the inhibitor. Considerable levels of zenarestat were confirmed in the sciatic nerve in the drug treated rats. These thereby suggested that ARI zenarestat might restore or prevent the alteration of endoneurial blood flow resulting from an impairment of nitric oxide function [101]. The dorsal root ganglia has been identified as the target tissue in diabetic somatosensory neuropathy. Recent study in streptozotocin-induced diabetic rats showed that the cell area of the dorsal root ganglia was smaller than that in normal rats, and a decrease in fiber size and a greater fiber density were apparent in the sural nerve. However, these morphological changes were reversed in diabetic rats treated with zenarestat. These functions of zenarestat in animal model also indicate that, in peripheral sensory diabetic neuropathy, hyperactivation of the polyol pathway may induce abnormalities not only in peripheral nerve fiber, but also in the dorsal root ganglia, which is an aggregate of primary sensory afferent cell bodies [102].

In an earlier study of randomized, placebo-controlled, double-blinded, multiple-dose, clinical trial, zenarestat was supplied for 52 weeks to patients with mild to moderate diabetic peripheral polyneuropathy. Dose-dependent increments in sural nerve zenarestat level and sorbitol suppression were observed along with significant improvement in nerve conduction velocity. Further analysis showed that zenalrestat doses producing >80% sorbitol suppression were associated with a significant increase in the density of small-diameter sural nerve myelinated fibers. Therefore, the slowing of nerve conduction velocity and the loss of small myelinated nerve fiber in diabetic peripheral polyneuropathy in humans could be improved by zenarestat treatment, but >80% suppression of nerve sorbitol content may be required [103].

In further studies of clinical trials, however, mixed results for effects of zenarestat on patiants were obtained. In a multicentered trial of zenarestat over 12 months, sural sensory velocity, median sensory amplitude, median distal motor latency, and cool thermal quantitative sensory testing declined significantly from baseline in the placebo group of patients [104]. After that, a larger size of multicenter trial of zenarestat treatment in 1100 patients was conducted but significant improvement could not be observed [105].

4.2.5. Sorbinil

Sorbinil has shown an effective approach for preventing peripheral nerve dysfunction and morphological abnormalities in nerves of diabetic animal models although it has the exact toxicity. Experimental diabetic neuropathy is characterized by sorbitol accumulation and myo-inositol depletion and usually also by enhanced turnover of particularly phosphatidylinositol-4,5-bisphosphate (PIP2). Nerves in the streptozotocin-diabetic rats exhibited 52% to 76% greater PIP2 labeling, markedly elevated sorbitol levels, and 30% less myo-inositol when compared with normal rats. In contrast, in nerves of diabetic rats that received the sorbinil-supplemented diet for either 4 or 8 weeks, both PIP2 labeling and myo-inositol levels were restored to normal [106]. Also in the streptozotocin-diabetic rats, the treatment with sorbinil at 65 mg/kg/day in the diet for 2 weeks resulted in complete inhibition of increased sorbitol pathway activity. The sorbinil-treatment improved diabetes-induced nerve functional changes; that is, decrease in endoneurial nutritive blood flow, motor and sensory nerve conduction velocities, and metabolic abnormalities including mitochondrial and cytosolic NAD+/NADH redox imbalances and energy deficiency. The treatment also restored nerve concentrations of two major non-enzymatic antioxidants, reduced glutathione and ascorbate, and completely arrested diabetes-induced lipid peroxidation [107].

Pressure-induced vasodilation, a neurovascular mechanism relying on the interaction between mechanosensitive C-fibers and vessels, allows skin blood flow to increase in response to locally nonnociceptive applied pressure that in turn may protect against pressure ulcers. In 8-week diabetic mice model, pressure-induced vasodilation, endothelial response, C-fiber threshold, and motor nerve conduction velocity were all altered in diabetic mice. The treatment with sorbinil for 2 weeks had a significant effect on motor nerve conduction velocity. Sorbinil restored acetylcholine-dependent vasodilation, C-fiber threshold, and pressure-induced vasodilation development. Therefore, sorbinil may improve vascular and C-fiber functions via the inhibition of AR and the polyol pathway [108].

Clinical investigations with sorbinil in patients with diabetic peripheral neuropathy showed an improvement both in motor and sensory nerve conduction velocities. Median nerve somatosensory evoked potential studies in patients showed significant sorbinil-related improvements in peripheral conduction and cortical responses. The incidence of sorbinil toxicity in 106 patients was 11.3 percent. Side effects were confined to rash, which was sometimes accompanied by fever, and disappeared rapidly after discontinuation of the drug [64].

4.2.6. Tolrestat

Tolrestat had proved to be an ARI with ability of treating diabetic complications, particularly nerve dysfunction although it was withdrawn because of its toxicity.

Patients with diabetic autonomic neuropathy have an increased cardiovascular mortality rate compared with diabetic patients without diabetic autonomic neuropathy. Heart rate variability time and frequency domain indices are strong predictors of malignant arrhythmias and sudden cardiac death. Treatment of the patients having diabetic autonomic neuropathy and diabetes mellitus by the administration of tolrestat at 200 mg/day for 12 months was evaluated in a randomised, double-blind, placebo-controlled trial. At the twelfth month, tolrestat, compared with placebo, had a beneficial effect on heart rate variability indices related to vagal tone. Heart rate variability indices remained less than that of patients with diabetes mellitus but without diabetic autonomic neuropathy, and healthy controls. The 12 patients of the 22 with moderate diabetic autonomic neuropathy benefited more than the 10 patients of the 22 with severe diabetic autonomic neuropathy. Moreover, no patient showed deterioration in heart rate variability indices with tolrestat as was seen with placebo [109]. Therefore, the effect of tolrestat on reduction in risk for malignant ventricular arrhythmias was suggested.

In an earlier study, the effects of tolrestat on chronic symptomatic diabetic sensorimotor neuropathy were evaluated during a placebo-controlled, randomised, 52-week multicenter trial. Of the four tolrestat doses investigated, only the highest dose group, 200 mg once daily, showed subjective and objective benefit over baseline and placebo. Significant improvements in both tibial and peroneal motor nerve conduction velocities were seen at 52 weeks. Tolrestat 200 mg once daily was significantly better than placebo in producing concordant improvements in both motor nerve conduction velocities and paraesthetic symptom scores at 24 weeks. Benefit lasting for 52 weeks was seen in 28% of treated patients indicating some sustained improvement in symptomatic diabetic neuropathy [110].

4.3. Nephropathy

Increased flux through the polyol pathway is accompanied by the depletion of myo-inositol, a loss of Na/K ATPase activity, and the accumulation of sodium in diabetic nerves. Supportive evidence linking these biochemical changes to the loss of nerve function has come from studies in which ARIs block polyol pathway activity, prevent the depletion of myo-inositol and the accumulation of sodium, and preserve Na/K ATPase activity as well as nerve function. However, the pathophysiologic mechanisms underlying diabetic neuropathy may be different from those of diabetic nephropathy. In the kidney cortex in diabetic rats, polyol levels, medulla, and red blood cells were found to increase 2-9 folds, whereas myo-inositol levels decreased by 30% only in the kidney cortex and Na/K ATPase activity by 59% only in red blood cells. In contrast, in the rats treated with ARI tolrestat, only Na/K ATPase activity in red blood cells was improved although myo-inositol levels, Na/K ATPase, and conduction velocity in the sciatic nerve were preserved [111].

Thickening and reduplication of the tubular basement membrane has been suggested as an early event in diabetic nephropathy. During the incubation of confluent monolayers of LLC-PK1 cells grown on tissue culture, D-glucose treatment induced significant fibronectin accumulation in the basolateral compartment. The increase in fibronectin concentration in response to glucose was inhibited by sorbinil [112]. Moreover, glucose activation of the polyol pathway may lead to renal arteriolar smooth muscle and glomerular mesangial cell hypocontractility. In the streptozotocin-induced diabetic rats, functional alterations including increase in glomerular filtration rate, raised glomerular permeability to albumin, and glomerular hypertrophy were prevented by administration of tolrestat. Endothelin-1-induced contraction of isolated glomeruli was normal in tolrestat-treated diabetic animals compared with the hypocontractile diabetic glomeruli. Fractional mesangial expansion was unchanged in tolrestat-treated diabetic rats compared with untreated animals [113].

Both increased AR activity and oxidative/nitrosative stress have been implicated in the pathogenesis of diabetic nephropathy. In vitro studies revealed that accumulation of nitrosylated and poly(ADP-ribosyl)ated proteins in cultured human mesangial cells was induced by D-glucose but stopped by L-glucose or D-glucose plus fidarestat. In animal experiments, concentrations of sorbitol and fructose were significantly increased in the renal cortex of streptozotocin-diabetic rats and then prevented by fidarestat-treatment. Fidarestat at least partially prevented diabetes-induced increase in kidney weight as well as nitrotyrosine (a marker of peroxynitrite-induced injury and nitrosative stress), and poly(ADP-ribose) (a marker of polymerase activation) accumulation in glomerular and tubular compartments of the renal cortex. These results indicate that fidarestat treatment counteracts nitrosative stress and polymerase activation in the diabetic renal cortex and high-glucose-exposed human mesangial cells [24].

Long-term clinical trial study has shown beneficial effect of epalrestat on the development of incipient diabetic nephropathy in type 2 diabetic patients. At the end of the study conducted for 5 years, urinary albumin excretion increased significantly in the control group whereas it remained unchanged in the epalrestat-treated group. However, the reduction rate of reciprocal creatinine in the epalrestat-treated group was significantly smaller than that in the control group [114].

4.4. Others

As described in the preceding section of this chapter, the increased flux of the polyol pathway by hyperglycemia is implicated in the pathogenesis of diabetic complications, and one of the linkages has been proposed to be an increase in oxidative stress mediated by ROS. Early, it was found that some of enzymes responsible for oxidative defense were altered by treatment of ARI imirestat, particularly in rabbit livers, although direct changes in lipid peroxidation within normal rat and rabbit livers were not detected [115]. Clinical trial study in patients with type 2 diabetes mellitus revealed that administration of epalrestat at 150 mg/day for 3 months prevented adverse alterations in the levels of oxidative stress markers and antioxidants including plasma thiobarbituric acid-reactive substances, malondialdehyde-modified low-density lipoprotein, and vitamin E or β-carotene. In addition, epalrestat significantly reduced lipid hydroperoxides in erythrocytes [116]. The role of ARIs in the reduction of oxidative stress associated with diabetic complications is receiving increasing attention.

Very recently, Srivastava and co-workers found that alcohols, products from the reduction of ROS-induced lipid peroxidation-derived lipid aldehydes such as 4-hydroxy-trans-2-nonenal (HNE) and their glutathione-conjugates, are generated by AR catalysis and mediate inflammatory signals. Therefore, ARI fidarestat significantly prevented tumor necrosis factor-alpha (TNF-α)-, growth factors-, lipopolysachharide (LPS)-, and environmental allergens-induced inflammatory signals that cause various inflammatory diseases. Moreover, inhibition of AR significantly prevented the inflammatory signals induced by cytokines, NF-kappa B, growth factors, endotoxins, high glucose, allergens, and auto-immune reactions in cellular as well as animal models. Also, it significantly ameliorated the diseases in animal models of inflammatory diseases such as diabetes, cardiovascular, uveitis, asthma, and cancer (colon, breast, prostate and lung) and metastasis. Thereby ROS-induced inflammatory response could be reduced with ARIs [117, 118].

On the other hand, beneficial effects of ARI zopolrestat at 500 or 1,000 mg/day for 1 year on asymptomatic cardiac abnormalities were identified in patients with diabetic neuropathy in a double-blind placebo-controlled clinical trial study. In the zopolrestat treatment group, there were significant increases in resting left ventricular ejection fraction, cardiac output, left ventricular stroke volume, and exercise left ventricular ejection fraction. The increase in exercise left ventricular ejection fraction was independent of blood pressure, insulin use, or the presence of baseline abnormal heart rate variability. In contrast, there were decreases in exercise cardiac output, stroke volume, and end diastolic volume in the control group [119].

Furthermore, the beneficial effects of AR inhibition has been shown on the esophageal dysfunction in diabetic patients. When type 2 diabetic patients with peripheral neuropathy were administered with the ARI epalrestat at 150 mg/day for 90 days, parameters related to the gastroesophageal acid reflux and the esophageal motility were remarkably improved. These parameters include % time of pH<4, DeMeester score, duration of the longest reflux episode, reflux episodes longer than 5 min, ratios of peristaltic waves with the amplitude greater than 25 mmHg, and ratios of effective peristalsis [120].

5. Summary and perspective

The increased activities of AR and the consequent polyol pathway are believed likely to be the mechanism of diabetic complications. They have been shown to be involved in the diabetic alterations including particularly diabetic neuropathy, nephropathy, retinopathy, and cataract. The relevance of AR inhibition to the improvements of diabetic changes suggests the design of drugs that specifically target the polyol pathway, particularly AR, the rate-limiting enzyme of the pathway. There has been a considerable effort to develop small molecules useful for the AR inhibition over the past decades and a number of potent ARIs have been identified. These ARIs have proven effective in studies in vitro and some of them have been advanced to late phases of clinical trials. In particular, epalrestat has been marked in Japan for years and recently approved to markets in China and India.

While AR and the polyol pathway are promising targets for the treatment of diabetic complications and pharmaceutical developments, some ARIs able to redress all aspects of the polyol pathway but they in vivo or in clinical trials give a poor or only a partial amelioration, and some show unacceptable toxicities. For example, a long-term AR inhibition in diabetic dogs prevented sorbitol accumulation in erythrocytes and even diabetic neuropathy, but showed no beneficial effect on renal structure or albuminuria. It failed to prevent retinopathy or thickening of the capillary basement membrane in the retina, kidney and muscle [121, 122]. The similar results were observed in a transgenic rat model with human AR cDNA. In this model, AR inhibition was without effect on microalbuminuria, which follows glomerular and tubular dysfunction [123]. Fidarestat seems clinically not very effective, although it has already undergone late phase clinical trial for diabetic neuropathy and found to be safe [117]. As a result, very few ARIs could be passed through late stage of clinical trials, and only epalrestat is on the markets.

Several reasons may be suggested for these inconsistent and adverse effects with ARIs or AR inhibition. First, knowledge of structure and particularly conformational shape of AR active site has yet to be sufficiently acquired for the discovery of more specific ARIs. Amino acid sequences of AR were suggested to have a relatively low sequence identity conserved among human, rat, and other animal species although the existence of tissue-specific isoforms for human AR has not been verified [124]. This could account for the species-dependent differences in the sensitivity of AR to some of the inhibitors. Moreover, the conformational shape of AR active center may be variable depending on animals and tissues, and accurate conformation remains to be identified. Second, the diverse complications may not share the same mechanisms. At least evidence for a uniform pathogenetic mechanism is far from established although a single unifiying mechanism for diabetic complications was suggested [23] and the polyol pathway has proved to be the most attractive.

Therefore, further studies regarding the structural features of AR and identification of more specific ARIs are of importance to the understanding of the mechanism of diabetic complications and the treatment of the diseases.

Author details

Changjin Zhu
Department of Applied Chemistry, Beijing Institute of Technology, Beijing, China

6. References

[1] Yang W, Lu J, Weng J, Jia W, Ji L, Xiao J, Shan Z, Liu J, Tian H, Ji Q, Zhu D, Ge J, Lin L, Chen L, Guo X, Zhao Z, Li Q, Zhou Z, Shan G, He J. Prevalence of Diabetes among Men and Women in China. New England Journal of Medicine 2010; 362(12) 1090-1101.

[2] Brownlee M. Biochemistry and Molecular Cell Biology of Diabetic Complications. Nature 2001; 414(6865) 813-820.

[3] Fowler MJ. Microvascular and Macrovascular Complications of Diabetes. Clinical Diabetes 2008; 26(2) 77-82.

[4] Nathan DM. Long-Term Complications of Diabetes Mellitus. New England Journal of Medicine 1993; 328(23) 1676-1685.

[5] Oates PJ. Aldose Reductase, Still a Compelling Target for Diabetic Neuropathy Current Drug Targets 2008; 9(1) 23.

[6] Hers HG. The Mechanism of the Transformation of Glucose in Fructose in the Seminal Vesicles. Biochimica et biophysica acta 1956; 22(1) 202-203.

[7] Van Heyningen R. Formation of Polyols by the Lens of the Rat with /`Sugar/' Cataract. Nature 1959; 184(4681) 194-195.

[8] Kinoshita JH. Cataracts in Galactosemia. The Jonas S. Friedenwald Memorial Lecture. Investigative ophthalmology 1965; 4(5) 786-799.

[9] KINOSHITA JH. Mechanisms Initiating Cataract Formation Proctor Lecture. Investigative Ophthalmology & Visual Science 1974; 13(10) 713-724.

[10] Sango K, Suzuki T, Yanagisawa H, Takaku S, Hirooka H, Tamura M, Watabe K. High Glucose-Induced Activation of the Polyol Pathway and Changes of Gene Expression Profiles in Immortalized Adult Mouse Schwann Cells Ims32. Journal of Neurochemistry 2006; 98(2) 446-458.

[11] Suzuki T, Mizuno K, Yashima S, Watanabe K, Taniko K, Suzuki T, Yabe-Nishimura C. Characterization of Polyol Pathway in Schwann Cells Isolated from Adult Rat Sciatic Nerves. Journal of Neuroscience Research 1999; 57(4) 495-503.

[12] Yagihashi S, Yamagishi SI, Wada R, Baba M, Hohman TC, Yabe-Nishimura C, Kokai Y. Neuropathy in Diabetic Mice Overexpressing Human Aldose Reductase and Effects of Aldose Reductase Inhibitor. Brain 2001; 124 2448-2458.

[13] Yang B, Hodgkinson A, Oates PJ, Millward BA, Demaine AG. High Glucose Induction of DNA-Binding Activity of the Transcription Factor Nf Kappa B in Patients with Diabetic Nephropathy. Biochimica Et Biophysica Acta-Molecular Basis of Disease 2008; 1782(5) 295-302.

[14] Derylo B, Babazono T, Glogowski E, Kapor-Drezgic J, Hohman T, Whiteside C. High Glucose-Induced Mesangial Cell Altered Contractility: Role of the Polyol Pathway. Diabetologia 1998; 41(5) 507-515.

[15] Cheung AKH, Fung MKL, Lo ACY, Lam TTL, So KF, Chung SSM, Chung SK. Aldose Reductase Deficiency Prevents Diabetes-Induced Blood-Retinal Barrier Breakdown, Apoptosis, and Glial Reactivation in the Retina of Db/Db Mice. Diabetes 2005; 54(11) 3119-3125.

[16] Ho ECM, Lam KSL, Chen YS, Yip JCW, Arvindakshan M, Yamagishi SI, Yagihashi S, Oates PJ, Ellery CA, Chung SSM, Chung SK. Aldose Reductase-Deficient Mice Are Protected from Delayed Motor Nerve Conduction Velocity, Increased C-Jun Nh2-Terminal Kinase Activation, Depletion of Reduced Glutathione, Increased Superoxide Accumulation, and DNA Damage. Diabetes 2006; 55(7) 1946-1953.

[17] Yagihashi S, Mizukami H, Ogasawara S, Yamagishi SI, Nukada H, Kato N, Hibi C, Chung SJ, Chung S. The Role of the Polyol Pathway in Acute Kidney Injury Caused by Hindlimb Ischaemia in Mice. Journal of Pathology 2010; 220(5) 530-541.

[18] Obrosova IG, Pacher P, Szabó C, Zsengeller Z, Hirooka H, Stevens MJ, Yorek MA. Aldose Reductase Inhibition Counteracts Oxidative-Nitrosative Stress and Poly(Adp-Ribose) Polymerase Activation in Tissue Sites for Diabetes Complications. Diabetes 2005; 54(1) 234-242.

[19] Huang P, Zhang YJ, Jiang T, Zeng WJ, Zhang N. Role of Aldose Reductase in the High Glucose Induced Expression of Fibronectin in Human Mesangial Cells. Molecular Biology Reports 2010; 37(6) 3017-3021.

[20] Nakamura J, Koh N, Sakakibara F, Hamada Y, Hara T, Sasaki H, Chaya S, Komori T, Nakashima E, Naruse K, Kato K, Takeuchi N, Kasuya Y, Hotta N. Polyol Pathway Hyperactivity Is Closely Related to Carnitine Deficiency in the Pathogenesis of Diabetic Neuropathy of Streptozotocin-Diabetic Rats. Journal of Pharmacology and Experimental Therapeutics 1998; 287(3) 897-902.

[21] Palm F, Hansell P, Ronquist G, Waldenstrom A, Liss P, Carlsson PO. Polyol-Pathway-Dependent Disturbances in Renal Medullary Metabolism in Experimental Insulin-Deficient Diabetes Mellitus in Rats. Diabetologia 2004; 47(7) 1223-1231.

[22] Yabe-Nishimura C. Aldose Reductase in Glucose Toxicity: A Potential Target for the Prevention of Diabetic Complications. Pharmacological Reviews 1998; 50(1) 21-34.

[23] Nishikawa T, Edelstein D, Brownlee M. The Missing Link: A Single Unifying Mechanism for Diabetic Complications. Kidney Int 2000; 58(S77) S26-S30.

[24] Drel VR, Pacher P, Stevens MJ, Obrosova IG. Aldose Reductase Inhibition Counteracts Nitrosative Stress and Poly(Adp-Ribose) Polymerase Activation in Diabetic Rat Kidney and High-Glucose-Exposed Human Mesangial Cells. Free Radical Biology and Medicine 2006; 40(8) 1454-1465.

[25] Mulhern ML, Madson CJ, Kador PF, Randazzo J, Shinohara T. Cellular Osmolytes Reduce Lens Epithelial Cell Death and Alleviate Cataract Formation in Galactosemic Rats. Molecular Vision 2007; 13 1397-1405.

[26] Schade SZ, Early SL, Williams TR, Kézdy FJ, Heinrikson RL, Grimshaw CE, Doughty CC. Sequence Analysis of Bovine Lens Aldose Reductase. Journal of Biological Chemistry 1990; 265(7) 3628-3635.

[27] Rondeau JM, Tete-Favier F, Podjarny A, Reymann JM, Barth P, Biellmann JF, Moras D. Novel Nadph-Binding Domain Revealed by the Crystal Structure of Aldose Reductase. Nature 1992; 355(6359) 469-472.

[28] Wilson D, Bohren K, Gabbay K, Quiocho F. An Unlikely Sugar Substrate Site in the 1.65 a Structure of the Human Aldose Reductase Holoenzyme Implicated in Diabetic Complications. Science 1992; 257(5066) 81-84.

[29] Sotriffer CA, Krämer O, Klebe G. Probing Flexibility and "Induced-Fit" Phenomena in Aldose Reductase by Comparative Crystal Structure Analysis and Molecular Dynamics Simulations. Proteins: Structure, Function, and Bioinformatics 2004; 56(1) 52-66.

[30] Urzhumtsev A, Tête-Favier F, Mitschler A, Barbanton J, Barth P, Urzhumtseva L, Biellmann JF, Podjarny AD, Moras D. A 'Specificity' Pocket Inferred from the Crystal Structures of the Complexes of Aldose Reductase with the Pharmaceutically Important Inhibitors Tolrestat and Sorbinil. Structure 1997; 5(5) 601-612.

[31] Steuber H, Zentgraf M, Gerlach C, Sotriffer CA, Heine A, Klebe G. Expect the Unexpected or Caveat for Drug Designers: Multiple Structure Determinations Using Aldose Reductase Crystals Treated under Varying Soaking and Co-Crystallisation Conditions. Journal of Molecular Biology 2006; 363(1) 174-187.

[32] Howard EI, Sanishvili R, Cachau RE, Mitschler A, Chevrier B, Barth P, Lamour V, Van Zandt M, Sibley E, Bon C, Moras D, Schneider TR, Joachimiak A, Podjarny A. Ultrahigh Resolution Drug Design I: Details of Interactions in Human Aldose Reductase–Inhibitor Complex at 0.66 Proteins: Structure, Function, and Bioinformatics 2004; 55(4) 792-804.

[33] El-Kabbani O, Ramsland P, Darmanin C, Chung RPT, Podjarny A. Structure of Human Aldose Reductase Holoenzyme in Complex with Statil: An Approach to Structure-Based Inhibitor Design of the Enzyme. Proteins: Structure, Function, and Bioinformatics 2003; 50(2) 230-238.

[34] El-Kabbani O, Darmanin C, Schneider TR, Hazemann I, Ruiz F, Oka M, Joachimiak A, Schulze-Briese C, Tomizaki T, Mitschler A, Podjarny A. Ultrahigh Resolution Drug Design. Ii. Atomic Resolution Structures of Human Aldose Reductase Holoenzyme Complexed with Fidarestat and Minalrestat: Implications for the Binding of Cyclic Imide Inhibitors. Proteins: Structure, Function, and Bioinformatics 2004; 55(4) 805-813.

[35] El-Kabbani O, Darmanin C, Oka M, Schulze-Briese C, Tomizaki T, Hazemann I, Mitschler A, Podjarny A. High-Resolution Structures of Human Aldose Reductase

Holoenzyme in Complex with Stereoisomers of the Potent Inhibitor Fidarestat: Stereospecific Interaction between the Enzyme and a Cyclic Imide Type Inhibitor. Journal of Medicinal Chemistry 2004; 47(18) 4530-4537.
[36] Van Zandt MC, Jones ML, Gunn DE, Geraci LS, Jones JH, Sawicki DR, Sredy J, Jacot JL, DiCioccio AT, Petrova T, Mitschler A, Podjarny AD. Discovery of 3-[(4,5,7-Trifluorobenzothiazol-2-Yl)Methyl]Indole-N-Acetic Acid (Lidorestat) and Congeners as Highly Potent and Selective Inhibitors of Aldose Reductase for Treatment of Chronic Diabetic Complications. Journal of Medicinal Chemistry 2005; 48(9) 3141-3152.
[37] Cosconati S, Marinelli L, La Motta C, Sartini S, Da Settimo F, Olson AJ, Novellino E. Pursuing Aldose Reductase Inhibitors through in Situ Cross-Docking and Similarity-Based Virtual Screening. Journal of Medicinal Chemistry 2009; 52(18) 5578-5581.
[38] Bohren KM, Grimshaw CE, Lai CJ, Harrison DH, Ringe D, Petsko GA, Gabbay KH. Tyrosine-48 Is the Proton Donor and Histidine-110 Directs Substrate Stereochemical Selectivity in the Reduction Reaction of Human Aldose Reductase: Enzyme Kinetics and Crystal Structure of the Y48h Mutant Enzyme. Biochemistry 1994; 33(8) 2021-2032.
[39] El-Kabbani O, Wilson DK, Petrash JM, Quiocho FA. Structural Features of the Aldose Reductase and Aldehyde Reductase Inhibitor-Binding Sites. Molecular Vision 1998; 4(19) 19-25.
[40] Bohren KM, Grimshaw CE, Gabbay KH. Catalytic Effectiveness of Human Aldose Reductase. Critical Role of C-Terminal Domain. Journal of Biological Chemistry 1992; 267(29) 20965-20970.
[41] Barski OA, Gabbay KH, Bohren KM. The C-Terminal Loop of Aldehyde Reductase Determines the Substrate and Inhibitor Specificity†. Biochemistry 1996; 35(45) 14276-14280.
[42] Barski OA, Gabbay KH, Grimshaw CE, Bohren KM. Mechanism of Human Aldehyde Reductase: Characterization of the Active Site Pocket. Biochemistry 1995; 34(35) 11264-11275.
[43] Carper DA, Wistow G, Nishimura C, Graham C, Watanabe K, Fujii Y, Hayashi H, Hayaishi O. A Superfamily of Nadph-Dependent Reductases in Eukaryotes and Prokaryotes. Experimental Eye Research 1989; 49(3) 377-388.
[44] Feather MS, Geoffrey Flynn T, Munro KA, Kubiseski TJ, Walton DJ. Catalysis of Reduction of Carbohydrate 2-Oxoaldehydes (Osones) by Mammalian Aldose Reductase and Aldehyde Reductase. Biochimica et Biophysica Acta (BBA) - General Subjects 1995; 1244(1) 10-16.
[45] Ratliff DM, Vander Jagt DJ, Eaton RP, Vander Jagt DL. Increased Levels of Methylglyoxal-Metabolizing Enzymes in Mononuclear and Polymorphonuclear Cells from Insulin-Dependent Diabetic Patients with Diabetic Complications: Aldose Reductase, Glyoxalase I, and Glyoxalase Ii--a Clinical Research Center Study. Journal of Clinical Endocrinology & Metabolism 1996; 81(2) 488-492.
[46] Kador PF, Kinoshita JH, Sharpless NE. Aldose Reductase Inhibitors: A Potential New Class of Agents for the Pharmacological Control of Certain Diabetic Complications. Journal of Medicinal Chemistry 1985; 28(7) 841-849.

[47] Suzen S, Buyukbingol E. Recent Studies of Aldose Reductase Enzyme Inhibition for Diabetic Complications Current Medicinal Chemistry 2003; 10(15) 33.

[48] Hayman S, Kinoshita JH. Isolation and Properties of Lens Aldose Reductase. Journal of Biological Chemistry 1965; 240(2) 877-882.

[49] Kikkawa R, Hatanaka I, Yasuda H, Kobayashi N, Shigeta Y, Terashima H, Morimura T, Tsuboshima M. Effect of a New Aldose Reductase Inhibitor, (E)-3-Carboxymethyl-5-[(2e)-Methyl-3-Phenylpropenylidene]Rhodanine (Ono-2235) on Peripheral Nerve Disorders in Streptozotocin-Diabetic Rats. Diabetologia 1983; 24(4) 290-292.

[50] Sestanj K, Bellini F, Fung S, Abraham N, Treasurywala A, Humber L, Simard-Dequesne N, Dvornik D. N-[[5-(Trifluoromethyl)-6-Methoxy-1-Naphthalenyl]Thioxomethyl]-N-Methylglycine (Tolrestat), a Potent, Orally Active Aldose Reductase Inhibitor. Journal of Medicinal Chemistry 1984; 27(3) 255-256.

[51] Ao S, Shingu Y, Kikuchi C, Takano Y, Nomura K, Fujiwara T, Ohkubo Y, Notsu Y, Yamaguchi I. Characterization of a Novel Aldose Reductase Inhibitor, Fr74366, and Its Effects on Diabetic Cataract and Neuropathy in the Rat. Metabolism 1991; 40(1) 77-87.

[52] Mylari BL, Larson ER, Beyer TA, Zembrowski WJ, Aldinger CE, Dee MF, Siegel TW, Singleton DH. Novel, Potent Aldose Reductase Inhibitors: 3,4-Dihydro-4-Oxo-3-[[5-(Trifluoromethyl)-2-Benzothiazolyl]Methyl]-1-Phthalazineacetic Acid (Zopolrestat) and Congeners. Journal of Medicinal Chemistry 1991; 34(1) 108-122.

[53] Stribling D, Mirrlees DJ, Harrison HE, Earl DCN. Properties of Ici 128,436, a Novel Aldose Reductase Inhibitor, and Its Effects on Diabetic Complications in the Rat. Metabolism 1985; 34(4) 336-344.

[54] Zenarestat: Fk 366, Fr 74366, Fr 901366. Drugs in R&D 2002; 3(4) 235-237.

[55] Da Settimo F, Primofiore G, La Motta C, Sartini S, Taliani S, Simorini F, Marini AM, Lavecchia A, Novellino E, Boldrini E. Naphtho[1,2-D]Isothiazole Acetic Acid Derivatives as a Novel Class of Selective Aldose Reductase Inhibitors. Journal of Medicinal Chemistry 2005; 48(22) 6897-6907.

[56] La Motta C, Sartini S, Salerno S, Simorini F, Taliani S, Marini AM, Da Settimo F, Marinelli L, Limongelli V, Novellino E. Acetic Acid Aldose Reductase Inhibitors Bearing a Five-Membered Heterocyclic Core with Potent Topical Activity in a Visual Impairment Rat Model. Journal of Medicinal Chemistry 2008; 51(11) 3182-3193.

[57] Chen X, Zhu C, Guo F, Qiu X, Yang Y, Zhang S, He M, Parveen S, Jing C, Li Y, Ma B. Acetic Acid Derivatives of 3,4-Dihydro-2h-1,2,4-Benzothiadiazine 1,1-Dioxide as a Novel Class of Potent Aldose Reductase Inhibitors. Journal of Medicinal Chemistry 2010; 53(23) 8330-8344.

[58] Chen X, Yang Y, Ma B, Zhang S, He M, Gui D, Hussain S, Jing C, Zhu C, Yu Q, Liu Y. Design and Synthesis of Potent and Selective Aldose Reductase Inhibitors Based on Pyridylthiadiazine Scaffold. European Journal of Medicinal Chemistry 2011; 46(5) 1536-1544.

[59] Yang Y, Zhang S, Wu B, Ma M, Chen X, Qin X, He M, Hussain S, Jing C, Ma B, Zhu C. An Efficient Synthesis of Quinoxalinone Derivatives as Potent Inhibitors of Aldose Reductase. ChemMedChem 2012; 7(5) 823-835.

[60] Hamada Y, Nakamura J. Clinical Potential of Aldose Reductase Inhibitors in Diabetic Neuropathy. Treatments in Endocrinology 2004; 3(4) 245-255.

[61] Costantino L, Rastelli G, Vianello P, Cignarella G, Barlocco D. Diabetes Complications and Their Potential Prevention: Aldose Reductase Inhibition and Other Approaches. Medicinal Research Reviews 1999; 19(1) 3-23.

[62] Fukushi S, Merola LO, Kinoshita JH. Altering the Course of Cataracts in Diabetic Rats. Investigative Ophthalmology & Visual Science 1980; 19(3) 313-315.

[63] Robison WG, Laver NM, Jacot JL, Glover JP. Sorbinil Prevention of Diabetic-Like Retinopathy in the Galactose-Fed Rat Model. Investigative Ophthalmology & Visual Science 1995; 36(12) 2368-2380.

[64] Jaspan JB, Herold K, Bartkus C. Effects of Sorbinil Therapy in Diabetic Patients with Painful Peripheral Neuropathy and Autonomic Neuropathy. The American Journal of Medicine 1985; 79(5, Supplement 1) 24-37.

[65] Spielberg SP, Shear NH, Cannon M, Hutson NJ, Gunderson K. In-Vitro Assessment of a Hypersensitivity Syndrome Associated with Sorbinil. Annals of Internal Medicine 1991; 114(9) 720-724.

[66] Negoro T, Murata M, Ueda S, Fujitani B, Ono Y, Kuromiya A, Komiya M, Suzuki K, Matsumoto J-i. Novel, Highly Potent Aldose Reductase Inhibitors: (R)-(−)-2-(4-Bromo-2-Fluorobenzyl)-1,2,3,4-Tetrahydropyrrolo[1,2-a]Pyrazine- 4-Spiro-3′-Pyrrolidine-1,2′,3,5′-Tetrone (as-3201) and Its Congeners. Journal of Medicinal Chemistry 1998; 41(21) 4118-4129.

[67] Asano T, Saito Y, Kawakami M, Yamada N. Fidarestat (Snk-860), a Potent Aldose Reductase Inhibitor, Normalizes the Elevated Sorbitol Accumulation in Erythrocytes of Diabetic Patients. Journal of Diabetes and its Complications 2002; 16(2) 133-138.

[68] Kurono M, Fujii A, Murata M, Fujitani B, Negoro T. Stereospecific Recognition of a Spirosuccinimide Type Aldose Reductase Inhibitor (as-3201) by Plasma Proteins: A Significant Role of Specific Binding by Serum Albumin in the Improved Potency and Stability. Biochemical Pharmacology 2006; 71(3) 338-353.

[69] Matsumoto T, Yoshiyuki, Kuromiya A, Toyosawa K, Ueda Y, Bril V. Long-Term Treatment with Ranirestat (as-3201), a Potent Aldose Reductase Inhibitor, Suppresses Diabetic Neuropathy and Cataract Formation in Rats. Journal of Pharmacological Sciences 2008; 107(3) 340-348.

[70] Miwa I, Hirano M, Inagaki K, Belbeoc'h C, Okuda J. Development of Potent Aldose Reductase Inhibitors Having a Hydantoin Structure. Biochemical Pharmacology 1987; 36(17) 2789-2794.

[71] Miwa I, Hirano M, Kanbara M, Okuda J. In Vivo Activities of Aldose Reductase Inhibitors Having a 1-(Arylsulfonyl)Hydantoin Structure. Biochemical Pharmacology 1990; 40(2) 303-307.

[72] Kato K, Nayama K, Mizota M, Miwa I, Okuda j. Properties of Novel Aldose Reductase Inhibitors, M16209 and M16287, in Comparison with Known Inhibitors, Ono-2235 and Sorbinil. CHEMICAL & PHARMACEUTICAL BULLETIN 1991; 39(6) 1540-1545.

[73] Mylari BL, Armento SJ, Beebe DA, Conn EL, Coutcher JB, Dina MS, O'Gorman MT, Linhares MC, Martin WH, Oates PJ, Tess DA, Withbroe GJ, Zembrowski WJ. A Novel Series of Non-Carboxylic Acid, Non-Hydantoin Inhibitors of Aldose Reductase with Potent Oral Activity in Diabetic Rat Models: 6-(5-Chloro-3-Methylbenzofuran-2-Sulfonyl)-2h-Pyridazin-3-One and Congeners. Journal of Medicinal Chemistry 2005; 48(20) 6326-6339.
[74] Sun W, Oates PJ, Coutcher JB, Gerhardinger C, Lorenzi M. A Selective Aldose Reductase Inhibitor of a New Structural Class Prevents or Reverses Early Retinal Abnormalities in Experimental Diabetic Retinopathy. Diabetes 2006; 55(10) 2757-2762.
[75] Alexiou P, Demopoulos VJ. A Diverse Series of Substituted Benzenesulfonamides as Aldose Reductase Inhibitors with Antioxidant Activity: Design, Synthesis, and in Vitro Activity. Journal of Medicinal Chemistry 2010; 53(21) 7756-7766.
[76] La Motta C, Sartini S, Mugnaini L, Simorini F, Taliani S, Salerno S, Marini AM, Da Settimo F, Lavecchia A, Novellino E, Cantore M, Failli P, Ciuffi M. Pyrido[1,2-a]Pyrimidin-4-One Derivatives as a Novel Class of Selective Aldose Reductase Inhibitors Exhibiting Antioxidant Activity. Journal of Medicinal Chemistry 2007; 50(20) 4917-4927.
[77] Kador PF, Betts D, Wyman M, Blessing K, Randazzo J. Effects of Topical Administration of an Aldose Reductase Inhibitor on Cataract Formation in Dogs Fed a Diet High in Galactose. American Journal of Veterinary Research 2006; 67(10) 1783-1787.
[78] Randazzo J, Zhang P, Makita J, Blessing K, Kador PF. Orally Active Multi-Functional Antioxidants Delay Cataract Formation in Streptozotocin (Type 1) Diabetic and Gamma-Irradiated Rats. Plos One 2011; 6(4).
[79] Drel VR, Pacher P, Ali TK, Shin J, Julius U, El-Remessy AB, Obrosova IG. Aldose Reductase Inhibitor Fidarestat Counteracts Diabetes-Associated Cataract Formation, Retinal Oxidative-Nitrosative Stress, Glial Activation, and Apoptosis. International Journal of Molecular Medicine 2008; 21(6) 667-676.
[80] Obrosova IG, Maksimchyk Y, Pacher P, Agardh E, Smith M-L, El-Remessy AB, Agardh C-D. Evaluation of the Aldose Reductase Inhibitor Fidarestat on Ischemia-Reperfusion Injury in Rat Retina. International Journal of Molecular Medicine 2010; 26(1) 135-142.
[81] Hattori T, Matsubara A, Taniguchi K, Ogura Y. Aldose Reductase Inhibitor Fidarestat Attenuates Leukocyte-Endothelial Interactions in Experimental Diabetic Rat Retina in Vivo. Current Eye Research 2010; 35(2) 146-154.
[82] Kim J, Kim C-S, Sohn E, Lee YM, Kim JS. Kiom-79 Inhibits Aldose Reductase Activity and Cataractogenesis in Zucker Diabetic Fatty Rats. Journal of Pharmacy and Pharmacology 2011; 63(10) 1301-1308.
[83] Sato S, Mori K, Wyman M, Kador PF. Dose-Dependent Prevention of Sugar Cataracts in Galactose-Fed Dogs by the Aldose Reductase Inhibitor M79175. Experimental Eye Research 1998; 66(2) 217-222.
[84] Sato S, Takahashi Y, Wyman M, Kador PF. Progression of Sugar Cataract in the Dog. Investigative Ophthalmology & Visual Science 1991; 32(6) 1925-1931.

[85] Kador PF, Webb TR, Bras D, Ketring K, Wyman M. Topical Kinostat (Tm) Ameliorates the Clinical Development and Progression of Cataracts in Dogs with Diabetes Mellitus. Veterinary Ophthalmology 2010; 13(6) 363-368.

[86] Schemmel KE, Padiyara RS, D'Souza JJ. Aldose Reductase Inhibitors in the Treatment of Diabetic Peripheral Neuropathy: A Review. Journal of Diabetes and its Complications 2010; 24(5) 354-360.

[87] Hotta N, Akanuma Y, Kawamori R, Matsuoka K, Oka Y, Shichiri M, Toyota T, Nakashima M, Yoshimura I, Sakamoto N, Shigeta Y, Group tAS. Long-Term Clinical Effects of Epalrestat, an Aldose Reductase Inhibitor, on Diabetic Peripheral Neuropathy. Diabetes Care 2006; 29(7) 1538-1544.

[88] Ramirez MA, Borja NL. Epalrestat: An Aldose Reductase Inhibitor for the Treatment of Diabetic Neuropathy. Pharmacotherapy 2008; 28(5) 646-655.

[89] Kawai T, Takei I, Tokui M, Funae O, Miyamoto K, Tabata M, Hirata T, Saruta T, Shimada A, Itoh H. Effects of Epalrestat, an Aldose Reductase Inhibitor, on Diabetic Peripheral Neuropathy in Patients with Type 2 Diabetes, in Relation to Suppression of N(Epsilon)-Carboxymethyl Lysine. Journal of Diabetes and Its Complications 2010; 24(6) 424-432.

[90] Sharma SR, Sharma N. Epalrestat, an Aldose Reductase Inhibitor, in Diabetic Neuropathy: An Indian Perspective. Annals of Indian Academy of Neurology 2008; 11(4) 231-235.

[91] Hotta N, Kawamori R, Atsumi Y, Baba M, Kishikawa H, Nakamura J, Oikawa S, Yamada N, Yasuda H, Shigeta Y, Grp AS. Stratified Analyses for Selecting Appropriate Target Patients with Diabetic Peripheral Neuropathy for Long-Term Treatment with an Aldose Reductase Inhibitor, Epalrestat. Diabetic Medicine 2008; 25(7) 818-825.

[92] Misawa S, Kuwabara S, Kanai K, Tamura N, Nakata M, Sawai S, Yagui K, Hattori T. Aldose Reductase Inhibition Alters Nodal Na+ Currents and Nerve Conduction in Human Diabetics. Neurology 2006; 66(10) 1545-1549.

[93] Ohi T, Saita K, Furukawa S, Ohta M, Hayashi K, Matsukura S. Therapeutic Effects of Aldose Reductase Inhibitor on Experimental Diabetic Neuropathy through Synthesis/Secretion of Nerve Growth Factor. Experimental Neurology 1998; 151(2) 215-220.

[94] Hotta N, Toyota T, Matsuoka K, Shigeta Y, Kikkawa R, Kaneko T, Takahashi A, Sugimura K, Koike Y, Ishii J, Sakamoto N, Gr SNKDNS. Clinical Efficacy of Fidarestat, a Novel Aldose Reductase Inhibitor, for Diabetic Peripheral Neuropathy - a 52-Week Multicenter Placebo-Controlled Double-Blind Parallel Group Study. Diabetes Care 2001; 24(10) 1776-1782.

[95] Kuzumoto Y, Kusunoki S, Kato N, Kihara M, Low PA. Effect of the Aldose Reductase Inhibitor Fidarestat on Experimental Diabetic Neuropathy in the Rat. Diabetologia 2006; 49(12) 3085-3093.

[96] Giannoukakis N. Drug Evaluation: Ranirestat - an Aldose Reductase Inhibitor for the Potential Treatment of Diabetic Complications. Current Opinion in Investigational Drugs 2006; 7(10) 916-923.

[97] Matsumoto T, Ono Y, Kurono M, Kuromiya A, Nakamura K, Bril V. Ranirestat (as-3201), a Potent Aldose Reductase Inhibitor, Reduces Sorbitol Levels and Improves Motor Nerve Conduction Velocity in Streptozotocin-Diabetic Rats Journal of Pharmacological Sciences 2008; 107(3) 231-237.
[98] Bril V, Buchanan RA, Ranirestat Study G. Long-Term Effects of Ranirestat (as-3201) on Peripheral Nerve Function in Patients with Diabetic Sensorimotor Polyneuropathy. Diabetes Care 2006; 29(1) 68-72.
[99] Bril V, Hirose T, Tomioka S, Buchanan R, Group ftRS. Ranirestat for the Management of Diabetic Sensorimotor Polyneuropathy. Diabetes Care 2009; 32(7) 1256-1260.
[100] Shimoshige Y, Ikuma K, Yamamoto T, Takakura S, Kawamura I, Seki J, Mutoh S, Goto T. The Effects of Zenarestat, an Aldose Reductase Inhibitor, on Peripheral Neuropathy in Zucker Diabetic Fatty Rats. Metabolism-Clinical and Experimental 2000; 49(11) 1395-1399.
[101] Kihara M, Mitsui Y, Shioyama M, Hasegawa T, Takahashi M, Takakura S, Minoura K, Kawamura I. Effect of Zenarestat, an Aldose Reductase Inhibitor, on Endoneurial Blood Flow in Experimental Diabetic Neuropathy of Rat. Neuroscience Letters 2001; 310(2-3) 81-84.
[102] Shimoshige Y, Minoura K, Matsuoka N, Takakura S, Mutoh S, Kamijo M. Thirteen-Month Inhibition of Aldose Reductase by Zenarestat Prevents Morphological Abnormalities in the Dorsal Root Ganglia of Streptozotocin-Induced Diabetic Rats. Brain Research 2009; 1247 182-187.
[103] Greene DA, Arezzo JC, Brown MB, Grp ZS. Effect of Aldose Reductase Inhibition on Nerve Conduction and Morphometry in Diabetic Neuropathy. Neurology 1999; 53(3) 580-591.
[104] Brown MJ, Bird SJ, Watling S, Kaleta H, Hayes L, Eckert S, Foyt HL. Natural Progression of Diabetic Peripheral Neuropathy in the Zenarestat Study Population. Diabetes Care 2004; 27(5) 1153-1159.
[105] Bird SJ, Brown MJ, Spino C, Watling S, Foyt HL. Value of Repeated Measures of Nerve Conduction and Quantitative Sensory Testing in a Diabetic Neuropathy Trial. Muscle & Nerve 2006; 34(2) 214-224.
[106] BertiMattera L, Day N, Peterson RG, Eichberg J. An Aldose Reductase Inhibitor but Not Myo-Inositol Blocks Enhanced Polyphosphoinositide Turnover in Peripheral Nerve from Diabetic Rats. Metabolism-Clinical and Experimental 1996; 45(3) 320-327.
[107] Obrosova IG, Van Huysen C, Fathallah L, Cao XC, Greene DA, Stevens MJ. An Aldose Reductase Inhibitor Reverses Early Diabetes-Induced Changes in Peripheral Nerve Function, Metabolism, and Antioxidative Defense. FASEB journal : official publication of the Federation of American Societies for Experimental Biology 2002; 16(1) 123-125.
[108] Demiot C, Tartas M, Fromy B, Abraham P, Saumet JL, Sigaudo-Roussel D. Aldose Reductase Pathway Inhibition Improved Vascular and C-Fiber Functions, Allowing for Pressure-Induced Vasodilation Restoration During Severe Diabetic Neuropathy. Diabetes 2006; 55(5) 1478-1483.

[109] Didangelos TP, Athyros VG, Karamitsos DT, Papageorgiou AA, Kourtoglou GI, Kontopoulos AG. Effect of Aldose Reductase Inhibition on Heart Rate Variability in Patients with Severe or Moderate Diabetic Autonomic Neuropathy. Clinical Drug Investigation 1998; 15(2) 111-121.

[110] Boulton A, Levin S, Comstock J. A Multicentre Trial of the Aldose-Reductase Inhibitor, Tolrestat, in Patients with Symptomatic Diabetic Neuropathy. Diabetologia 1990; 33(7) 431-437.

[111] Raccah D, Coste T, Cameron NE, Dufayet D, Vague P, Hohman TC. Effect of the Aldose Reductase Inhibitor Tolrestat on Nerve Conduction Velocity Na/K Atpase Activity, and Polyols in Red Blood Cells, Sciatic Nerve, Kidney Cortex, and Kidney Medulla of Diabetic Rats. Journal of Diabetes and its Complications 1998; 12(3) 154-162.

[112] Morrisey K, Steadman R, Williams JD, Phillips AO. Renal Proximal Tubular Cell Fibronectin Accumulation in Response to Glucose Is Polyol Pathway Dependent. Kidney International 1999; 55(6) 2548-2548.

[113] Donnelly SM, Zhou XP, Huang JT, Whiteside CI. Prevention of Early Glomerulopathy with Tolrestat in the Streptozotocin-Induced Diabetic Rat. Biochemistry and Cell Biology-Biochimie Et Biologie Cellulaire 1996; 74(3) 355-362.

[114] Iso K, Tada H, Kuboki K, Inokuchi T. Long-Term Effect of Epalrestat, an Aldose Reductase Inhibitor, on the Development of Incipient Diabetic Nephropathy in Type 2 Diabetic Patients. Journal of Diabetes and its Complications 2001; 15(5) 241-244.

[115] Thomas T, Rauscher F, Sanders R, Veltman J, Watkins JB. Effects of Aldose Reductase Inhibitors on Antioxidant Defense in Rat and Rabbit Liver. Toxicological Sciences 2000; 53(1) 145-149.

[116] Ohmura C, Watada H, Azuma K, Shimizu T, Kanazawa A, Ikeda F, Yoshihara T, Fujitana Y, Hirose T, Tanaka Y, Kawamori R. Aldose Reductase Inhibitor, Epalrestat, Reduces Lipid Hydroperoxides in Type 2 Diabetes. Endocrine Journal 2009; 56(1) 149-156.

[117] Srivastava SK, Yadav UCS, Reddy ABM, Saxena A, Tammali R, Shoeb M, Ansari NH, Bhatnagar A, Petrash MJ, Srivastava S, Ramana KV. Aldose Reductase Inhibition Suppresses Oxidative Stress-Induced Inflammatory Disorders. Chemico-Biological Interactions 2011; 191(1-3) 330-338.

[118] Yadav UCS, Ramana KV, Srivastava SK. Aldose Reductase Inhibition Suppresses Airway Inflammation. Chemico-Biological Interactions 2011; 191(1-3) 339-345.

[119] Johnson BF, Nesto RW, Pfeifer MA, Slater WR, Vinik AI, Chyun DA, Law G, Wackers FJT, Young LH. Cardiac Abnormalities in Diabetic Patients with Neuropathy - Effects of Aldose Reductase Inhibitor Administration. Diabetes Care 2004; 27(2) 448-454.

[120] Kinekawa F, Kubo F, Matsuda K, Fujita Y, Kobayashi M, Funakoshi F, Uchida N, Watanabe S, Tomita T, Uchida Y, Kuriyama S. Effect of an Aldose Reductase Inhibitor on Esophageal Dysfunction in Diabetic Patients. Hepato-Gastroenterology 2005; 52(62) 471-474.

[121] Kern TS, Engerman RL. Aldose Reductase and the Development of Renal Disease in Diabetic Dogs. Journal of Diabetes and Its Complications 1999; 13(1) 10-16.

[122] Engerman R, Kern T, Larson M. Nerve Conduction and Aldose Reductase Inhibition During 5 Years of Diabetes or Galactosaemia in Dogs. Diabetologia 1994; 37(2) 141-144.

[123] Dunlop M. Aldose Reductase and the Role of the Polyol Pathway in Diabetic Nephropathy. Kidney international Supplement 2000; 77 S3-12.

[124] Nishimura C, Yamaoka T, Mizutani M, Yamashita K, Akera T, Tanimoto T. Purification and Characterization of the Recombinant Human Aldose Reductase Expressed in Baculovirus System. Biochimica et Biophysica Acta (BBA) - Protein Structure and Molecular Enzymology 1991; 1078(2) 171-178.

Chapter 3

Behavioral Problems and Depressive Symptoms in Adolescents with Type 1 Diabetes Mellitus: Self and Parent Reports

Nienke M. Maas- van Schaaijk, Angelique B.C. Roeleveld-Versteegh, Roelof R.J. Odink and Anneloes L. van Baar

Additional information is available at the end of the chapter

http://dx.doi.org/10.5772/50667

1. Introduction

Children and adolescents with chronic diseases are at higher risk for mental health problems. Especially in adolescence, which involves a multitude of physical, cognitive and emotional developmental changes, a chronic disease such as diabetes mellitus type 1 (T1DM) that requires daily, careful attention, may influence social and emotional functioning. Adolescents with T1DM must deal with disease-specific stressors, in addition to age-specific stressors (Reid, Dubow, Carey, & Dura, 1994). Stress, in itself, may dysregulate diabetes through psycho-physiological processes or associated changes in self-management behaviors (Snoek, 2000). Therefore, diabetic treatment guidelines include metabolic goals, as well as facilitation of normal social and emotional development (Grey & Boland, 1996). Problems in social-emotional functioning are reflected in the occurrence of internalizing or externalizing behavior problems. Diabetes has been found to form a risk factor for psychiatric disorders in adolescence, especially for internalizing behavior problems like depression Kovacs, Obrosky, Goldston & Drash, 1997; Northam, Matthews, Anderson, Cameron & Werther, 2005). Several studies have found that diabetes and depression frequently co-occur in adolescence Anderson, Freedland, Clouse & Lustman, 2001; Lin et al., 2004; Hood et al., 2006; Lawrence et al., 2006; McGrady & Hood, 2010, although this is not always the case (DeWit, 2007).

Externalizing problems may also be important among adolescents with T1DM. Externalizing behavior problems have been found to result in poorer glycemic control (Cohen, Lumley, Naar-King, Partridge & Cakan, 2004), and diagnoses of pre-existing externalizing behavior problems were associated with poorly controlled diabetes and externalizing behaviors in adolescence (Northam et al., 2005).

The kind of mental health problems experienced by adolescents with T1DM needs to be clarified, in order to improve guidelines for treatment of diabetes. To this end, researchers should rely upon both adolescent-reported measures that might be applied in regular care, as well as parent-reported measures. Comparing answers of these youths to those from healthy peers can indicate the extent to which differences exist between these groups.

We studied whether Dutch adolescents with T1DM had increased levels of behavior problems in comparison to peers without T1DM, both according to their self-reports and reports from their mothers and fathers. We studied depressive symptoms, and detailed clusters of behavioral problems. Additionally, we examined the extent to which metabolic control is related to depressive symptoms and specific behavior problems.

2. Design and methods

2.1. Sample

Patients with T1DM between 12 and 18 years of age (n=302) and their parents were recruited for participation. They were treated by a multidisciplinary team at nine hospitals in The Netherlands. A total of 151 adolescents agreed to participate, as did their parents. Informed consent was obtained from 135 mothers and 114 fathers (see table 1). Medical information (most recent HbA1c, duration of the disease, and treatment regimen) was recorded from the hospital charts. HbA1c was analyzed with similar assays, using gas chromatography, in the different hospitals.

Schools were approached for cooperation in the same time period in order to recruit the comparison group. Healthy adolescents without T1DM and their parents were invited to participate, matching school type, age, and gender to that of the adolescents with T1DM. The comparison group comprised 122 adolescents without T1DM; In formation was also collected from 114 of these mothers and 61 of the fathers. Exclusion criteria for both groups were no participation of a parent, and comorbid medical or psychiatric illness of the adolescent. All participants in both groups were of Northern European ethnicity.

2.2. Measures

2.2.1. The children's depression inventory

The Children's Depression Inventory (CDI) was developed to measure self-reported depressive symptoms in children and adolescents aged 7 to 17 years (Kovacs, 1992). The inventory assesses a variety of self-reported depressive symptoms, including disturbance in mood, self-evaluation, and interpersonal behaviors. The overall scale gives an indication for the extent of depressive feelings, with a mean (sd) of 7.69 (4.9) for boys and 10.46 (6.5) for girls. Higher scores reflect more depressive feelings. A cutoff score of 13 was used to indicate a serious level of depressive complaints, at risk for a clinical depression (Kovacs, 1992). Psychometric characteristics are sufficient (Evers, Vliet-Mulder & Groot, 2000).

2.2.2. The child behavior checklist (CBCL) and youth self-report (YSR)

The presence of behavior problems was studied using information from different sources, namely the adolescent themselves (YSR), and their mothers (CBCL) and fathers (CBCL). The Child Behavior Checklist (CBCL) measures behavior problems and competencies of children and adolescents between the ages of 6 to 18, as reported by their parents (Achenbach & Rescorla, 2001). The Youth Self-Report (YSR) is a self-report derivative of the CBCL for adolescents between 11 and 18 years. A detailed clustering of behavior problems is provided in the syndrome scale, which consist of anxious/depressed behaviors, withdrawn/depressed behaviors, somatic complaints, social problems, thought problems, attention problems, rule-breaking behavior, and aggressive behavior. The CBCL and YSR questionnaires have been shown to have adequate reliability and validity (Evers et al., 2000).

2.3. Procedure

The adolescents with T1DM answered the questionnaires when they visited the diabetes team, or at home. The parents were sent questionnaires by mail. For the control group, the questionnaires were sent to the adolescents and their parents at home. The study was approved by the medical ethical committees of the Catharina hospital in Eindhoven and all participating hospitals.

According to protocol, adolescents who answered in the positive to the critical item on the CDI concerning suicidality, or who scored above the clinical range for depression on both YSR and CDI, were approached to verify whether they received psychological treatment and to offer it when necessary.

2.4. Data analyses

Potential differences in group characteristics were analyzed using chi-square or t-tests. Group differences were examined using multivariate and univariate analyses of variances. All tests were two-sided. Within the T1DM group, a regression analysis was conducted to study the relationship between HbA1c and the depressive symptoms and behavior syndrome scales.

3. Results

3.1. Group characteristics

A description of baseline group characteristics can be found in table 1. The total group of adolescents with T1DM did not differ from the comparison group in age, gender, or education level, as expected in light of the matching procedure.

Variable	Controls (n=122)	T1DM (n=151)
Age :mean (SD)	14.62 (1.66)	14.89 (1.71)
Range	12-18	12-18
Gender		
male	50 (41%)	65 (43%)
female	72 (59%)	86 (57%)
School level		
lower	51 (41.8%)	42 (27.8%)
vocational	12 (9.8%)	19 (12.6%)
higher	27 (22.1%)	46 (30.5%)
pre-university	32 (26.2%)	40 (26.5%)
unknown		4 (2.6%)
Treatment		
Injections		71 (47%)
Pump		80 (53%)
HbA1c: mean (SD)		8.3 (1.46)
Range		5.1-13.0
Age at diagnose: mean (SD)		9.43 (3.82)
range		0-18
Years T1DM: mean (SD)		5.74 (3.92)
range		0-15

*Group differences are not significant

Table 1. Baseline group characteristics*.

3.2. Depressive symptoms

The adolescents with T1DM (mean=7.32, sd=5.32) did not differ from the comparison group (mean=6.55, sd=5.94) in number of depressive complaints according to the CDI (F(1,265)=1.100, p=0.295). In the group with T1DM, 18 adolescents (12.4% of a total 145 with complete data) were identified as being at risk for a clinical depression, as were18 adolescents in the control group (14,8% of in total 122 with complete data). These proportions did not not differ (χ^2 (1, N =270) =0.197, p = 0.66), see figure 1.

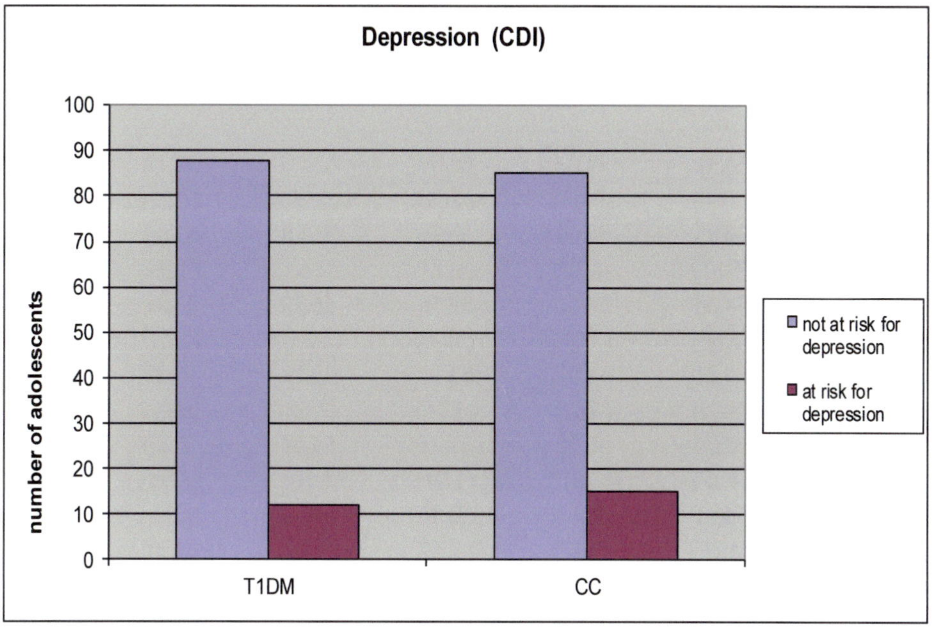

Figure 1. Depression in adolescents with and without T1DM

3.3. Behavior problems

Means and standard deviations for the YSR (as assessed by the adolescents) are presented in table 2, as are CBCL behavioral syndromes (as assessed by mothers and fathers). This table also indicates significant differences found with univariate analyses of variance. Mean factor scores (internalizing, externalizing, and total behavior problems,) and mean scores for the behavioral syndrome scales for adolescents with and without T1Dm, are presented in figures 2 and 3.

For adolescents' self reports on the YSR for the behavioral syndromes, a multivariate analysis of variance showed a significant overall difference ($F(8,239)=2.37$, $p=0.018$). One behavioral syndrome scale differed significantly between the groups, reflecting Thought problems, ($F(1,247)=11,63$, $p=0.001$), see table 2. The adolescents with T1DM reported more problems than the comparison group on this subscale, which refers to questions such as: 'can't get my mind off certain thoughts'; 'have twitches'; 'have sleeping problems'. Adolescents with T1DM also reported more Thought problems in the borderline and clinical range (n=27) than did the comparison group (n=4) (χ^2 (2)= 14.450, p=.001).

The difficulties concerning Thought problems were corroborated by the CBCL reports from mothers, which showed a significant difference on this syndrome scale ($F(1,231)=6.64$, $p=0.01$). The fathers' CBCL reports also showed a significant difference for Thought problems ($F(1,155)=4.37$, $p=0.04$). Overall, however, mothers of adolescents with T1DM did not differ significantly from mothers of healthy peers in their CBCL reports concerning behavioral syndromes ($F(8,223)=1.80$, $p=0.08$), nor did the fathers ($F(8,147)=1.27$, $p=0.26$).

CBCL/YSR	Adolescents		Mothers		Fathers	
	Controls N=111	T1DM N=140	Controls N= 104	T1DM N=128	Controls N=59	T1DM N=99
anxious/ depressed	53.11 (5.50)	53.37 (9.03)	52.55 (4.61)	53.78 (7.27)	52.12 (4.12)	52.91 (8.04)
withdrawn/ depressed	53.15 (5.61)	54.84 (8.34)	53.76 (4.97)	55.58 (7.40)	52.90 (4.39)	54.52 (9.31)
somatic complaints	54.60 (5.86)	56.04 (7.59)	54.76 (5.52)	56.72 (7.53)*	53.37 (4.29)	55.18 (6.48)
social problems	54.21 (5.89)	54.37 (6.62)	53.37 (5.16)	53.22 (7.57)	53.22 (5.09)	53.61 (6.15)
thought problems	52.86 (4.47)	55.74 (8.13)**	52.76 (4.34)	54.81 (7.10)*	52.08 (3.55)	54.01 (6.79)*
attention problems	54.01 (4.98)	54.83 (6.32)	53.46 (4.23)	54.12 (5.88)	52.97 (4.08)	53.79 (5.06)
rule-breaking behav.	53.98 (4.49)	54.65 (6.65)	52.24 (4.04)	52.61 (4.79)	51.59 (3.24)	53.41 (5.18)*
aggressive behavior	52.21 (3.61)	52.87 (5.54)	52.21 (3.96)	52.94 (8.26)	51.83 (4.12)	53.11 (5.51)

Univariate analyses: * p< 0.05; ** p< 0.01

Table 2. Means and standard deviations for YSR (adolescents) and CBCL (mothers and fathers)

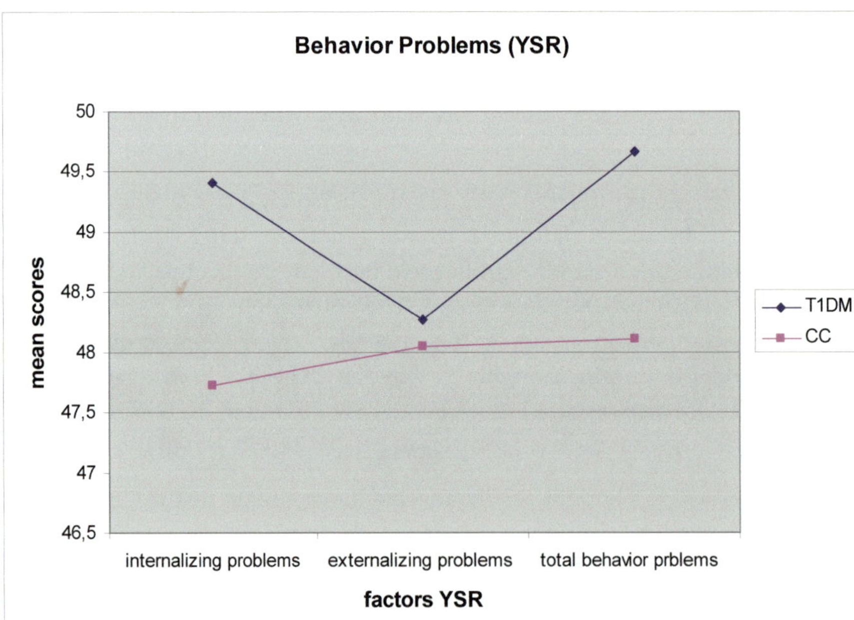

Figure 2. Behavioral problems in adolescents with and without diabetes (YSR)

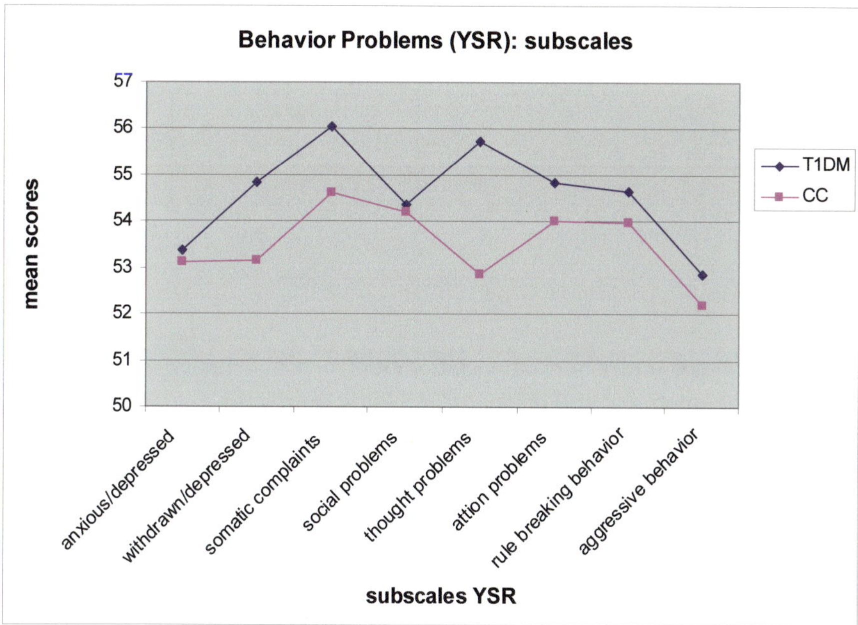

Figure 3. Specific behavioral problems in adolescents with and without diabetes (subscales YSR)

3.4. Glycemic control and social emotional functioning

A regression analysis, using the enter procedure, was conducted in order to study the relationship between glycemic control and social-emotional functioning of adolescents with T1DM, as represented by their CDI score and the scores on the eight behavioral syndromes of the YSR (see table 3). This model was significant ($F(9,121)=2.17$ $p=.029$), explaining 14% of the variance in the HbA1c levels. Children with more depressive symptoms and rule breaking behavior were found to have higher HbA1c levels.

	B	p
anxious/depressed	.086	.554
withdrawn/depressed	-.092	.587
somatic complaints	.214	.120
social problems	-.281	.052
thought problems	-.252	.071
attention problems	-.021	.883
rule-breaking behavior	.392	.013
CDI	.301	.009
R^2	14%	
R^2 *change*	14%	
F	(9,121)=2.17	.029

Table 3. Relationships between depressive symptoms, behavior problems and HbA1c

4. Discussion

Our study on the types and extent of social-emotional problems among adolescents with T1DM revealed that emotional and behavior problems are related to glycemic control. Blood glucose regulation was found to be related specifically to depressive symptoms and rule breaking behavior among the adolescents with T1DM. The adolescents with poor blood glucose regulation experienced difficulties, in general, as well as problems followng rules; This likely also extends to difficulties in following the rules of their treatment for diabetes. The problems adolescents with T1DM experienced in social emotional functioning could be specifically related to diabetes and diabetes management tasks. The questionnaires used in this study were not diabetes-specific, however, so we cannot indicate diabetes-specific burdens yet.

We also found a remarkable difference, in that the adolescents with DM1 reported more thought problems than the comparison group. The results of our comparison group were in the same range as those of the original norm group of the YSR (Achenbach & Rescorla, 2001). The reports of both mothers and fathers did not show an overall significant difference, but looking univariately at the dimension, a difference in thought problems also appeared in mothers' and fathers' reports of youths' functioning, with parents of adolescents with T1DM reporting more thought problems than the parents of healthy adolescents. The fact that mothers and fathers of youths with T1DM agreed with their children regarding the higher prevalence of Thought problems may underline the importance of these kinds of behavioral difficulties. This result is not easy to interpret, however. Thought problems refer to a variety of problems in learning behavior and information processing. These adolescents more often ruminate on certain thoughts, and have twitches, strange thoughts, or sleeping problems. An explanation for such group differences may be found in subtle neuropsychological effects of diabetes. Both hypo- and hyperglycemia affect cognitive functioning, but in different ways (Periantie et al., 2006). In a recent meta-analysis, Naguib and colleagues (Naguib, Kulinskaya, Lomax & Garralda, 2009) found mild cognitive impairments in adolescents with T1DM, especially poorer visuospatial ability, motor speed, writing, and sustained attention. This was independent of a history of hypoglycemic episodes. The relationship between thought problems and blood glucose regulation was only marginally significant in our study. It is conceivable, however, that the fluctuating blood glucose levels that all patients with diabetes experience, and the high blood glucose regulation in our group (mean 8.3%), may influence thinking and perception. Our findings are also in line with Nardi (Nardi et al., 2008), who found more thought problems among adolescents in the age of 14 to 18 with T1DM, relative to a comparison group.

Another important finding is a lack of group differences in other syndromes. Further, although depressive symptoms are often associated with T1DM, we found that the incidence of depressive symptoms among adolescents with T1DM was similar to that of adolescents without T1DM. This corroborates findings of the SEARCH study (Lawrence et al., 2006). Our findings indicate that one in eight youths with T1DM met the clinical cut off for depression. This level of depressive symptoms is comparable with the results of Hood (Hood et al., 2006), who reported that one in seven adolescents with T1DM met the same criteria for depression as used in our study. Hood, however, concluded that this level nearly doubles that of the highest estimate of depression among youths in general, but this was based on prior reports and not in comparison with a control group (Fleming, Boyle & Offord, 1993; Anderson & McGee, 2006).

4.1. Clinical implications

In view of the elevated thought problems, and the important associations that blood glucose regulation held with both depressive symptoms and rule breaking behaviors, routine screening for behavioral problems in adolescents with T1DM is recommended.

Increased attention should be devoted to the large group of adolescents who have poor metabolic control. Although strict diabetic treatment management is necessary to maintain adequate levels of HbA1c, this may indicate greater interference with daily life. Adolescents need to be stimulated by their parents and health care professionals to find intrinsic motivation for their own disease management, and to maintain their mental health. Thought problems may need special consideration, and it seems useful to investigate whether and how these problems interfere with diabetes management and daily living. To optimize glycemic levels, specific attention should be paid to adolescents reporting depressive symptoms or rule breaking behavior, in general, because they may experience the most adaptation problems when it comes to treatment rules.

4.2. Strengths, limitations, and future directions

A strength of our study is that we examined a relatively large group of 151 adolescents with T1DM. Many eligible patients refused to participate, however. Although a participation rate of 50% is comparable to other studies (Lawrence et al., 2006; Lin et al., 2004; De Wit et al., 2007), our research may have been biased in that our results reflect data of relatively well functioning adolescents. The self-selection evolving from voluntary participation may have led to an underestimation of the number of adolescents with depressive symptoms in the group with T1DM. Nevertheless, the group differences found in a behavioral syndrome like thought problems need further study, as it may be important to consider for treatment improvements.

5. Conclusion

One in eight Dutch youths with T1DM met the clinical cut off for depression. The adolescents with T1DM did not differ from healthy peers in their number of depressive complaints. However, the combination of depressive symptoms and rule breaking behavior was related to metabolic control. Further, elevated thought problems were found among adolescents with T1DM, in comparison to healthy peers. This finding warrants further attention in research, as well as in clinical practice.

Author details

Nienke M. Maas- van Schaaijk, Angelique B.C. Roeleveld-Versteegh and Roelof R.J. Odink
Catharina hospital, Division of Paediatrics, Eindhoven, The Netherlands

Anneloes L. van Baar
Utrecht university, Department of Pedagogics and Educational Sciences, Utrecht, The Netherlands

6. References

Achenbach, T.M., & Rescorla, L.A. (2001). *Manual for the ASEBA school-age forms profiles.* University of Vermont: Research Center for Children, Youth and Families: Burlington.

Anderson, R.J., Freedland, K.E., Clouse, R.E., & Lustman, P.J. (2001). The prevalence of comorbid depression in adults with diabetes. *Diabetes Care,* 24, 1069-1078.

Anderson, J., & McGee, R. (2006). Comorbidity of depression in children and adolescents. In: Reynolds WM, Johnson HF (ed.) *Handbook of depression in Children and Adolescents.* New York: Plenum, 581-601.

Cohen, D.M., Lumley, M.A., Naar-King, S., Partridge, T., & Cakan, N. (2004). Child behavior problems and family functioning as predictors of adherence and glycemic control in economically disadvantaged children with type 1 diabetes: a prospective study. *Journal of Pediatric Psychology,* 29, 171-184.

De Wit, M., Delemarre-van de Waal, H.A., Bokma, J.A., Haasnoot, K., Houdijk, M.C., Gemke, R.J., & Snoek, F.J. (2007). Self-report and parent-report of physical and psychosocial well-being in Dutch adolescents with type 1 diabetes in relation to glycemic control. *Health and Quality of Life Outcomes,* 16, 5-10.

Evers, A., Vliet-Mulder, J.C., & Groot, C.J. (2000) *Documentatie van tests en testresearch in Nederland*. Boom.

Fleming, J.F., Boyle, M.H., & Offord, D.R. (1993). The outcome of adolescent depression in the Ontario Child Health Study follow-up. *Journal of the American Academy of Child Psychiatry*, 32, 28-33.

Grey, M., & Boland, E.A. (1996). Diabetes Mellitus (Type I). In: Jackson PL (ed.) *Primary Care of the Child with a Chronic Condition*. St. Louis: C.V, Mosby, 350-370.

Hood, K.K., Huestis, S.H., Maher, A., Butler, D., Volkening, L., & Laffel, L.M. (2006). Depressive symptoms in children and adolescents with type 1 diabetes. *Diabetes Care, 29*, 1389-1391.

Kovacs, M. (1992). *The Childrens Depression Inventory (CDI)*. Multi-Health Systems, New York.

Kovacs, M., Obrosky, D.S., Goldston, D., & Drash, A. (1997). Major depressive disorder in youth with IDDM: a controlled prospective study of course and outcome. *Diabetes Care*, 20, 45-51.

Lawrence, J.M., Standiford, D.A., Loots, B., Klingensmith, G.J., Williams, D.E., Ruggiero, A., Liese, A.D., Bell, R.A., Waitzfelder, B.E., & McKeown, R.E. (2006). Prevalence and correlates of depressed mood among youth with diabetes: the SEARCH for Diabetes in Youth study. *Pediatrics*, 117,1348-1358.

Lin, E.H.B., Katon, W., Von Korff, M., Rutter, C., Simon, G.E., Oliver, M., Ciechanowski, P., Ludman, E.J., Bush, T., & Young, B. (2004). Relationship of depression and diabetes self-care, medication adherence, and preventive care. *Diabetes Care*, 27, 2154-2160.

McGrady, M.E., & Hood, K.K. (2010) Depressive symptoms in adolescents with type 1 diabetes: associations with longitudinal outcomes. *Diabetes Research and.Clinical Practice*, 88, e35-e37.

Naguib, J.M., Kulinskaya, E., Lomax, C.L., & Garralda, M.E. (2009). Neuro-cognitive performance in children with type 1 diabetes--a meta-analysis. *Journal of Pediatric Psychology*, 34, 271-282.

Nardi, L., Zucchinni, S., Dálberton, F., Salardi, S., Maltoni, G., Bisacchi, N., Elleri, D., & Cicognani, A. (2008). Quality of life, psychological adjustment and metabolic control in youth with type 1 diabetes : a study with self- and parent-report questionnaires. *Pediatric Diabetes*, 9, 496-503.

Northam, E.A., Matthews, L.K., Anderson, P.J., Cameron, F.J., & Werther, G.A. (2005). Psychiatric comorbidity and health outcome in type 1 diabetes; perspectives from a prospective longitudinal study. *Diabetic Medicine*, 22, 152-157.

Periantie, D.C., Lim, A., Wu, J., Weaver,,P., Warren, S.L., Sadler, M., White, N.H., & Hershey, T. (2008). Effects of prior hypoglycemia and hyperglycemia on cognition in children with type 1 diabetes mellitus. *Pediatric Diabetes*, 9, 87-95.

Reid, G.J., Dubow, E.F., Carey, T.C., & Dura, J.R. (1994). Contribution of coping to medical adjustment and treatment responsibility among children and adolescents with diabetes. *Journal of Developmental and Behavioral Pediatrics*, 15, 327-325.

Snoek, F.J. (2000). *Psychosociale zorg aan mensen met diabetes*. Nederlandse Diabetes Federatie: Leusden.

Chapter 4

GPR119 Agonists: A Novel Strategy for Type 2 Diabetes Treatment

Xiaoyun Zhu, Wenglong Huang and Hai Qian

Additional information is available at the end of the chapter

http://dx.doi.org/10.5772/48444

1. Introduction

Type 2 diabetes (T2DM), also known as non-insulin-dependent diabetes mellitus (NIDDM), manifests with an inability to adequately regulate blood-glucose levels. T2DM may be characterized by a defect in insulin secretion or by insulin resistance, namely those that suffer from T2DM have too little insulin or cannot use insulin effectively. Insulin resistance which refers to the inability of body tissues to respond properly to endogenous insulin develops because of multiple factors, including genetics, obesity, increasing age, and having high blood sugar over long periods of time[1].

Current therapies for diabetes mellitus include: glucose-lowering effectors, such as metformin which reduces glucose production from the liver; insulin; insulin secretagogues, such as sulphonylureas, which increase insulin production from pancreatic β-cells; activators of the peroxisome proliferator-activated receptor-γ (PPAR-γ), such as the thiazolidinediones, which enhance insulin action; and α-glucosidase inhibitors which interfere with gut glucose production. There are, however, deficiencies associated with currently available treatments, including hypoglycemicepisodes, weight gain, loss in responsiveness to therapy over time, gastrointestinal problems, and edema[2]. Glucagon-like peptide 1 (GLP-1) analogs and dipeptidyl peptidase 4 (DPP-4) inhibitors are also widely used in clinical therapy for T2DM. GLP-1 analogs, which require parenteral administration, appear not to be associated with hypoglycemia but cause a relatively high frequency of gastrointestinal side effects[3]. Small molecule DPP-4 inhibitors enhance glucose-dependent insulin release by inhibiting the degradation of endogenous GLP-1[4]. Several nonpeptide, except DPP-4 inhibitors, binding G protein-coupled receptors (GPCRs) have been deorphanized recently and are currently being evaluated as candidate GLP-1 secretagogues for T2DM[5, 6]. Among these, the G protein-coupled receptor 119 (GPR119) has received considerable attention from the pharmaceutical industry in recent years. GPR119 may present an attractive drug target for treating T2DM, and its agonists may therefore represent potential new insulin secretagogues free of the risk of causing hypoglycemia.

GPR119 has been described as a class A (rhodopsin-type) orphan GPCR without close primary sequence relative in the human genome[7]. The activation of GPR119 increases the intracellular accumulation of cAMP, leading to enhanced glucose-dependent insulin secretion from pancreatic β-cells and increased release of the gut peptides GLP-1 (glucagon-like peptide 1), GIP (glucose-dependent insulinotropic peptide) and PYY (polypeptide YY)[8]. Preclinical and clinical studies with GPR119 agonists in type 2 diabetes support that GPR119 agonists have been proposed as a novel therapeutic strategy for diabetes. These investigations indicate that orally available, potent, selective, synthetic GPR119 agonists: a) lower blood glucose without hypoglycemia; b) slow diabetes progression; and c) reduce food intake and body weight. This review provides an overview of the recent progress made in the discovery of orally active GPR119 agonists[9], and outlines the current clinical trial landscape and paints a detailed illustration of the key structural information realized from GPR119 agonist campaigns.

2. GPR119: A historical perspective

2.1. Discovery and characteristics of GPR119

After the discovery of GPR119 in 1999 using data afforded by the Human Genome Project, it was subsequently described in the peer-reviewed literature as a Class A receptor with no close relatives. Independently, this receptor has been studied and described in the literature under various synonyms, including SNORF25 [10, 11], RUP3 [12], GPCR2 [13] , 19AJ [14] , OSGPR116 [15], MGC119957, HGPCR2 and glucose-dependent insulinotropic receptor (GDIR) [9]. This potentially confusing nomenclature has now been largely rationalized in favor of the designation "GPR119".

The human receptor is encoded by a single exon with introns located on the short arm of X-chromosome (Xp26.1) (Figure 1). GPR119 homologs have been identified in several vertebrate species, including the rat, mice, hamster, chimpanzee, rhesus monkey, cattle and dog[14]. Fredriksson et al. (2003) report the rat isoform of GPR119 (accession number AY288429) as being 133 amino acids longer than the mouse and human receptors (468 vs. 335 amino acids)[16]. In contrast, Bonini et al. (accession number AR240217) and Ohishi et al. give identical sequences for the rat receptor, which are 335 amino acids in length and have 96% amino-acid identity with mouse GPR119[10, 11, 17].

2.2. GPR119 Receptor Expression

Using methods to detect receptor GPR119 mRNA, it has been proposed that, in human tissues, the pancreas and foetal liver have been consistently identified as major sites of GPR119 mRNA expression, with high expression also being noted in the gastrointestinal tract in several studies, while, in rodents, mRNA was detected in most of the tissues examined [9-11] , with the pancreas [12, 18] and gastrointestinal tract, in particular the colon and small intestine, again appearing as major sites of expression. GPR119 expression has also been described in certain regions of the rat brain.

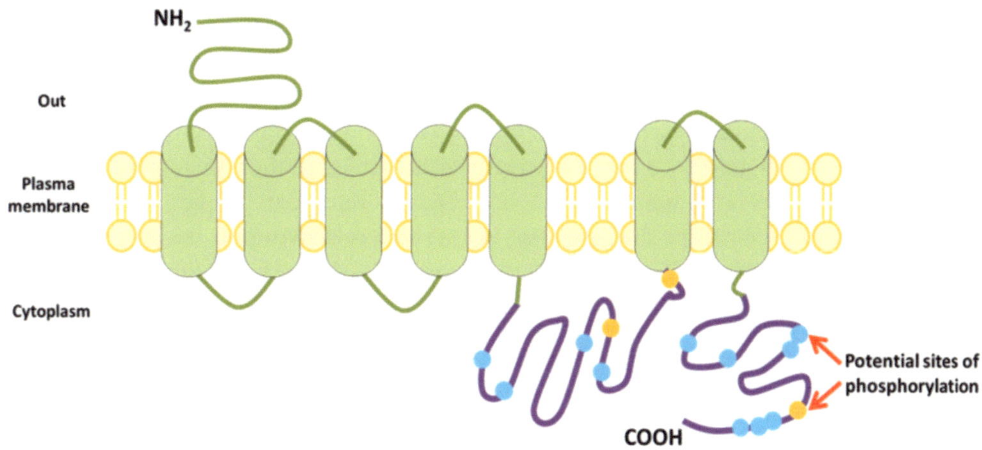

Figure 1. Schematic summary of Human GPR119 membrane topology model. Clusters of serine (S) and threonine (T) residues are highlighted in blue orange circles in the third intracellular loop and the C-terminus domain, and could represent potential sites of phosphorylation.

In situ reveals that pancreatic β cells are the main site of GPR119 expression in pancreatic islets[19]. High expression levels in pancreatic β cell lines NIT-1, MIN6 and RIN5 supports this observation[18, 20, 21]. Consistent with its expression in gut tissues, GPR119 mRNA was strongly expressed in several rodent GLP-1 secreting L-cell lines-including STC-1, FRIC, Hnci-h716 and GLUTag line[21, 22]. GPR119 mRNA has also been found in glucose-dependent insulinotropic peptide (GIP)-producing murine intestinal K cells[23].

2.3. GPR119 signaling and de-orphanization

High-level expression of GPR119 in transfected HEK293 cells led to an increase in intracellular cAMP levels via activation of adenylate cyclase [10, 11, 19], indicating that this receptor couples efficiently to $G\alpha_s$. In support of these data, potential endogenous ligands and synthetic small molecule agonists of GPR119 have been shown to increase cAMP levels (Figure 2).

Lysophosphatidylcholine (LPC, Figure 3, **1**) was the first proposed endogenous ligand for GPR119, based on its ability to stimulate glucose-dependent insulin release and increase cAMP in GPR119-transfected cells. Overton et al. have reported that the fatty-acid amide oleoylethanolamide (OEA, Figure 3, **2**) promotes a concentration-dependent increase in cAMP levels in stably transfected and endogenous GPR119-expressing cell lines with potency that was greater than LPC[24]. The identification of OEA as a potential endogenous ligand for GPR119 was of particular interest, since this compound has been reported to produce a number of pharmacological effects in rodent studies[25], including: a) reducing food intake and body weight gain through interacting with the nuclear receptor peroxisome proliferator-activated receptor α (PPAR-α)[16, 26]; b) increasing fatty acid uptake by adipocytes and enterocytes through increased fatty acid translocase expression[27]; and c) altering feeding behaviour and motor activity through activation of an ion channel, the transient receptor potential channel, subfamily V, member 1 (TRPV1)[28]. The endovanilloid compounds *N*-oleoyl dopamine (OLDA, Figure 3, **3**) and olvanil have recently been described as GPR119 agonists with in vitro potencies similar to that of OEA. Moreover, in vivo studies demonstrated that oral administration of OLDA (100 mg/kg) increased GIP release and improved oral glucose tolerance in mice; these effects were absent or attenuated in GPR119 null mice. These fatty acid amides, OEA and OLDA, represent the best candidates for endogenous ligands, although they are less potent and selective than the natural ligands identified for many other GPCRs. Nonetheless, this work raises the possibility that other lipid amides may play a physiological role via GPR119 signaling[23, 25].

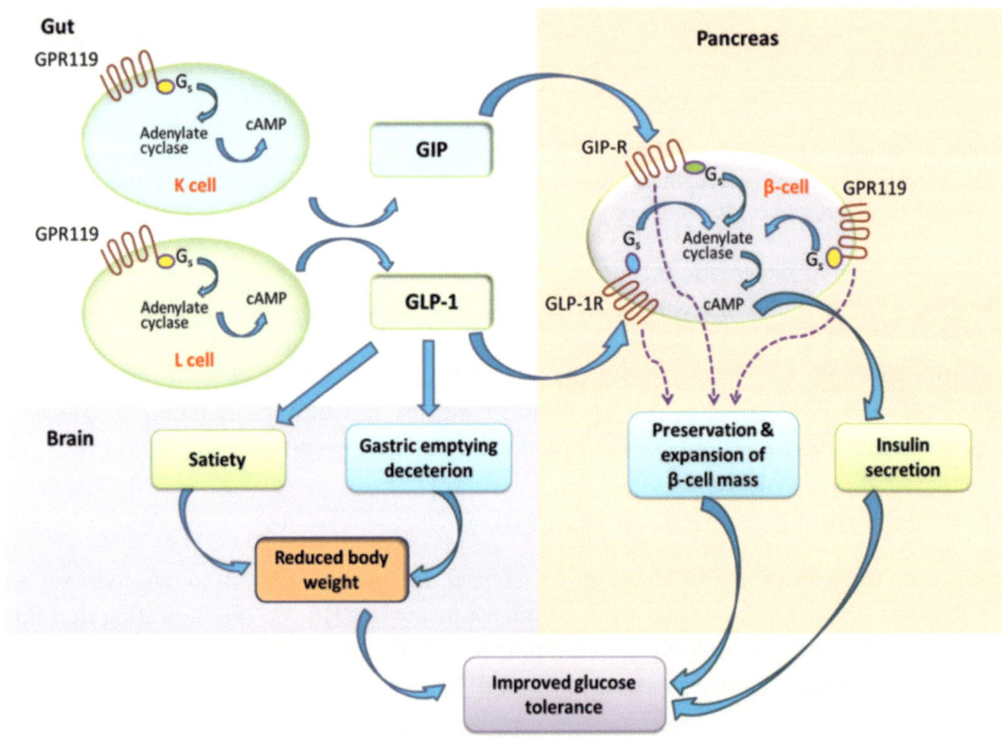

Figure 2. Schematic diagram illustrating the possible actions of GPR119 agonists[23]. GPR119 is expressed on certain enteroendocrine cells (L and K cells) in the small intestine and by β-cells within the islets of Langerhans of the pancreas. In all three cell types, ligation of GPR119 by an agonist leads to the activation of adenylate cyclase and a rise in cAMP. This triggers the release of glucagon-like peptide 1 (GLP-1), and glucose-dependent isulinotropic peptide (GIP) or insulin from L, K and β-cells, respectively. Addtitionally, GLP-1 and GIP can both interact with their cognate receptors on the β-cell to elicit insulin secretion. Thus, GPR119 agonists lead to a rise in insulin release by both direct mechanisms. Since GLP-1 (and probably GIP) also promotes β-cell viability, it is possible that orally acting GPR119 agonists may influence both the secretory activity and the viability of β-cells, leading to improved glucose homeosetasis in patients with T2DM.

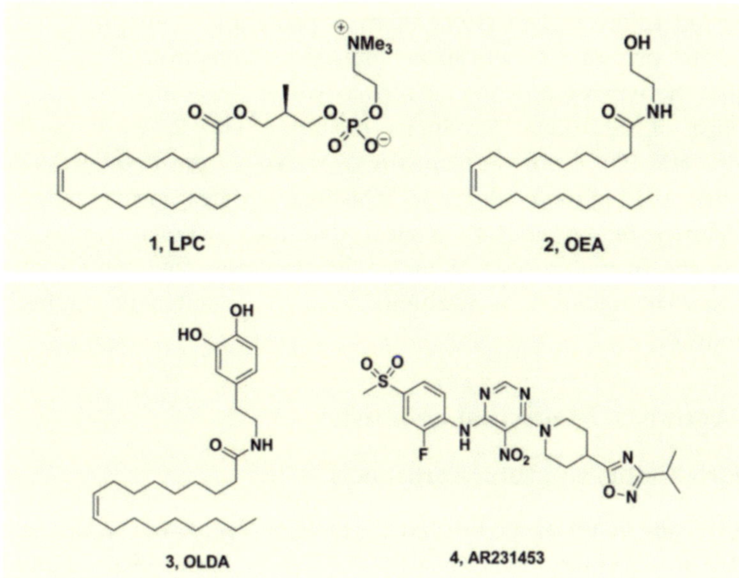

Figure 3. Proposed ligands of GPR119.

3. GPR119 regulation of insulin and incretin secretion

3.1. GPR119 regulation of insulin secretion

Based on the expression profile and coupling properties of GPR119, it stands to reason that activation of the receptor in pancreatic β cells might lead to enhanced glucose-dependent insulin release. Although the mechanism by which insulin secretion is increase following the activation of GPR119 involves a rise in cAMP, Ning et al. have demonstrated that potentiation of insulin secretion is also dependent on the closure of ATP-sensitive K^+ channels and the consequent gating of voltage sensitive calcium channels[29]. The potent, selective GPR119 agonist discovered at Arena Pharmaceuticals, Inc., AR231453 (Figure 3, 4), significantly increased insulin release in HIT-T15 cells (a hamster insulinoma-derived line with robust GPR119 expression) and in rodent islets. By contrast, no effect of this compound could be seen in islets isolated from GPR119-deficient mice, confirming that its effects were indeed mediated by GPR119[25].

3.2. GPR119 regulation of incretin secretion

GPR119 stimulates the release of GIP, GLP-1 and at least one other L-cell peptide, peptide YY (3-36) (PYY)[30]. GPR119 mRNA was found to be expressed at significant levels in intestinal sub-regions that produce GIP and GLP-1. Cellular expression studies have extended these observations by showing that most GLP-1 producing L cells in the ileum and colon also contain GPR119 [30]. This is consistent with data showing high GPR119 expression in most *in vitro* L-cell models[30, 31]. GIP, the other major insulinotropic hormone of the gut, is produced primarily in the duodenal K cells (Figure 2).

In considering the actions of GPR119 agonists as pontential mediators of GLP-1 and GIP secretion, and the potential beneficial actions that derive from this, it should not be overlooked that the enteroendocrine cells from which these incretins are released, also secrete a range of additional products, including GLP-2, oxyntomodulin (OXM), cholecystokinin, and PYY from L cells, as well as xenin from K cells. So far, very little attention has been paid to these additional intestinal peptides during analysis of GPR119-mediated responses *in vivo*, but it is clear that their actions may be important in determining of the overall profile of metabolic responses following administration of GPR119 agonists. The role of these additional hormonal agents will required to clarify in the further study[23].

4. GPR119 Agonists: Medicinal chemistry

4.1. Clinical trial status and future prospects

It is hardly surprising that, based on the strong biological proof of concept generated using the potent, selective agonist molecule 4[19, 30, 32]. In recent years, numerous patents describing GPR119 agonists have been disclosed, and several companies have advanced GPR119 agonists into the clinic for the treatment of type 2 diabetes (Table 1, Figure 4): Ortho-McNeil/Arena (APD-668 and APD-597; both discontinued), Sanofi-Aventis/Metabolex (SAR-260093/MBX-2982; Phase 2), Glaxo-SmithKline (GSK-1292263; Phase 2), Astellas/Prosidion (PSN-821; Phase 2) and Bristol-Meyers Squibb (Phase 1). The following sections provide an overview of the multiple classes of GPR119 agonists, along with the available biological data, reported by various pharmaceutical organizations. Each section is categorized according to applicant.

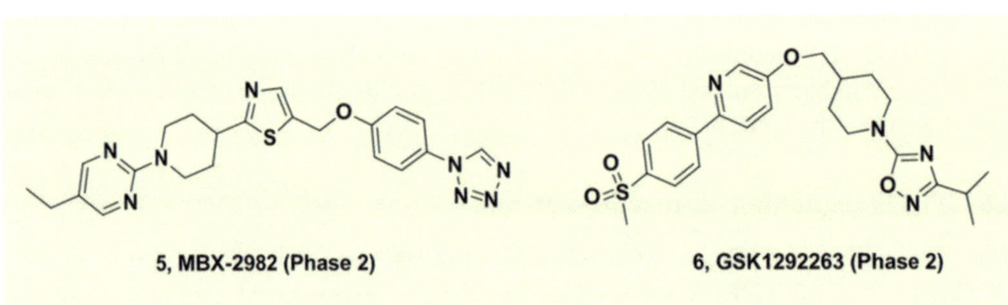

Figure 4. Structures of GPR119 agonists (MBX-2982 [5] and GSK1292263 [6]).

Drug	Company	Highest development status	ClinicalTrials.gov identifier
SAR-260093 /MBX-2982	Sanofi-Aventis /Metabolex	Phase 2	NCT01035879
GSK-1292263	GlaxoSmithKline	Phase 2	NCT01119846, NCT01218204, NCT01128621, NCT00783549, NCT01101568
PSN-821	Astellas/Prosidion	Phase 2	NCT01386099
APD-668	Ortho-McNeil/Arena	Discontinued	
APD-597	Ortho-McNeil/Arena	Discontinued	

Table 1. GPR119 agonists currently in development.

4.2. Available structures of GPR119 agonists

4.2.1. Arena pharmaceuticals

Arena Pharmaceuticals has been actively pursuing two GPR119 modulators, derived from 4 that were both considered for progression into human clinical, studies as potential drug candidates after the discovery and validation of this receptor as a viable target for the treatment of metabolic disorders. In December 2004, Arena announced a collaboration agreement with Ortho-McNeil Pharmaceutical, Inc., under which two Arena-discovered GPR119 agonists were selected for preclinical development (Arena Pharmaceuticals, Inc., Press Release, December 23, 2004, http://arna.client.shareholder.com/releasedetail.cfm?ReleaseID=320778). The first compound, APD668 (also known as JNJ28630355), displayed high GPR119 potency across various species (hEC50 = 0.47 nM, mEC50 = 0.98 nM, rEC50 = 2.51 nM; melanophore dispersion assay) and demonstrated good in vivo activity (3–30 mg/kg, p.o.) in rat and mouse oGTT studies. Compared to a known DPP-IV inhibitor, APD668 (Figure 5, **7**) was found to be more potent at a dose of 30 mg/kg. In addition to delaying the onset of hyperglycemia, APD668 delayed elevation of HbA1c and also decreased the levels of triglycerides and free fatty acids. Furthermore, APD668 demonstrated a reduction in food intake (30mg/kg) causing a slight decrease in body weight[8, 33]. However, APD668 was a potent inhibitor of CYP2C9 (IC50 = 0.1 μM), a hydroxylated metabolite **8** (Figure 5) was shown to accumulate to a much greater extent than was expected based on observations in preclinical species that showed such accumulation only at very high doses (>300 mg/kg). Though **8** showed only 80–90% of the exposure of **7** after 24 h, as a result of its significantly longer half-life (41–50 h) compared to **7** this ratio was increased to 4.3- to 5.1-fold after 14 days of dosing. Although this metabolite did not have significant activity at the target receptor (either in agonist or antagonist assays), the high concentration and long half-life were considered a potential liability for the further development of APD668 (Arena Pharmaceuticals, Inc., Press Release, January 07, 2008; http://arna.client.shareholder.com/releasedetail.cfm?ReleaseID=320208).

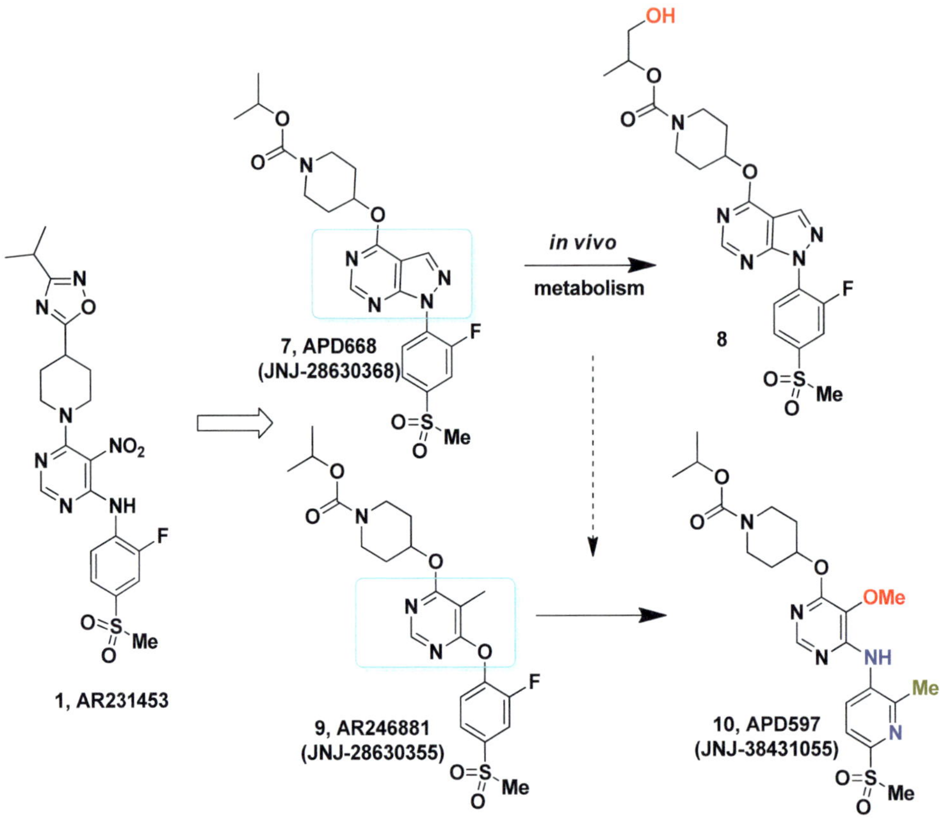

Figure 5. Early clinical candidates for GPR119 derived from the tool compound AR231453 and the structure of the major hydroxylated metabolite of APD668[34].

To tackle the CYP2C9 inhibition we elected to focus primarily on our alternative scaffold, as exemplified by **9** (Figure 5), which generally had significantly lower CYP2C9 inhibition than the pyrazolopyrimidine series (CYP2C9 IC50 for 9 = 5.3 μM) without bringing other obvious liabilities into play[34]. Therefore, they were encouraged that switching to this scaffold may also be the best approach to try to increase the range of possible sites of metabolism, without greatly increasing clearance. Then APD597 (JNJ-38431055, Figure 5, **10**) was then developed, which described the second generation trisubstituted pyrimidine agonists with improved solubility, pharmacokinetic and metabolism characteristics and excellent in vivo activity. In the anesthetized Guinea Pig, treatment with APD597 (hGPR119 EC50 = 46 nM) did not produce any dose-related, statistically significant effects on mean arterial blood pressure (MAP), heart rate (HR) or on the electrocardiogram (ECG) at cumulative doses up to 5 mg/kg IV, when compared to vehicle controls. Preliminary safety studies in rat (14-day) and dog (7-day) revealed no obvious liabilities that would prevent further development[34]. In December 2008, Ortho-McNeil–Janssen Pharmaceuticals, Inc., put APD668 on hold to initiated phase 1 clinical trials of the second Arena-discovered GPR119 agonist, APD597 for the treatment of T2DM (Arena Pharmaceuticals, Inc., Press Release, December 15, 2008; http://arna.client.shareholder.com/releasedetail.cfm?ReleaseID=354391).

4.2.2. Astellas

Compounds effective in stimulating insulin secretion and inhibiting the increase of blood sugar levels have been reported by Astellas. These were derived from a bicyclic scaffold in which a pyrimidine ring was fused to an aromatic (e.g., thiophene, thiazole, and pyridine) or a nonaromatic (e.g., dihydrothiophene, dihydrofuran, and cycloalkyls) heterocycle[8]. Detailed pharmacological data on two disclosed GPR119 agonists from Astellas have been presented. The first generation analog, AS1535907 (Figure 6, **11**), increased intracellular cAMP levels in GPR119 transfected HEK293 cells (EC50 = 1.5 μM) and enhanced insulin secretion in the mouse NIT-1 pancreatic β-cell line and rat perfused pancreas. *In vivo* studies in normal and *db/db* mice suggested improved glucose tolerance following oral treatment with this compound (10 mg/kg). Gene expression studies also revealed that AS1535907 upregulated PC-1 mRNA, thus suggesting possible involvement in insulin biosynthesis[8, 35].

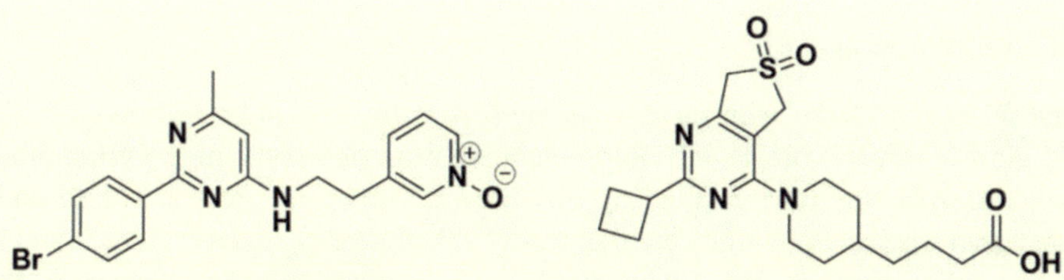

Figure 6. Compounds AS1535907 and AS1907417 from Astellas.

Further SAR optimization resulted in the second generation compound, AS1907417 (hEC50 = 1.1 μM, Figure 6, **12**), which improved upon the metabolism and efficacy liabilities associated with AS1535907, AS1907417 effectively reduced glucose levels in normal and diabetic mice. Significant increases in insulin secretion, were observed in vitro at concentrations of 0.3μM and in vivo after oral administration at doses of 3 mg/kg. The potential long term pharmacological efficacy of AS1907417 for preserving pancreatic β-cell function and insulin production was suggested by the reduction of plasma TG and NEFA levels in several diabetic animal models[8, 36].

4.2.3. Biovitrum

Biovitrum has several published patent applications identifying GPR119 agonists which differ in the nature of the central aromatic ring (compounds 13–15)[8, 32]. The central heterocyclic ring consisted of a pyridine[37], pyradazine[38], pyrimidine[39], or pyrazine[40] nucleus, which was connected to the piperidine ring via an optionally substituted amino methylene (e.g., Figure 7, **13**) or an oxymethylene linker. Compounds 13, 14, and 15 (Figure 7) were reported to have EC50 values of 22, 46, and 14 nM, respectively, in a human GPR119 cAMP HTRF (homogenous timeresolved fluorescence) assay.

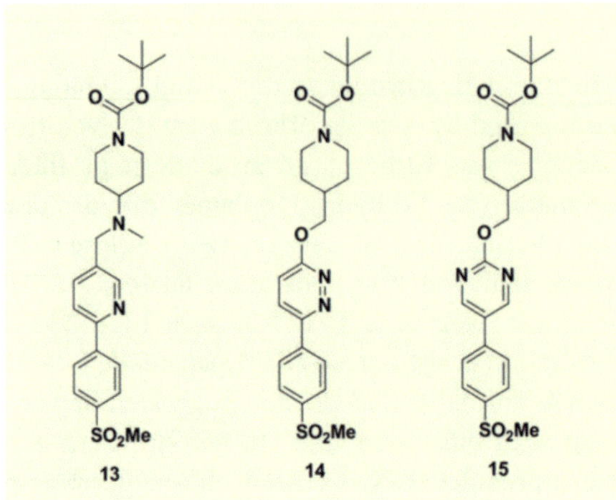

Figure 7. Compounds 13-15 from Biovitrum.

4.2.4. *Bristol-Myers squibb*

The first series of GPR119 agonists reported by Bristol–Myers Squibb featured a [6,5], [6,6], or [6,7] bicyclic central core[41, 42]. Representative examples containing pyrimidine-fused pyrrazole, triazole, and morpholine ring systems are shown in Figure 8. The second BMS series featured a pyridone central core that was N-substituted with the aryl motif and linked to the piperidine motif at the 4-position through an oxygen linker (Figure 8, 19, 20;); pyridazone analogs have also been claimed as GPR119 modulators[43, 44]

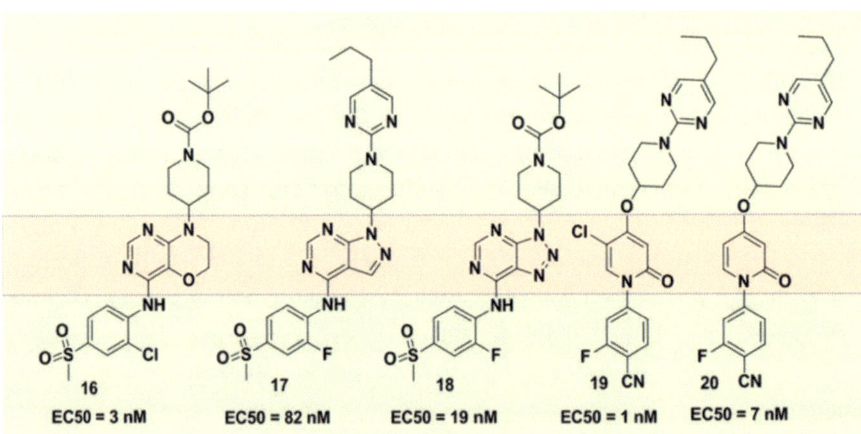

Figure 8. Compounds 16-20 from Bristol-Myers Squibb.

4.2.5. *GlaxoSmithKline*

Replacement of Arena's pyrazolopyrimidine ring system with a dihydropyrrolopyrimidine scaffold was shown to be successful by researchers at GlaxoSmithKline[45, 46]. The two initial filings, from July 2006, describe agonists that retain a 6,7-dihydro-5H-pyrrolo[2,3-

d]pyrimidine core unit (Figure 9). The third patent application contains compounds with a benzene, pyridine, pyrazine or pyridazine central core (e.g., **23**, **24**). The prototypical compound **21** (Figure 9) demonstrated an EC50 of 40 nM in a CHO6CRE reporter assay. In an oGTT, **21** reduced the glucose AUC by 28% (30 mg/kg) and 38% (10 mg/kg), respectively, in mice and rats. In addition, hyperinsulinemic clamp experiments in normal rats showed that compound **21** enhances whole body insulin sensitivity[8]. In these filings, compounds are described as having therapeutic value for diabetes and associated conditions, particularly T2DM, obesity, glucose intolerance, insulin resistance, metabolic syndrome X, hyperlipidemia, hypercholesterolemia and atherosclerosis.

In addition to the pyrrolopyrimidine scaffold, a series of GPR119 agonists based on monocyclic six-membered aryl and heteroaryl cores have also been reported by GlaxoSmithKline[47]. GSK1292263 (Phase 2, hGPR119 pEC50 = 6.9 nM, rat GPR119 pEC50 = 6.7 nM) augmented insulin secretion and decreased glucose AUC in rodent glucose tolerance tests; an increased incretin secretion (GLP-1 and GIP) was also observed[8]. The safety, tolerability, pharmacokinetics and pharmacodynamics of single and multiple oral doses of GSK-1292263 were evaluated in a completed randomized, placebo-controlled clinical trial in healthy volunteers (ClinicalTrials.gov Identifier NCT00783549). A total of 69 subjects received single escalating doses of GSK-1292263 (10-400 mg) prior to administration of a 250mg dose given once daily for 2 and 5 days, which was also evaluated in combination with sitagliptin (100 mg). Treatment with GSK-1292263 at all doses was described as well tolerated, with the most common drug-related effects being mild headache, dizziness, hyperhidrosis, flushing and post-oGTT hypoglycemia. Coadministration with sitagliptin increased plasma active GLP-1 concentrations and lowered total GLP-1, GIP and PYY levels; no effects on gastric emptying were observed with GSK1292263. The data support further evaluation of GSK-1292263 for the treatment of T2DM[48].

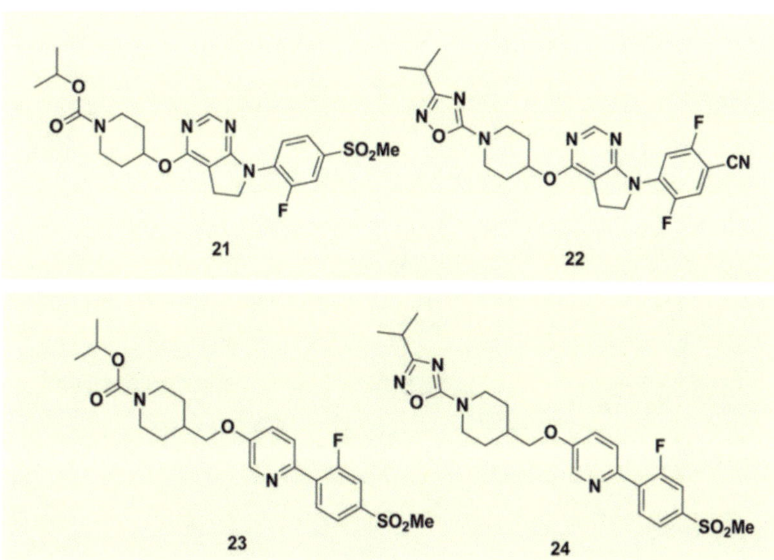

21

22

23

24

Figure 9. Compounds 21-24 from GlaxoSmithKline.

4.2.6. Merck

Merck has two published patent applications describing GPR119 agonists which retain a 4,4′-bipiperidine scaffold (Figure 10; **25** and **26**)[49, 50]. Compound **26** depicts one such example containing a 5-fluoro pyrimidine. Although the data for specific Merck analogs are not available, several compounds have been claimed to exhibit an EC50 < 10 nM in the cAMP homogeneous time-resolved fluorescence (HTRF) assay[8].

In 2006, Schering–Plough filed several patents describing spiro-azetidine and spiro-azetidinone derivatives, which are described as T-calcium channels blockers, GPR119 receptor agonists and Niemann-Pick C1-like protein-1 antagonists, with utility for the treatment of pain, diabetes and disorders of metabolism (Figure 10, **27**) [32, 51, 52]. Compound 28 was described as a modest GPR119 agonist (cAMP IC50 = 1922 nM); replacement of the amide functionality with a urea resulted in a potent T-type calcium channel blocker, 29 (IW hCav3.2 IC50 = 23nM).

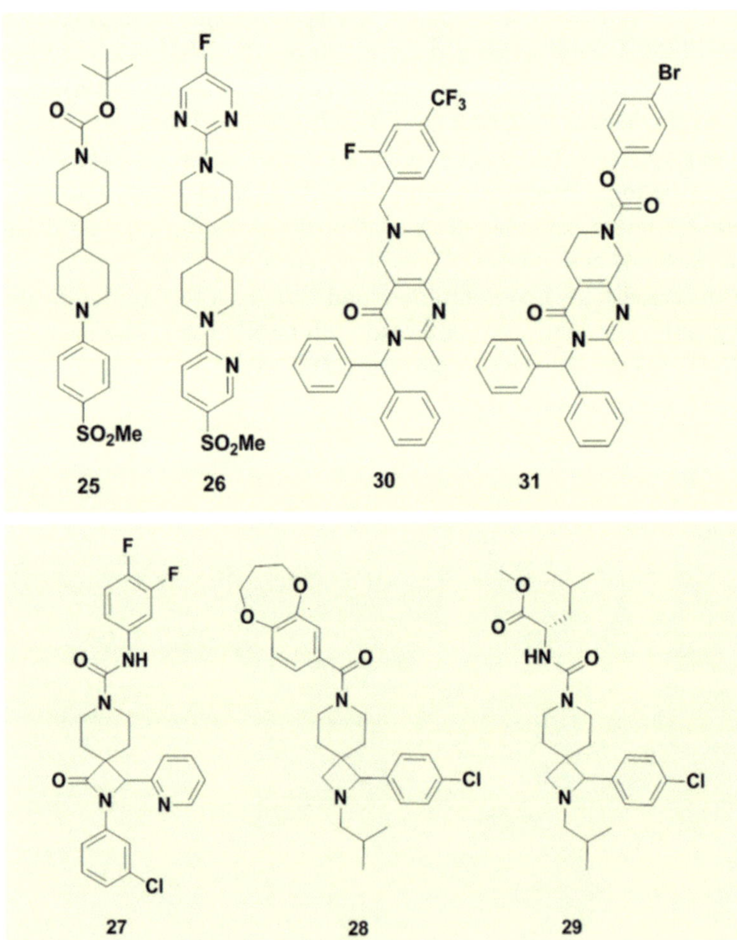

Figure 10. Compounds 25-29 from Merck.

More recent published patent filings from Schering describe selective GPR119 modulators comprised of a fused pyrimidinone core (compounds **30** and **31**)[53]. The patent application pertaining to 30 discloses a series of 6-substituted 5,6,7,8-tetrahydropyrido[4,3-d]pyrimidin-4(3H)-ones and the patent application associated with 31 describes a closely related chemical series of 7-substituted 5,6,7,8-tetrahydropyrido[3,4-d]pyrimidin-4(3H)-ones[54]. Both of these series of GPR119 modulators, which were reported to exhibit EC50 values ranging from about 50 nM to about 14,000 nM, are described as being useful for treating or preventing obesity, diabetes, metabolic disease, cardiovascular disease or a disorder related to the activity of GPR119 in a patient[32].

4.2.7. Metabolex

GPR119 agonists from Metabolex are based on a five-membered central heterocyclic core that is linked directly to the piperidine motif at its C4 position and to the aryl motif through an oxymethylene spacer[55-58] (Figure 11). Most examples in this application showed agonist activity at 10 μM in the fluorescence resonance energy transfer (FRET) assay corresponding to increased intracellular cAMP levels. Glucose stimulated insulin secretion experiments using isolated rat islets are described and compound **32** showed 1.78-fold stimulation of insulin secretion at 16 mM glucose. oGTTs in mice are described and both compounds **32** and **33** significantly reduce glucose AUC[8].

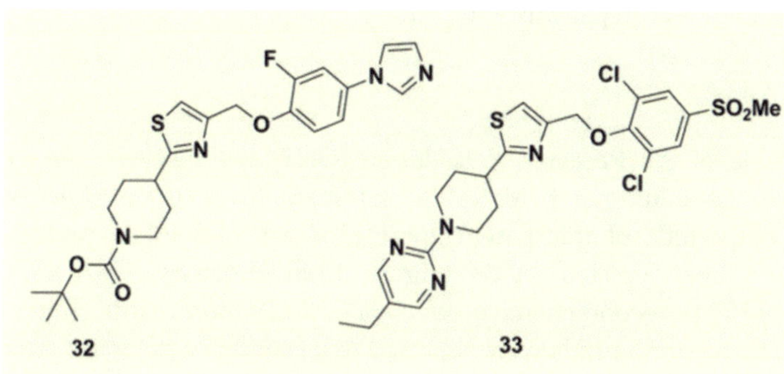

Figure 11. Compounds 32 and 33 from Metabolex.

Metabolex advanced their orally available GPR119 agonist MBX-2982 (Figure 4, **5**) into clinical trials of T2D (Phase 2, completed)[59, 60]; rights to this compound were recently acquired by Sanofi-aventis. In preclinical studies, MBX-2982 was shown to increase cAMP levels in CHO cells expressing human GPR119 (EC50 = 3.9 nM) and to stimulate GSIS from isolated islets. Metabolex has recently completed two additional Phase 1 studies of MBX-2982 in subjects with pre-diabetes. In both studies, subjects with either impaired fasting glucose or impaired glucose tolerance were enrolled. The first study investigated the effect of four consecutive once daily doses (100 or 300 mg) of MBX-2982 on the pharmacokinetics of the drug as well as its effect on glucose excursions following a mixed meal (Metabolex, Inc., Press Release, November 12, 2008 http://www.metabolex.com/news/nov122008.html). In addition, the effect of MBX-2982 on insulin secretion during a graded glucose infusion was examined. MBX-2982 was rapidly absorbed and its exposure at both doses approximately doubled on day four compared to day one, consistent with a terminal half-life of ~18 hr and supporting once daily dosing. The glucose excursions (area under the curve) following a mixed meal were reduced relative to baseline by 26% and 37%, respectively, for the 100 and 300 mg cohorts. During the graded glucose infusions, the exposure to glucose was reduced relative to baseline by 11% and 18% for the 100 and 300 mg cohorts, respectively. This was attributable to increases in insulin secretion. These results were all statistically significant. The second study in a pre-diabetic population was a five-day placebo-controlled multiple ascending dose study with an alternate formulation of MBX-2982 at doses of 25, 100, 300 and 600 mg (Metabolex, Inc., Press Release, October 13, 2009; http://www.metabolex.com/news/oct132009.html). Once daily dosing provided markedly enhanced exposures and improved dose proportionality, giving sustained levels of MBX-2982 predicted to be maximally effective. The effect of each dose on the glucose excursions following a mixed meal and an oral glucose challenge was investigated. All four doses of MBX-2982 produced statistically significant decreases in the glucose excursion following a mixed meal ranging from 34% to 51%. Similar decreases were also observed following the glucose challenge. In both studies, MBX-2982 was safe and generally well tolerated with no serious adverse events, adverse event trends or dose-limiting toxicities. These results provide continued clinical validation of the potential therapeutic benefits of MBX-2982 in the treatment of type 2 diabetes. Phase 2 trials for MBX-2982 has been completed in evaluating its efficacy, safety, tolerability, and pharmacokinetics following daily administration for 4 weeks in patients with T2D.

4.2.8. Novartis/IRM

Genomics Institute of the Research Foundation (GNF) has disclosed an extensive set of GPR119 agonists containing a heterocyclic sulfonamide as a novel left-side structural motif[61-63]. Compounds of this patent application are defined in part by the terminal tetrahydroisoquinoline depicted in **34** (Figure 12)in February 2007. Compound **35** is representative of IRM's second chemical series of GPR119 modulators which was filed later in 2007[32, 64]. These compounds were reported to be similarly potent in stimulating cAMP in Flp-In-CHO-hGPR119 cells, and are purported to be useful for the treatment or prevention of disorders associated with this receptor.

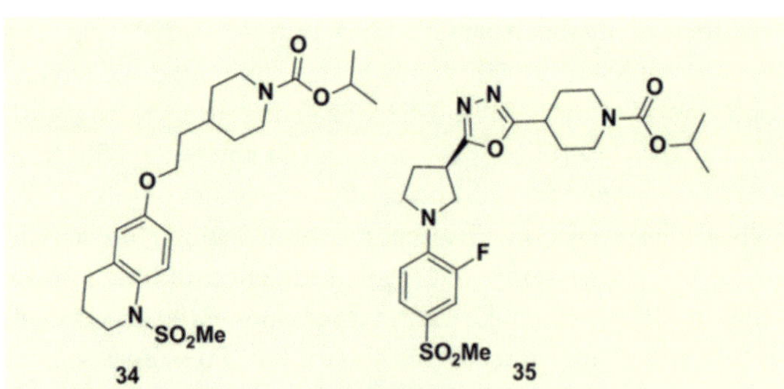

Figure 12. Compounds 34 and 35 from Novartis/IRM.

4.2.9. *Prosidion Ltd.*

The GPR119 agonist program at Prosidion evolved from their earlier lead PSN632408 (Figure 13, EC50 = 5.6 μM, E_{max} = 110%). Replacement of the left-side pyridine ring with the more commonly employed methanesulfonyl phenyl motif (Figure 13), while retaining the oxadiazole core, was shown to be tolerated (e.g., **37**: EC50 = 3.8 μM, E_{max} = 243%)[8, 65]. Refer to Arena analogs, introducing a fluoro substituent *meta* to the sulfone, moving the fluoro group adjacent to the sulfone moiety, as well as incorporating an (*R*)-methyl group to the methyleneoxy linker provided a more potent analog, PSN119-2 (EC50 = 0.4 μM, E_{max} = 358%), a potent GPR119 agonist that stimulated insulin secretion from HIT-T15 cells (EC50 = 18 nM) and GLP-1 release from GLUTag cells (EC50 = 8 nM)[65]. In rats, this compound improved oral glucose tolerance (10, 30 mg/kg, p.o.), delayed gastric emptying, and reduced food intake, thus supporting the premise that PSN119-2 as a GPR119 agonist could be effective oral antidiabetic agents that have the added potential to cause weight loss[8].

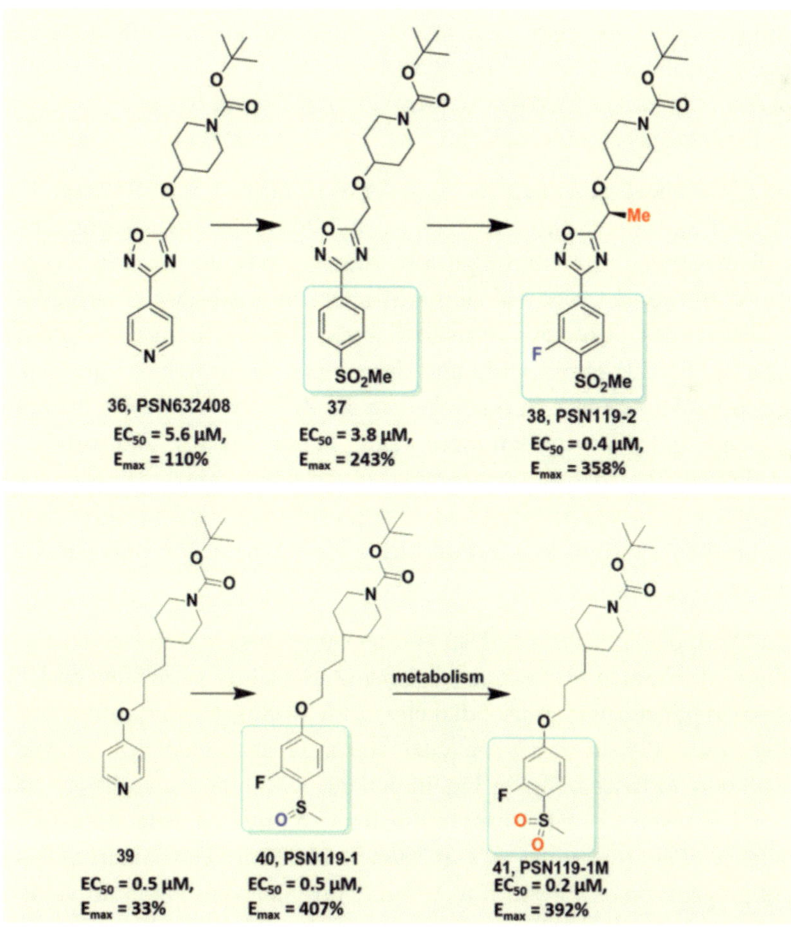

Figure 13. Compounds 36-41 from Prosidion Ltd.

Applications were filed in 2007 disclosed GPR119 agonists by Prosidion containing a central acyclic alkoxylene or alkylene spacer instead of the oxadiazole core. Compound **39** was the initial hit[66] (Figure 13), which demonstrated good potency (EC50 = 0.5 μM) but poor efficacy (E_{max} = 33%). replacing the pyridine ring with the 3-fluoro-4-methanesulfoxide phenyl moiety provided analogs with superior potency and efficacy (e.g., PSN119-1, EC50 = 0.5 μM, Emax = 407%). In several rodent models of obesity and type 2 diabetes, PSN119-1 reduced food intake and improved oral glucose tolerance, giving credence to the premise that GPR119 agonists have the makings of effective oral antidiabesic agents. When administered orally to rats, this compound achieved high plasma concentrations, as did its active sulfone metabolite PSN119-1M (EC50 = 0.2 μM, E_{max} = 392%)[67] (Figure 13).

More recently, the Prosidion group described GPR119 agonists in which the potentially labile tert-butylcarbamate functionality was replaced with bioisosteric heteroaryl groups, in particular with an oxadiazole similar to Arena's AR231453. Several azetidine-based GPR119 agonists (Figure 14) have also been disclosed by Prosidion [8, 68, 69]. These analogs featured an appropriately substituted biaryl moiety five-membered heterocycle connected to the azetidine through an oxygen atom (e.g., **42**, **43**). Preferred analogs within these inventions were claimed to exhibit an EC50 of less than 1 μM (HIT-T15 Camp and insulin secretion assays), to statistically reduce glucose excursion in rat oGTTs (≤ 10 mg/kg, p.o.), as well as to demonstrate a statistically significant hypophagic effect at a dose of ≤ 100 mg/kg.

Optimization of the above described chemical series resulted in identification of the clinical candidate PSN821[8], the structure of which has not been disclosed. In pre-clinical studies, PSN821 has demonstrated pronounced glucose lowering in rodent models of type 2 diabetes with no loss of efficacy on repeated administration, and substantial reductions of body weight in rodent models of obesity. In male diabetic ZDF rats, both acute and chronic oral administration of PSN821, significantly and dose-dependently reduced glucose excursions in an oral glucose tolerance test. In prediabetic male ZDF rats, weeks significantly lowered nonfasting blood glucose concentrations and HbA1c levels compared to vehicle. Furthermore, in weight-stable, dietary-induced obese (DIO) female Wistar rats, daily oral dosing of PSN821 for 4 weeks reduced body weight substantially and significantly by 8.8%, approaching the 10.6% weight loss induced by a high dose of the prescribed anti-obesity agent sibutramine[70].

In the double-blind, placebo-controlled, ascending single dose first-in-human study, PSN821 was generally well tolerated at doses up to 3000mg in healthy volunteers and 1000mg (the top dose tested) in patients with type 2 diabetes, with no clinically important adverse effects on laboratory tests, 12-lead ECGs or vital signs. Pharmacokinetics showed a profile consistent with once or twice daily dosing. In patients with type 2 diabetes, PSN821 showed substantial and statistically significant reductions in glucose responses to a standard nutrient challenge of approximately 30% at 250mg and 500mg. The data from this study was supportive of progression of PSN821 into a 14-day dosing ascending multiple dose study in healthy subjects and patients with type 2 diabetes and will be submitted for presentation at a scientific meeting together with the data from the multiple ascending dose study.

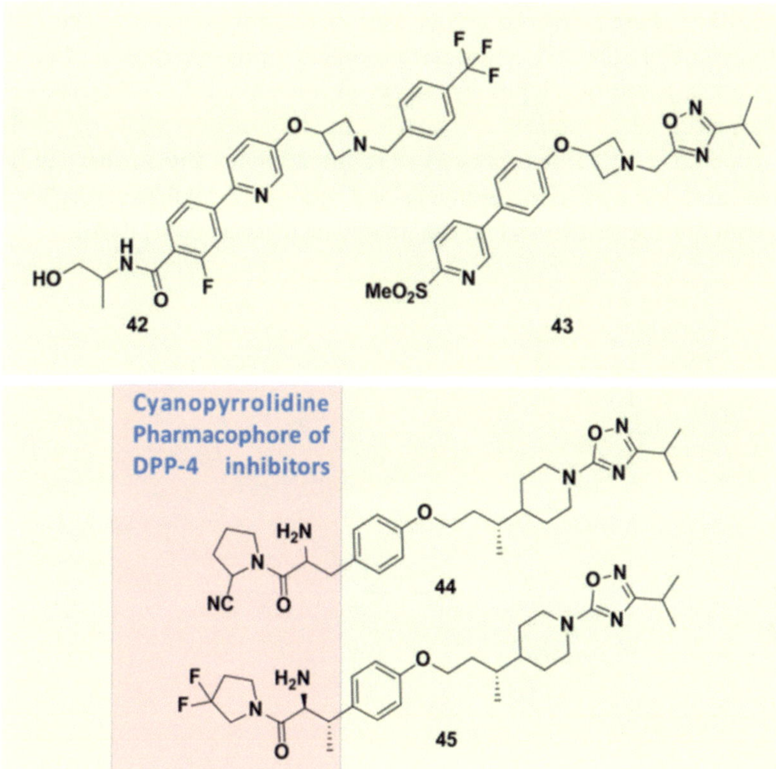

Figure 14. Compounds 42-45 from Prosidion Ltd.

The discovery team at Prosidion has explored a unique approach of combining DPP-4 inhibition and GPR119 agonism in a single molecule[71]. Introduction of the cyanopyrrolidine pharmacophore of known DPP-4 inhibitors on the aryl motif of their GPR119 agonists provided compounds, which displayed dual activity as agonists of GPR119 and inhibitors of DPP-IV (Figure 14, **44** and **45**). Limited biological data are available from this SAR effort. PSN-IV/119-1 (structure not disclosed) was recently reported to exhibit a GPR119 EC50 of 2.24mmol/L and DPP-4 IC50 of 0.2mmol/L[72]. Oral administration of PSN-IV/119-1 at a dose of 30mg/kg in diabetic ZDF rats led to a greater reduction in glucose AUC compared to the DPP-IV inhibitor sitagliptin (58% vs. 22%); at a lower dose of 10 mg/kg, the activity was comparable to sitagliptin (20 mg/kg).

4.3. The pharmacophore model for potent GPR119 agonists

Xiaoyun Zhu et al. have generated pharmacophore models using Discovery Studio V2.1 for a diverse set of molecules as GPR119 agonist with an aim to obtain the pharmacophore model that would provide a hypothetical picture of the chemical features responsible for activity[73]. The best hypothesis (Figure 15) consisting of five features, namely, two hydrogen bond acceptors and three hydrophobic features, has a correlation coefficient of 0.969, cost difference of 62.68, RMS of 0.653, and configuration cost of 15.24, suggesting that a highly predictive pharmacophore model was successfully obtained. The Fit-Value and Estimate activity of GSK-1292263, which have completed phase II clinical trials as a GPR119 agonist (Figure 15), based on Hypo1 in Decoy set are 8.8 and 7.7 (nM), respectively. The validated pharmacophore generated can be used to evaluate how well any newly designed compound maps on the pharmacophore before undertaking any further study including synthesis, and also used as a three-dimensional query in database searches to identify compounds with diverse structures that can potentially agonist GPR119[73].

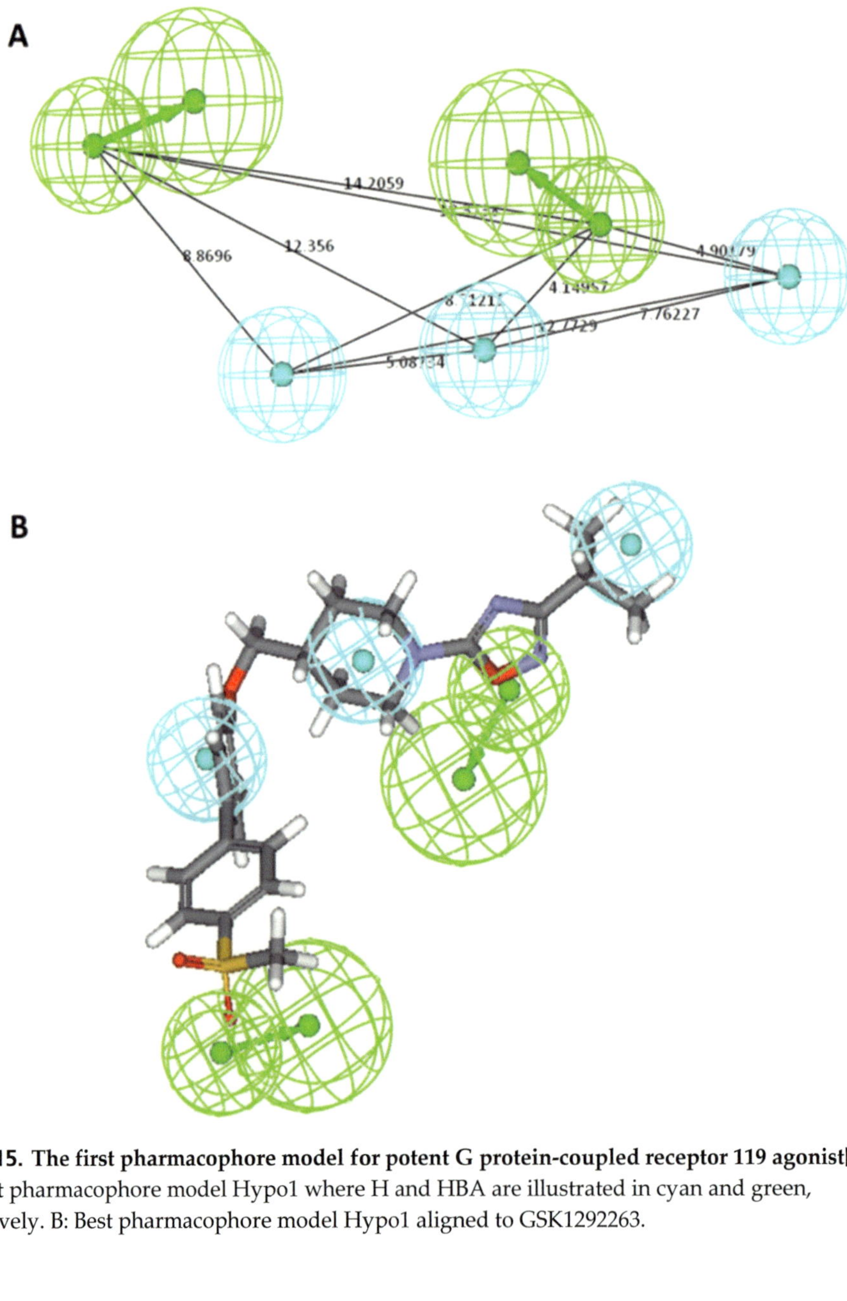

Figure 15. The first pharmacophore model for potent G protein-coupled receptor 119 agonist[73]. A: The best pharmacophore model Hypo1 where H and HBA are illustrated in cyan and green, respectively. B: Best pharmacophore model Hypo1 aligned to GSK1292263.

5. Future directions and concluding remarks

In summary, GPR119 agonists seem to provide a completely novel and previously unexplored approach to incretin therapy in patients with T2DM, increasing glucose-dependent insulin secretion through two complementary mechanisms: directly, through actions on the β cell, and indirectly, through enhancement of GLP-1 and GIP release from the GI tract. It is also worth pointing out the obvious potential advantages that could theoretically be obtained by the co-administration of a GPR119 agonist (with a mechanism as a GLP-1 secretagogue) and a DPP-4 inhibitor (with a mechanism to protect secreted GLP-1), and some preliminary and recent published data support this attractive concept. Such a strategy may not only provide improved glycemic control, but also induce weight loss, a feature observed with GLP-1 mimetics but not with DPP-4 inhibitors. Following the recent entry of the GPR119 agonists MBX-2982, GSK-1292263 and PSN821 into clinical development, the value of these compounds as a new class of therapeutics for type 2 diabetes and associated obesity is likely to be determined within the next few years.

Author details

Xiaoyun Zhu, Wenglong Huang* and Hai Qian*
Centre of Drug Discovery, State Key Laboratory of Natural Medicines,
China Pharmaceutical University, Nanjing,China

Acknowledgement

This study was supported by the National Natural Science Foundation of China (No. 81172932) and the Fundamental Research Funds for the Central Universities of China (No. 2J10023 and JKY2011009).

6. References

[1] Rayburn WF (1997) Diagnosis and classification of diabetes mellitus: highlights from the American Diabetes Association. J Reprod Med. j. 42:585-586.
[2] Collins FM (2002) Current treatment approaches to type 2 diabetes mellitus: successes and shortcomings. Am J Manag Care. j. 8:S460-471.
[3] Tourrel C, Bailbe D, Meile MJ, Kergoat M, Portha B (2001) Glucagon-like peptide-1 and exendin-4 stimulate beta-cell neogenesis in streptozotocin-treated newborn rats resulting in persistently improved glucose homeostasis at adult age. Diabetes. j. 50:1562-1570.
[4] Ross SA, Ekoe JM (2010) Incretin agents in type 2 diabetes. Can Fam Physician. j. 56:639-648.

---

* Corresponding Authors

[5] Ahren B (2009) Islet G protein-coupled receptors as potential targets for treatment of type 2 diabetes. Nat Rev Drug Discov. j. 8:369-385.
[6] Mohler ML, He Y, Wu Z, Hwang DJ, Miller DD (2009) Recent and emerging anti-diabetes targets. Med Res Rev. j. 29:125-195.
[7] Fredriksson R, Hoglund PJ, Gloriam DE, Lagerstrom MC, Schioth HB (2003) Seven evolutionarily conserved human rhodopsin G protein-coupled receptors lacking close relatives. FEBS Lett. j. 554:381-388.
[8] Shah U, Kowalski TJ (2010) GPR119 agonists for the potential treatment of type 2 diabetes and related metabolic disorders. Vitam Horm. j. 84:415-448.
[9] Fyfe (2008) GPR119 agonists as potential new oral agents for the treatment of type 2 diabetes and obesity. Expert Opin Drug Discov. j. 3:403-413.
[10] Bonini JA, Borowsky BE (2001) DNA encoding SNORF25 receptor. p. US6221660.
[11] Bonini JA, Borowsky BE (2002) Methods of identifying compounds that bind to SNORF25 receptors. p. US6468756.
[12] Jones RM (2004) 1,2,3-trisubstituted aryl and heteroaryl derivatives as modulators of metabolism and the prophylaxis and treatment of disorders related thereto such as diabetes and hyperglycaemia. p. WO2004065380.
[13] Takeda S, Kadowaki S, Haga T, Takaesu H, Mitaku S (2002) Identification of G protein-coupled receptor genes from the human genome sequence. FEBS Lett. j. 520:97-101.
[14] Davey J (2004) G-protein-coupled receptors: new approaches to maximise the impact of GPCRS in drug discovery. Expert Opin Ther Targets. j. 8:165-170.
[15] Griffin G (2006) Methods for identifi cation of modulators of OSGPR116 activity. p. US7083933.
[16] Fu J (2003) Oleoylethanolamide regulates feeding and body weight through activation of the nuclear receptor PPAR-α. Nature. j. 425:90-93.
[17] Ohishi T (2003) Method of screening remedy for diabetes. p. EP1338651.
[18] Soga T, Ohishi T, Matsui T, Saito T, Matsumoto M, Takasaki J, Matsumoto S, Kamohara M, Hiyama H, Yoshida S, Momose K, Ueda Y, Matsushime H, Kobori M, Furuichi K (2005) Lysophosphatidylcholine enhances glucose-dependent insulin secretion via an orphan G-protein-coupled receptor. Biochem Biophys Res Commun. j. 326:744-751.
[19] Chu ZL, Jones RM, He H, Carroll C (2007) A role for beta-cell-expressed G protein-coupled receptor 119 in glycemic control by enhancing glucose-dependent insulin release. Endocrinology. j. 148:2601-2609.
[20] Ohishi T, Yoshida S (2012) The therapeutic potential of GPR119 agonists for type 2 diabetes. Expert Opin Investig Drugs. j. 21:321-328.
[21] Chu Z-L (2006) Combination therapy for the treatment of diabetes and conditions related thereto and for the treatment of conditions ameliorated by increasing a blood GLP-1 level. p. WO2006076231

[22] Drucker DJ, Jin T, Asa SL, Young TA, Brubaker PL (1994) Activation of proglucagon gene transcription by protein kinase-A in a novel mouse enteroendocrine cell line. Mol Endocrinol. j. 8:1646-1655.

[23] Dhayal S, Morgan NG (2010) The significance of GPR119 agonists as a future treatment for type 2 diabetes. Drug News Perspect. j. 23:418-424.

[24] Overton HA, Babbs AJ, Doel SM, Fyfe MC, Gardner LS, Griffin G, Jackson HC, Procter MJ, Rasamison CM, Tang-Christensen M, Widdowson PS, Williams GM, Reynet C (2006) Deorphanization of a G protein-coupled receptor for oleoylethanolamide and its use in the discovery of small-molecule hypophagic agents. Cell Metab. j. 3:167-175.

[25] Overton HA, Fyfe MC, Reynet C (2008) GPR119, a novel G protein-coupled receptor target for the treatment of type 2 diabetes and obesity. Br J Pharmacol. j. 153 Suppl 1:S76-81.

[26] Rodriguez de Fonseca F, Navarro M, Gomez R, Escuredo L, Nava F, Fu J, Murillo-Rodriguez E, Giuffrida A, LoVerme J, Gaetani S, Kathuria S, Gall C, Piomelli D (2001) An anorexic lipid mediator regulated by feeding. Nature. j. 414:209-212.

[27] Yang Y, Chen M, Georgeson KE, Harmon CM (2007) Mechanism of oleoylethanolamide on fatty acid uptake in small intestine after food intake and body weight reduction. Am J Physiol Regul Integr Comp Physiol. j. 292:R235-241.

[28] Proulx K, Cota D, Castaneda TR, Tschop MH, D'Alessio DA, Tso P, Woods SC, Seeley RJ (2005) Mechanisms of oleoylethanolamide-induced changes in feeding behavior and motor activity. Am J Physiol Regul Integr Comp Physiol. j. 289:R729-737.

[29] Ning Y, O'Neill K, Lan H, Pang L, Shan LX, Hawes BE, Hedrick JA (2008) Endogenous and synthetic agonists of GPR119 differ in signalling pathways and their effects on insulin secretion in MIN6c4 insulinoma cells. Br J Pharmacol. j. 155:1056-1065.

[30] Chu Z-L, Carroll C, Alfonso J, Gutierrez V, He H, Lucman A, Pedraza M, Mondala H, Gao H, Bagnol D, Chen R, Jones RM, Behan DP, Leonard J (2008) A role for intestinal endocrine cell-expressed g protein-coupled receptor 119 in glycemic control by enhancing glucagon-like Peptide-1 and glucose-dependent insulinotropic Peptide release. Endocrinology. j. 149:2038-2047.

[31] Lauffer LM, Iakoubov R, Brubaker PL (2009) GPR119 is essential for oleoylethanolamide-induced glucagon-like peptide-1 secretion from the intestinal enteroendocrine L-cell. Diabetes. j. 58:1058-1066.

[32] Jones RM, Leonard JN, Buzard DJ, Lehmann J (2009) GPR119 agonists for the treatment of type 2 diabetes. Expert Opin Ther Pat. j. 19:1339-1359.

[33] Gharbaoui T (2006) Processes for preparing aromatic ethers. p. US20060155129.

[34] Semple G, Lehmann J, Wong A, Ren A, Bruce M (2012) Discovery of a second generation agonist of the orphan G-protein coupled receptor GPR119 with an improved profile. Bioorg Med Chem Lett. j. 22:1750-1755.

[35] Yoshida S, Ohishi T, Matsui T, Tanaka H, Oshima H, Yonetoku Y, Shibasaki M (2011) The role of small molecule GPR119 agonist, AS1535907, in glucose-stimulated insulin secretion and pancreatic beta-cell function. Diabetes Obes Metab. j. 13:34-41.
[36] Yoshida S, Tanaka H, Oshima H, Yamazaki T, Yonetoku Y, Ohishi T, Matsui T, Shibasaki M (2010) AS1907417, a novel GPR119 agonist, as an insulinotropic and beta-cell preservative agent for the treatment of type 2 diabetes. Biochem Biophys Res Commun. j. 400:745-751.
[37] Brandt P, Emond R (2008) Pyridine compounds for treating GPR119 related disorders. p. WO2008025798.
[38] Brandt P, Johansson G (2008) Pyridazine compounds for treating GPR119 related disorders. p. WO2008025799.
[39] Brandt P, Johansson G (2008) Pyrimidine compounds for treating GPR119 related disorders. p. WO2008025800.
[40] Bremberg U, Johansson G (2009) Agonists of GPR119. p. WO2009106565.
[41] Fevig JM (2008) [6, 6] and [6, 7]-Bicyclic GPR119 G proteincoupled receptor agonists. p. WO2008137435.
[42] Fevig JM, Wacker DA (2008) [6, 5]-Bicyclic GPR119 G protein-coupled receptor agonists. p. WO2008137436.
[43] Wacker DA, Rossi KA (2009) Pyridone GPR119 G protein-coupled receptor agonists. p. WO2009012275.
[44] Wacker DA, Rossi KA (2010) Pyridone and pyridazone analogues as GPR119 modulators. p. WO2010009183.
[45] Ammala C, Briscoe C (2008) GPR119 agonists for the treatment of diabetes and related disorders. p. WO2008008895.
[46] Katamreddy SR, Caldwell RD (2008) Chemical compounds. p. WO2008008887.
[47] Carpenter AJ, Fang J (2010) Chemical compounds and uses. p. WO2010014593.
[48] Nunez DJ (2010) Diabetes [70th Annu Meet Sci Sess Am Diabetes Assoc (ADA) (June 25-29, Orlando) 2010] 2010, 59(Suppl. 1): Abst 80-OR).
[49] Wood HB, Adams AD (2008) Acyl bipiperidinyl compounds, compositions containing such compounds and methods of treatment. p. WO2008076243.
[50] Wood HB, Adams AD (2008) Bipiperidinyl compounds, compositions containing such compounds and methods of treatment. p. WO2008085316.
[51] Harris J (2008) Spiro-condensed azetidine derivatives useful in treating pain, diabetes and disorders of lipid metabolism. p. WO08033456.
[52] Harris J (2008) Azetidinone derivatives and methods of use thereof p. WO08033464.
[53] Harris J (2008) Pyrimidinone derivatives and methods of use thereof. p. WO08130584.
[54] Harris J (2008) Pyrimidinone derivatives and methods of use thereof. p. WO08130581.

[55] Chen X, Cheng P (2008) Heterocyclic receptor agonists for the treatment of diabetes and metabolic disorders. p. WO2008083238.

[56] Ma J, Rabbat CJ (2009) N-linked heterocyclic receptor agonists for the treatment of diabetes and metabolic disorders. p. WO2009014910.

[57] Song J, Ma J (2010) Aryl GPR119 agonists and uses thereof. p. WO2010008739.

[58] Wilson ME, Johnson J (2009) Oxymethylene aryl compounds and uses thereof. p. WO2009123992.

[59] McWherter C (2010) The discovery of novel agonists of GPR119 receptor for the treatment of type 2 diabetes. In "32nd Annual National Medicinal Chemistry Symposium," Minneapolis, MN, USA, 6-9 June.

[60] Roberts B, Karpf DB (2010) MBX-2982, a novel GPR119 agonist, shows greater efficacy in patients with the most glucose intolerance: Results of a phase I study with an improved formulation. In "American Diabetes Association 70th Annual Scientific Sessions," Orlando, FL, USA, 25-29 June, Abstract 603-P.

[61] Alper P, Azimioara M (2008) Compounds and compositions as modulators of GPR119 activity. p. WO2008097428.

[62] Alper P, Azimioara M (2009) Compounds and compositions as modulators of GPR119 activity. p. WO2009038974.

[63] Azimioara M, Cow C (2009) Compounds and compositions as modulators of GPR119 activity. p. WO2009105717.

[64] IRM L (2008) Compounds and compositions as modulators of GPR119 activity. p. WO08109702.

[65] Fyfe M, Babbs AJ (2008) Discovery of PSN119-2, a novel oxadiazole-containing GPR119 agonist. In "236th American Chemical Society National Meeting," Philadelphia, PA, USA, 17-21 August 2008, MEDI 197.

[66] Fyfe M (2007) Synthesis, SAR, and in vivo efficacy of novel GPR119 agonists with a 4-[3-(4-methanesulfinylphenoxy)propyl]-1-Boc-piperidine core. In "234th American Chemical Society National Meeting," Boston, MA, USA, 19-23 August 2007, MEDI 062.

[67] Fyfe M (2007) GPR119 agonists are potential novel oral agents for the treatment of diabesity. In "American Diabetes Association 67th Annual Scientific Sessions," Chicago, IL, USA, 22-26 June 2007, Abstract 0532-P.

[68] Fyfe M (2009) Azetidinyl G-protein coupled receptor agonists. p. WO2009050522.

[69] Fyfe M (2009) Azetidinyl G-protein coupled receptor agonists. p. WO2009050523.

[70] Fyfe M, Mccormack, J., Overton, H., Procter, M., and Reynet, C. (2008) PSN821: A novel oral GPR119 agonist for the treatment of type 2 diabetes producing substantial glucose lowering and weight loss in rats. In "American Diabetes Association 68th Annual Scientific Sessions," San Francisco, CA, USA, 6-10 June 2008, Abstract 297-OR.

[71] Barba O, Bradley SE (2009) Compounds for the treatment of metabolic disorders. p. WO2009034388.

[72] Swain S, Cock TA, and Wong-Kai-In, P. (). (2009) A novel dual DPP-IV inhibitor and GPR119 agonist that exhibits superior glucose lowering to sitagliptin in diabetic ZDF rats. In "American Diabetes Association 69th Annual Scientific Sessions," New Orleans, LA, USA, 5-9 June 2009, Abstract 453-P.

[73] Zhu X, Huang D, Lan X, Tang C, Zhu Y, Han J, Huang W, Qian H (2011) The first pharmacophore model for potent G protein-coupled receptor 119 agonist. Eur J Med Chem. j. 46:2901-2907.

Chapter 5

The Role of Nutrition in the Management of Diabetes Mellitus

Olabiyi Folorunso and Oluwafemi Oguntibeju

Additional information is available at the end of the chapter

http://dx.doi.org/10.5772/48782

1. Introduction

Scientific evidence abound to show that the prevalence of diabetes mellitus(DM) is increasing around the world at a rate that appears dramatic as to have been characterized as an epidemic[1]. Among several factors that have been postulated to contribute to DM epidemic, environmental factors have drawn particular attention because of the rapidity of the increase in type 2 or the so called 'maturity on- set' diabetes mellitus. Nobuko Seike, Mitsuhiko Noda and Takashi Kadowaki [2] evaluated the association between alcohol consumption and the risk of type 2 DM, it was pointed out that type 2 diabetes mellitus is closely related to life style factors including diet, physical activities, alcohol and smoking as well as obesity and a family history of diabetes. According to the researchers, in Japan the prevalence of diabetes mellitus both for men over age 50 and women over 60 well exceeds 10% and most have type 2 DM which is associated with excessive energy intake, lack of physical exercise and obesity. In addition, Mayes and Botham[3] revealed that obesity – particularly, abdominal obesity(a diet related disorder) is a risk factor for increased mortality, hypertension, type 2 DM, hyperlipidaemia and various endocrine dysfunctions.

On the other hand, type 1 DM, or 'Juvenile DM' or 'insulin-dependent' diabetes is less common than type 2. Only 10% of all diabetics have type 1.

Type 1 diabetes occurs when the pancreas produces no insulin at all. It tends to emerge in childhood or early adulthood (before the age of 40) and must be regulated by regularly injecting insulin. Although the exact cause of type 1 diabetes is currently unknown, it is widely believed that majority of type 1 diabetes is of the immune-mediated nature, where beta cell loss is a T-cell mediated autoimmune attack [4].

With type 1 diabetes, the immune system attacks cells in the pancreas. This destroys or damages them enough to stop the production of insulin. A number of experts attribute this occurrence to a viral infection.

Genetics are also thought to play a part in the cause of type 1 diabetes; it has often been seen to run in families.

People who have a close relative (parent or sibling) with type 1 diabetes have a 6% chance of developing type 1 diabetes too.

In some instances, type 1 diabetes can be caused by a condition of the pancreas known as 'chronic pancreatitis'. Chronis pancreatitis causes an inflammation of the pancreas and can cause serious damage to the cells that produce insulin [5].

It is a well known fact that DM being a metabolic, endocrine disorder is directly connected to carbohydrate, lipid and protein metabolism. As a result, nutrition therapy forms an integral part of diabetes management and diabetes self - management education. It is also well established that diabetes is caused by either a lack of Insulin secretion or by insulin resistance. The resultant disease or metabolic disturbance leads to hyperglycaemia and dyslipidemia in the short term, as well as long term complications such as retinopathy, neuropathy and nephropathy. Besides, persons with diabetes are 2 to 4 times more likely to develop coronary artery disease or to suffer a stroke. Findings from the diabetic control and complication trials (DCCT) and the United Kingdom prospective Diabetes study(UKPDS) clearly indicate that the maintenance of near normal blood glucose level dramatically reduces the chronic complications associated with this disorder. In addition, reducing elevated blood lipids levels has been shown to lower the incidence of acute coronary events in other at-risk populations. Research have shown that before the advent of insulin therapy in the early 20th century, medical nutrition therapy (MNT) was the only form of therapy for DM[6].

However, there are many misconceptions concerning nutrition and diabetes [7]. Moreso, most diabetics are confused with conflicting nutrition advice and opinions. And it is commonly believed that diabetes cannot be completely cured , but it may be more easily regulated and controlled with the right diet . With strict adherence to nutritionist's advice, diabetic patients may be able to significantly improve their quality of life. There is little data on the role nutrition played in diabetes management in our environment, hence, the need for a review like this.

2. Diabetes mellitus and nutrition

A number of nutritional factors have been found to influence the development of type 1 diabetes or type 1-related autoimmunity. One study has found, for example, that eating vegetables daily during pregnancy reduced the risk of a child's developing type 1-associated autoimmunity [8]. Another found that higher iron intake (via infant formula or supplements) in the first four months of life was associated with a higher risk of developing type 1 diabetes[9]. However, other studies have not found associations between diet and type 1 diabetes development. For example, Virtanen et al.[10] found only a weak protective effect of a few foods eaten during pregnancy and the development of type 1 related autoimmunity in the offspring (those foods were butter, low-fat margarine, berries, and coffee; most foods showed no association).

2.1. Omega-3 fatty acids

Norris et al.[11] found that dietary intake of omega-3 fatty acids, found in fish, flax seeds, walnuts, soy, canola, and greens, is protective against the development of type 1 diabetes-related autoantibodies in children at genetic risk of type 1 diabetes. Omega-3s can reduce inflammation, and the lack of omega-3s in Western diets may predispose people to inflammation. Yet the same authors later found that omega-3 levels were not associated with later development of type 1 in these children [12]. So, it is possible that omega-3s may be protective against type 1 autoantibody development, but be less significant later in the disease process.

An earlier study of the same children found that the mother's dietary intake of omega-3 fatty acids during pregnancy did not affect the risk of autoimmunity in children [13]. Cod liver oil, however, taken during pregnancy, has been associated with a reduced risk of type 1 diabetes in offspring. Both omega-3 fatty acids and vitamin D are present in this oil, and either or both may play a role [14].

Virtanen et al.[15] found that the fatty acids associated with milk and ruminant meat fat consumption were associated with an increased risk of type 1 related autoimmunity. Linoleic acid, however, was associated with lower levels of autoimmunity, in children genetically at risk of type 1 diabetes.

A group of people with metabolic syndrome (a group of conditions common in people with type 1 or 2 diabetes) were given omega-3 fatty acid supplements or a placebo for six months. Those taking the supplements were found to have lower markers of autoimmunity and inflammation, as well as more weight loss, compared to people who did not take the supplements [16].

Adequate intake of omega-3s during pregnancy may also decrease the risk of obesity in the offspring. Higher levels of omega-6 fatty acids in relation to omega-3s in umbilical cord blood has been associated with higher obesity in children at age 3 [17].

2.2. Chemicals and omega-3s

The presence of environmental contaminants in food may also play a role in the effects of nutritional factors. Some contaminants may interfere with the beneficial effects of foods. For example, in a study linking insulin resistance to persistent organic pollutants, the researchers concluded that beneficial aspects of omega-3 fatty acids in salmon oil could not counteract the harmful effects caused by the persistent organic pollutants in that oil [18].

Fish is one source of omega-3 fatty acids, but according to an editorial in the *American Journal of Clinical Nutrition* (AJCN), it may be better to rely on plant-based sources instead [19]. Studies on fish consumption and type 2 diabetes are inconsistent: some show that higher dietary intake of omega 3s decreases the risk of type 2, some show no connection, and some even show that higher fish consumption increases the risk of type 2 diabetes [20,21]. It may be that the chemicals in fish can explain these inconsistencies. A study shows that plant-based omega 3s have different effects than marine-based omega 3s in relation to type 2 diabetes [22], it was opined that this may be possibly due to the contaminants present in fish.

A high fat diet, especially one high in saturated fats, has been linked to type 2 diabetes and insulin resistance. It appears that saturated fatty acids (but not unsaturated fats) activate immune cells, which produce an inflammatory protein, which in turn then makes cells more insulin resistant [23].Mothers who consumed higher levels of trans fats had an increased risk of excess body fat, and so did their breastfed infants [24].

Can the effects of a high fat diet be passed down to subsequent generations? In animal studies, a high-fat diet that causes obesity in mothers can affect the metabolism and weight of her offspring. But what about a high fat diet in fathers? In one study, the female offspring of heavier father rats (fed a high-fat diet) had defects in their insulin and glucose levels, like their fathers. Unlike their fathers, they were not heavier than the controls [25]. Other researchers fed mice a high fat diet with fat composition similar to a standard Western diet, and then bred them and fed them the same diet for multiple generations. Over four generations, the offspring became gradually heavier, and developed higher insulin levels, despite not eating more calories. The diet was associated with changes in gene expression [26].

2.3. Glycemic index and sweeteners

The glycemic index(GI) is a measurement of how high a certain food raises blood glucose levels after it is eaten. Foods that have a high glycemic index will cause blood glucose to rise more, triggering insulin production (in people who still produce insulin), then leading to falling blood glucose levels. One prospective study has found that a higher glycemic index diet leads to a faster progression to type 1 diabetes. The group of people on this diet, however, did not have higher levels of autoantibodies, showing that the diet may affect disease progression but not disease initiation. The mechanisms involved may include oxidative stress, caused by high blood glucose levels after meals, or perhaps insulin resistance. Whatever the mechanism, a high glycemic index diet may place additional stress on beta cells that are already under an autoimmune attack [27].

Evidence favouring the active reduction of blood lipids continues to accumulate and several major diabetes associations now recommend that diabetic patients should reduce fat intake and increase carbohydrate intake to approximately 50% of total calories[1]. High fibre foods has been advocated [28]. It was highlighted that, although before detailed advice can be given, comparative data on the physiological effects of carbohydrate foods may be required.

The consumption of sugar-sweetened beverages has been associated with type 2 diabetes, obesity, and metabolic syndrome. A meta-analysis of a 11 prospective studies (of over 300,000 people) found that those who consumed 1-2 sweetened beverages per day had a 26% greater risk of developing type 2 diabetes than those who consumed fewer than one serving per month. The risk was 20% higher for developing metabolic syndrome. Sugar-sweetened beverages include soft drinks, fruit drinks, iced tea, and energy/vitamin water drinks [29].

High-fructose corn syrup is another sweetener linked to obesity. Rats given access to high-fructose corn syrup gained more weight than those given access to sucrose, despite eating the same number of calories [30].

2.4. Zinc

A few studies have found that higher zinc levels in drinking water may be protective against type 1 diabetes. For example, Zhao et al. [31], found that higher levels of zinc and magnesium were associated with lower rates of type 1 diabetes in southwest England. In Norway, a study found that higher zinc levels in water was associated with a lower risk of type 1 diabetes, but the association was not statistically significant [32]. In Finland, a study found that low zinc levels in drinking water was associated with a higher incidence of type 1 diabetes [33].

2.5. Nicotinamide and other antioxidants

Nicotinamide, is a component of vitamin B_3 that has been shown to protect against diabetes in animals, and prevent beta cell damage [34]. Even better, one study found that it prevented the development of type 1 diabetes in children with type 1-associated autoantibodies [35].

On the basis of these and other studies, a large, double-blind, placebo-controlled trial was conducted in Europe, the U.S. and Canada, called the European Nicotinamide Diabetes Intervention Trial (ENDIT). This trial gave nicotinamide to first degree relatives of people with type 1 diabetes who already had developed type 1-associated autoantibodies. Unfortunately, it found no difference in the development of diabetes between the two groups during the 5 year follow-up period. The study gave high doses of the vitamin, up to 3 g/day (30-50 times higher than the RDA) [34].

Another double-blind, placebo controlled study in Sweden gave high doses of anti-oxidants (including nicotinamide, vitamin C, vitamin E, Beta-carotene, and selenium) to people after they were already diagnosed with type 1 diabetes and also found that they had no effect in protecting the beta cells against the damage of free radicals [36]. There is no evidence linking the anti-oxidants alpha- or beta-carotene levels and the development of type 1 related autoimmunity in another study as well [37].

Uusitalo et al. [38] also found that if pregnant women took anti-oxidants and trace minerals (including retinol, beta-carotene, vitamin C, vitamin E, selenium, zinc, or manganese) during pregnancy, there was no effect on the risk of the child's developing type 1-related autoimmunity.

Czernichow et al.[39] found that anti-oxidant supplements were not protective against metabolic syndrome, a group of conditions common in people with type 1 or 2 diabetes. Yet they also found that the people who had the highest levels of some anti-oxidants (beta-carotene, vitamin C, and vitamin E) in the beginning of the study, presumably due to a diet rich in plant foods, did have a lower risk of developing metabolic syndrome.

While these studies did not find promising results concerning anti-oxidant supplements, they also did not find that these supplements did any harm.

Free radicals may play a role in the inflammatory process that destroys the beta cells in type 1 diabetes [36]. Therefore, anti-oxidants have been thought to protect the body from oxidative stress due to the production of free radicals. But, there is some animal evidence that anti-oxidant supplements may also increase insulin resistance, showing that the relationship may not be so simple. When the researchers gave certain mice an anti-oxidant, they were more likely to become insulin resistant [40]. Perhaps this finding could help explain why anti-oxidant supplements have not been found to be protective against type 1 diabetes.

3. Food processing: AGEs

Advanced Glycation End products (AGEs)are found in heat processed foods and have been linked to type 1 and type 2 diabetes in animal studies. They appear to predispose people to oxidative stress and inflammation, and may affect the fetus if the mother consumes them during pregnancy. A study has found that the level of AGEs that a mother eats are correlated with insulin levels in the baby. It found that if mothers have high AGE levels, and infant food is high in AGEs, it may raise the risk of diabetes in the offspring [41].

3.1. Protein

Researchers fed mother rats a diet that was deficient in protein, and found higher rates of diabetes in the offspring. They also found that one of the offspring's genes was "silenced"-- a gene associated with type 2 diabetes development. Nutrition, then, may have effects on gene expression that are linked to type 2 diabetes development [42].

3.2. Nutritional management of DM

In contemporary time, Medical Nutrition Therapy (MNT) is used to describe dietary prescriptions [43] .

MNT for diabetes aim to achieve the following objectives:

1. Achieve and maintain near normal blood glucose goals
2. Achieve and/ or maintain optimal blood lipid levels
3. Achieve and/ or maintain normal blood pressure
4. Prevent, delay or treat nutrition related complications
5. Provide adequate kcalories for achievement of reasonable body weight
6. Provide optimal nutrition for maximizing health and for growth, development, pregnancy, and lactation

Body of knowledge shows that, with respect to carbohydrates, the key emphasis of MNT for diabetes mellitus is on the total amount of carbohydrate in terms of energy intake [44].As far as the type of carbohydrates to be ingested is concerned, the guidelines for MNT in DM clearly stress the value of selecting vegetables, fruits and grains , so that the starches consumed will include adequate amounts of both fibre and micronutrients[43].

Research findings shows specific interests in the role that dietary fiber may play in the nutritional management of DM. Benefit of fiber were found with regard to glycaemic control, HDL and LDL cholesterol and triacylglycerols [45]. However, a 3- month study by Jenkins et al.[46] did not find a metabolic advantage of high fiber over low fiber cereals. Also, a study carried out by Erasmus et al. [47],showed that treatment with guar gum does not lower the postprandial glucose level in both non- diabetic and diabetic Nigerian subjects.

3.3. Dietary principles for diabetes mellitus

The American Diabetes Association [7] gave the following guidelines:

3.3.1. Type 1 DM

Which can achieve much if the following dietary principles are observed ;

i. Integrate and syncronise with the time of action of insulin treatment – patient on insulin therapy should eat at consistent time simultaneously with the time of action of insulin preparation used. This will help to minimize the peak of blood glucose as well as incidence of hypoglycaemia.
ii. Reduce saturated fat because diabetics are prone to having coronary heart disease and dietary restriction may reduce the risk.
iii. Keep salt intake low: salt intake must be reduced by diabetics because it has high risk of developing hypertension. However, intake of essential nutrients should be adequate among growing patients.
iv. Exercise: For planned exercise, reduction in insulin dosage may be the preferred choice to prevent hypoglycemia. Additional carbohydrate may be needed for unplanned exercise. Moderate-intensity exercise increases glucose uptake by 2–3 $mg \cdot kg^{-1} \cdot min^{-1}$ above usual requirements. Thus, a 70-kg person would need 8.4–12.6 g (10–15) carbohydrate per hour of moderate physical activity. More carbohydrate would be needed for intense activity.
v. Metabolic profile: Improved glycaemic control with insulin therapy is often associated with increased body weight. Because of the potential for weight gain to adversely affect glycaemia, lipids, blood pressure, and general health, prevention of weight gain is desirable.

3.3.2. Type 2 DM

A change in dietary regimen has a greater potential to improve type 2 diabetes , therefore, the following guidelines will serve a useful purpose.

Because many persons with type 2 diabetes are overweight and insulin resistant, medical nutrition therapy should emphasize lifestyle changes that result in reduced energy intake and increased energy expenditure through physical activity. Therefore, reducing body weight by eating few calories and taking regular exercise. Also, increased physical activity can lead to improved glycaemia, decreasing insulin resistance, and reduced cardiovascular risk factors.

i. Reduce saturated fat and maintaining a reduced plasma low density lipoprotein cholesterol levels.

ii. Eating low glycaemic index foods such as soya beans, apple, grapefruits, peas(groundnuts), increase intake of vegetables, fruits, legumes and whole grain cereal that may mostly have low glycaemic indices.
iii. Keep salt intake low
iv. Fried food is not good for diabetes patients . Wheat bread, lean meat, game meat (bush meat), green, leafy vegetables, garden egg, all these should be encouraged for DM patients.
v. Physical activity: Increased physical activity can lead to improved glycaemia, decreased insulin resistance, and reduced cardiovascular risk factors.

4. Epidemiological and laboratory studies

From the review by Kayode et al.(1), epidemiological studies (48) have reported that as nations become more affluent, the nature of the people's carbohydrate consumption changes such that the ratio of complex (starches) to simple carbohydrates decreases. It has been suggested that this change in dietary pattern is responsible for the occurrence of various diseases, such as atherosclerosis, diabetes and hyperlipidaemia. One proposed physiological basis underlying such suggestions is a traditionally held tenet that simple carbohydrates are more readily available for immediate absorption by the gut than are more complex carbohydrates and that they therefore produce a greater and faster rise in postprandial plasma glucose and insulin responses than do the supposedly more gradually digested and absorbed complex carbohydrate. Consequently, diets restricted in simple carbohydrates have been recommended in disease states in which control of plasma glucose and/or insulin is felt to be important. However, there is dearth of sufficient laboratory data to substantiate the role nutrition plays in the management of diabetes mellitus.

4.1. Recommendations and further studies

To be able to effectively manage diabetes with the aid of dietary control, patient's education, understanding, and participation is vital since the complications of diabetes are far less common and less severe in people who have well- managed blood glucose levels. Also, there is reduction in expenses incurred due to this metabolic disorder which research shows was a major drain on health and productivity – related resources of government and other employers of labour.

Given the associated higher risks of cardiovascular disease, lifestyle modifications(which includes smoking habits, sedentary life, lack of regular exercise etc,) are strongly recommended. Besides, regular exercise, coupled with blood pressure , cholesterol levels, body weight , HbA1C measurements is advocated among people with diabetes.

Omega-3 fatty acids may be protective against type 1 diabetes, but more studies would be necessary to confirm this finding. Eating high glycemic-index foods may accelerate the progression of type 1 diabetes, but this association should also be confirmed. Taking anti-oxidant supplements does not appear to reduce the risk of type 1 diabetes, but it is possible that a diet high in anti-oxidants may still be protective.

More research is highly imperative on the epidemiological and laboratory aspects of the role of nutrition in the management of diabetes mellitus.

Author details

Olabiyi Folorunso
Chemical Pathology Unit, Department of Medical Laboratory Science, Achievers University, Owo, Nigeria

Oluwafemi Oguntibeju
Department of Biomedical Sciences, Faculty of Health & Wellness Sciences, Cape Peninsula University of Technology, Bellville, South Africa

Acknowledgement

Our sincere appreciation goes to Professors S.A Shoyinka and J.I Anetor, for their invaluable contributions.

5. References

[1] J. Kayode, A. Sola, A. Adelani, A. Adeyinka, O. Kolawole, O. Bashiru (2009): The role of carbohydrate in diabetic nutrition: A review. The internet Journal of Laboratory Medicine. Volume 3 Number 2.

[2] Nobuko Seike, Mitsuhiko Noda, Takashi Kadowaki (2009): Alcohol consumption and the risk of type 2 diabetes mellitus in Japanese. A systematic review. Asia Pac J Clin Nutr 17(4):545 – 551.

[3] Peter A. Mayes, Katleen M. Botham (2003): Lipid transport and storage . Harpers illustrated Biochemistry. 26th Ed. Mc Graw Hill. 25: 205.

[4] Rother KI., (2007): ''Diabetes Treatment – bridging the divide ''. The New England Journal of Medicine. 356(15):1499-501.

[5] Narendran P, Estella E, Fourlanos S, (2005): Immunology of type 1 diabetes.QJM. 547 -56.

[6] Blades M., Morgan J., Dickerson J., (1997) : Dietary advice in the management of diabetes mellitus. history and current practice. J. R. Soc. Health 117: 143 – 150.

[7] American Diabetes Association (2004): Nutrition Principles and Recommendation in Diabetes. Diabetic Care. Volume 27 no suppl 1536.

[8] Brekke HK., and Ludviqsson J., (2009) :Daily vegetable intake during pregnancy negatively associated to islet autoimmunity in the offspring … the ABIS study. Pediatr Diabetes. 4 : 244-50.

[9] Ashraf AP., Easson NB., Kabagambe EK., Haritha J., Meleth S., McCormic KL., (2010):Dietary iron intake in the first 4 months of infancy and the development of type 1 diabetes : a pilot study. Diabetol Metab Syndr 2:58.

[10] Virtanen SM., Uusitalo L., Kenwaed MG., Nevalainen J., Uusitalo U., Kronberg –Kippila C., Ovaskainen ML., Arkkola T., Niinisto S., Hakulinen T., Ahonen S., Simeli O.,

IlonenJ., Veijola R., Knip M., (2011) : maternal food consumption during pregnancy and risk of advanced β-cell autoimmunityin the offspring. Pediatr Diabetes 12(2) : 95-9.

[11] Norris JM., Yin X., Lamb MM., Barriga K., Seifert J., Hoffman M., Orton HD., Baron AE., Clare-Salzler M., Chase HP., Szabo NJ., Erlich H., Eisenbarth GS., Rewers M., (2007): Omega -3 polyunsaturated fatty acid intake and islet autoimmunity in children at increased risk for type 1 diabetes. JAMA. 298(12):1420 -8.

[12] Miller MR., Yin X., Seifert J., Clare –Salzler M., Eisenbarth GS., Rewers M., Norris JM., (2011): Erythrocyte membrane omega-3 fatty acid levels and omega -3 fatty acid intake are not associated with conversion to type 1 diabetes in children with autoimmunity :the Diabetes Autoimmunity Study in the young (DAISY). Pediatr Diabetes 12(8):669 -75.

[13] Fronczak CM., Baron AE., Chase HP., Ross C., Brady HL., Hoffman M., Eisenbarth GS., Rewers M., Norris JM., (2003) : In utero dietary exposures and risk of islet autoimmunity in children. Diabetes Care. 26(12): 3237 - 42.

[14] Stene LC., Ulriksen J., Magnus P., Joner G., (2000) : Use of cod liver oil during pregnancy associated with lower risk of type 1 diabetes in the offspring. Diabetologia. 43(9):1093 – 8.

[15] Virtanen SM., Niisisto S., Nevalainen J., Salminen I., Takkinen HM., Kaaria S., Uusitalo L., Alfthan G., Kenward MG., Veijola R., Simeli O., Ilonen J., Knip M., (2010) : Serum fatty acids and risk of advanced β-cell autoimmunity :a nested case – control study among children with HLA – conferred susceptibility to type 1 diabetes. Eur J Clin Nutr 64(8) : 792 – 9.

[16] Ebrahimi M., Ghanyour –Mobarhan M., Rezaiean S., Hoseini M., Parizade SM., Farhoudi F., Hosseininezhad SJ., Tavallaaei S., Vejdani A., Azimi – Nezhad M., Shakeri MT., Rad M., Mobara N., Kazemi – Bajestani SM., Ferns GA., (2009) : Omega – 3 fatty acid supplements improve the cardiovascular risk profile of subjects with metabolic syndrome including markers of inflammation and autoimmunity . Acta Cardiol 64(3) :321 -7.

[17] Donahue SM., Rifas – Shiman SL., Gold DR., Jouni ZE., Gillman MW., Oken E., (2011) :Prenatal fatty acid status and child adiposity at age 3y : results from a US pregnancy cohort. Am J Clin Nutr 93(4):780 – 8.

[18] Ruzzin J., Petersen R., Mengnier E., Madsen L., Lock EJ., Lillefosse H., Ma T., Pesenti S., Soone SB., Marstrand TT., Malde MK., Du ZY., Chavey C., Fajas L., Lundebye AK., Brand CL., Vidal H., Kristiansen K., FrØyland L (2010) : Persistent organic pollutant exposure leads to insulin resistance syndrome. Environ Health Perspect 18(4) : 465 -71.

[19] Feskens EJ., (2011):The prevention of type 2 diabetes. Should we recommend vegetable oils instead of fatty fish? Am J Clin Nutr 94(2):369 -70.

[20] Djoussé L., Biggs ML., Lemaitre RN., Kings IB., Song X., Ix JH., Mukamal KJ., Siscovick DS., Mozaffarian D.,(2011) :Plasma omega -3 faaty acids and incident diabetes in older adults. Am J Clin Nutr 94(2) :527 – 33.

[21] Villegas R., Xiang YB., Elasy T., Li HL., Yang G., Cai H., Ye F., Gao YT., Shyr Y., Zheng W., Shu XO., (2011) :Fish, shellfish, and long –chain n-3 fatty acid consumption and risk of incident type 2 diabetes in middle –aged Chinese men and women. Am J Clin Nutr 94(2) :543- 51.

[22] Brostow DP., Odegaard AO., Koh WP., Duval S., Gross MD., Yuan JM., Pereira MA., (2011): Omega – 3 fatty acids and incident type 2 diabetes : the Singapore Chinese Health Study . Am J Clin Nutr 94(2): 520– 6.
[23] Wen H., Gris D., Lei Y., Jha S., Zhang L., Huang MT., Brickey WJ., Ting JP., (2011): Fatty acid –induced NLRP3-ASC inflammation activation interferes with insulin signalling. Nat Immunol 12(5):408 – 15.
[24] Anderson AK., McDougald DM., Steiner-Asiedu M., (2010) :Dietary trans fatty acid intake and maternal and infant adiposity. Eur J Clin Nutr 64(11);1308 – 15.
[25] Ng SF., Lin RC., Laybutt DR., Barres R., Owens JA., Morris MJ., (2010): Chronic high – fat diet in fathers programs β – cell dysfunction in female rat offspring. Nature. 21; 467(7318): 963 -6.
[26] Massiera F., Barbry P., Guesnet P., Joly A., Lugnet S., Moreilhon –Brest C., Mohsen – Kanson T., Amri EZ., Ailhaud G.,(2010) : A Western – like fat diet is sufficient to induce a gradual enhancement in fat mass over generations. J Lipid Res 51(8):2352-61.
[27] Lamb MM.,Yin X., Barriga K., Hoffman MR., Barón AE., Eisenbarth GS., Rewers M., Norris JM., (2008) : Dietary glycemic index , development of islet autoimmunity and subsequent progression to type 1 diabetes in young children . J Clin Endocrinol metab 93(10):3936 -42.
[28] Jenkins DJA, Wolever TMS, Jenkins AL, Wong GS, Josse R. (1984): Glycaemic response to carbohydrate foods. Lancet.388 -391.
[29] Malik VS.,Popkins BM., Bray GA., Pesprés JP., Willett WB., Hu FB., (2010):Sugar – sweetened beverages and risk of metabolic syndrome and type 2 diabetes : a meta-analysis. Diabetes Care. 33(11)2477 -83.
[30] Bocarsly ME., Powell ES., Avena NM., Hoebel BG., (2010): High fructose corn syrup causes characteristic obesity in rats: increased body weight, body fat and triglyceride levels. Pharmacol Biochem Behav 97(1):101 – 6.
[31] Zhao HX., Mold MD., Stenhouse EA., Bird SC., Wright DE., Demaine AG., Millward BA., (2001): Drinking water composition and childhood – onset type 1 diabetes mellitus in Devon and Cornwall England. Diabet Med 18(9): 709 - 17.
[32] Stene LC,Hongve D, Magnus P, RØnningen KS, Joner G (2002):Acidic drinking water and risk of childhood –onset type 1 diabetes. Diabetes Care. 25(9) :1534 -8.
[33] Ulf S., Oikarinen S., Hyöty H., Ludvigsson J., (2011): Low Zinc in drinking water is associated with the risk of type 1 diabetes in children. Pediatr Diabetes. 12(3 pt 1):156 – 64.
[34] Gale EA., Bingley PJ., Emmett CL., Collier T. (2004): European Nicotinamide Diabetes Intervention Trial(ENDIT): a randomized controlled trial of intervention before the onset of type 1 diabetes. Lancet. 363(9413):925 -31.
[35] Elliott RB., Pilcher CC., Fergusson DM., Stewart AW., (1996) :A population – based strategy to prevent insulin –dependent diabetes using nicotinamide. J Pediatr Endocrinol Metab 9(5): 501-9.
[36] Ludvigsson J., Samuelsson U., Johansson C., Sterhammar L., (2001) :Treatment with antioxidant at onset of type 1 diabetes in children : a randomised double- blind placebo-controlled study. Diabetes Metab Res Rev 17(2):131 -6.

[37] Prassad M., Takkinen HM., Nevalainen J., Ovaskainen ML., Alfthan G., Uusitalo L., Kenward MG., Veijola R., Simell O., Ilonen J., Knip M., Virtanen SM., (2011): Are serum α- anb β- carotene concentrations associated with the development of advanced β-cell autoimmunity in children with increased genetic susceptibility to type 1 diabetes? Diabetes Metab 37(2):162-7.

[38] Uusitalo L. Kenward MG. Virtanen SM., Uusitalo U., Nevalainen J., Niinistö S., Kronberg –Kippilä C., Ovaskainen ML., Marjamäki L., Simell O.,Ilonen J., Veijola R., Knip M.,(2008):Intake of antioxidant vitamins and trace elements during pregnancy and risk of advanced beta cell autoimmunity in the child. Am J Clin Nutr 88(2):458-64.

[39] Czernichow S., Vergnaud AC., Galan P., Arnaud J., Favier A., Faure H., Huxley R., Hercberg S., Ahluwalia N., (2009): Effects of long term antioxidant supplementation and association of serum antioxidant concentrations with risk of metabolic syndrome in adults. Am J Clin Nutr 90(2):329 – 35.

[40] Loh K., Deng H., Fukushima A., Cai X., Boivin B., Galic S., Bruce C., Shields BJ., Skiba B. Ooms LM., Stepto N., Wu B., Mitchell CA., Tonks NK., Watt MJ., Febbraio MA., Crack PJ., Andrikopoulos S., Tiganis T., (2009) :Reactive oxygen species enhance insulin sensitivity . Cell Memb 10(4) :260 -72.

[41] Mericq V., Piccardo C., Cai W., Chen X., Zhu L., Striker GE., Viassara H., Uribarri J., (2010): Maternally transmitted and food derived glycotoxins: a factor preconditioning the young to diabetes? Diabetes Care. 33(10):2232-7.

[42] Sandovici I., Smith NH., Nitert MD., Ackers-Johnson M., Uribe-Lewis S., Ito Y., Jones RH., Marguez VE., Cairns W., Tadayyon M., O'Neill Lp., Morrell A., Ling C., Constância M., Ozanne SE., (2011): Maternal diet and aging alter the epigenetic control of a promoter enhancer interaction at the Hnf4a gene in rat pancreatic islet. Proc natl Acad Sci 108(13):5449-54.

[43] American Diabetes Association (2002) :Evidence based Nutrition principles and recommendations for the treatment and prevention of diabetes and related complications. Diabetes Care. 25(suppl.): S50 -60.

[44] Kelly DE., (2003): Sugar and starch in the nutritional management of diabetes mellitus. Am. J. Clin. Nutr. 78(suppl) :858S -864S.

[45] Chandalia M.,Garg A., Lutjohann D., Bergmann K., Grundy S., Brinkley L., (2000) : Beneficial effects of high dietary fibre intake in patients with type 2 diabetes mellitus . N.Eng. J. Med; 342: 1392 -1398.

[46] Jenkins D., Kendall C., Augustine L., Martini M., Axelsen M., Faulker D et al (2002): Effect of wheat bran on glycaemic control and risk factors for cardiovascular disease in type 2 diabetes .Diabetes Care;25:1522 – 1529.

[47] Erasmus RT., Adelowo D., Olukoga D., Okesina K., Medubi A., Adewoye H., (1988) :Effect of guar gum on glucose and lipid levels in healthy and non- insulin dependent Nigerian diabetics. West Afr J Med; 7:45 -50.

[48] Crapo PA, Reaven G, Olefsky JM.(1977): Postprandial glucose and insulin responses to different complex carbohydrates. *Diabetes*; 26:1178-1183.

Chapter 6

Can Lifestyle Factors of Diabetes Mellitus Patients Affect Their Fertility?

Guillaume Aboua, Oluwafemi O. Oguntibeju and Stefan S. du Plessis

Additional information is available at the end of the chapter

http://dx.doi.org/10.5772/47838

1. Introduction

An increase in the number of diabetics diagnosed at a young age has coincided with worldwide concerns over the fertility status of these individuals. Infertility is already a major health problem in both the developed and developing world, with up to one in six couples requiring specialist investigation or treatments in order to conceive (Agbaje et al., 2007). Diabetes mellitus (DM) has impacted directly and indirectly on the fertility of couples (Glenn et al., 2003). It may affect both male and female reproductive function at multiple levels as a result of its effects on the endocrine system as well as on vasculature (Sexton and Jarow, 1997).

In a report released by the World Health Organization (WHO, 2004) indicated that the worldwide prevalence of diabetes was estimated to be 2.8% in 2000; furthermore, it was predicted to increase to 4.4% by 2030. The total number of people with diabetes was projected to rise from 171 million in 2000 to 366 million in 2030. It was also evident that the prevalence of diabetes is higher in men than in women, but there are more women with diabetes than men as females tend to have an increased life expectancy. These findings indicate that the "diabetes epidemic" will continue (Wild et al., 2004).

When a person has diabetes or insulin resistance, it may generate a hormone imbalance which can trigger a domino-like effect with the remaining hormones, including estrogen, progesterone and testosterone levels. These hormone imbalances can cause a wide variety of side effects, ranging from ovarian cysts to ED and infertility. The neuroendocrine effects may potentiate the adverse effects of diabetes on other organ systems and, in the case of reproductive function, are often of major patient concern (Steger and Rabe, 1997).

A recent study (Agbaje et al., 2007) strongly suggests that DM impairs male fertility, and the rising rates of diabetes may well pose a significant problem to human fertility. Male infertility problems may become more widespread as diabetes rates rise. Already the frequency of defective spermatogenesis and accompanying decreases in sperm parameters such as sperm count and motility appear to be on the increase. Arguably one of the most compelling reasons for this phenomenon is the contributing influence of environmental and lifestyle factors on male reproduction.

Lifestyle factors have had a dramatic impact on general health and the capacity to procreate. Cigarette smoking has been associated with adverse effects on fertility (Roth and Taylor, 2001). Poor diet and obesity are known to be key factors in the increase in Type 2 DM which has led to the increased risk for infertility. Despite the lack of conclusive studies, it is evident that there are enough compelling reasons to believe that the future of male and female fertility may be actively affected and impaired by DM, lifestyle and environmental factors.

In this review not only the effects of DM will be discussed, but also several lifestyle factors and occupational exposure that can impinge on the process of fertility. If and how lifestyle changes can positively impact on the diabetic patient's fertility status will also be investigated.

2. Lifestyle effects on fertility

Infertility is an increasingly prevalent issue; researchers point towards changing environmental and lifestyle conditions as arguably the most significant causes of this phenomenon. Environmental and lifestyle exposure to a wide variety of factors may stress the male reproductive system throughout a man's lifespan, from gestation to advanced adult age. Various environmental contaminants have been shown to impair sperm function through oxidative damage to sperm membranes. Reactive oxygen species (ROS)-mediated damage of sperm membranes has been reported to be responsible for impaired sperm motility (Archibong et al., 2008, de Lamirande and Gagnon, 1992). DNA damage, sperm head abnormalities (Kumar et al., 2002) as well as abnormal sperm function (Archibong et al., 2008) and impaired (?)sperm DNA integrity (Saleh et al., 2002) have been proven to be caused by the effects of environmental contaminants on the epididymis. Ultimately, male infertility may be the result of exposure to any combination of factors such as chemical toxins, smoking and alcohol abuse, poor diet and a lack of exercise and obesity, different types of stress, and the increasing prevalence of cellphone and ionizing radiation.

Despite the lack of conclusive studies tracking effects of the environment and lifestyle of an individual throughout life, there is enough reason to believe that the environment and lifestyle play significant roles in the quality of male gamete production and thus male fertility as a whole. This argument is supported by the fact that over the last 50 years mean sperm counts in the general population have decreased by 50% while dramatic environmental and lifestyle changes have occurred during this same period.

The prevalence of DM2 is increasing at a high rate, and the economic costs of caring for patients with diabetic complications are high. The increase in DM2 is closely associated with the epidemic of obesity in industrialized countries (Bruns and Kemnitz, 2004). Reduced physical activity is a contributing factor as sedentary lifestyles become more common.

Increased body fat, particularly in the visceral compartment, is a strong risk factor for the development of DM2. Elucidation of such risk factors will lead to interventions that can delay the onset or protect against the development of DM2 (Bruns and Kemnitz, 2004). Diabetes mellitus, whether due to lack of insulin secretion or resistance to insulin action, has adverse effects on all organ systems.

3. Brief overview of diabetes mellitus

Diabetes mellitus is a disorder in which blood levels of glucose are abnormally high because of the body's inability to release or to respond to insulin adequately. As the oxidation or metabolism of these sugars from carbohydrates is the major source of energy for the human body, diabetes can lead to major systemic problems.

Insulin, a hormone released from the pancreas, allows glucose to be transported into cells so that they can produce energy or store the glucose until it is needed. Scientists believe that an environmental factor (possibly a viral infection or a nutritional factor in childhood or early adulthood) could cause the immune system to destroy the insulin-producing cells in the pancreas. Some genetic predisposition is most likely needed for this to happen(Thorsby and Lie, 2005).

Whatever the cause, in Type 1 diabetes more than 90 percent of the insulin-producing beta cells of the pancreas are permanently destroyed. This results in severe insulin deficiency and approximately 10 percent of people with diabetes have Type 1 diabetes. Most people who have Type 1 diabetes develop the disease before the age of 30; and, in order to survive, a person with Type 1 diabetes must regularly inject him- or herself with insulin. In Type 2 diabetes mellitus (non-insulin-dependent diabetes), the pancreas continues to manufacture insulin, sometimes at even higher than normal levels. However, the body develops resistance to its effects, resulting in a relative insulin deficiency(Ferrannini, 1998).

Type 2 diabetes may occur in children and adolescents but usually begins after the age of 30 and becomes progressively more common with age: ninety percent of people with diabetes have Type 2 and about 15 percent of people over age 70 have Type 2 diabetes. Type 2 diabetes occurs when the pancreas does not produce enough insulin or when the body does not use the insulin that is produced effectively due to the development of insulin resistance(Ferrannini, 1998). DM2 is associated with a sedentary lifestyle and obesity. Obesity is a risk factor for Type 2 diabetes; 80 to 90 percent of the people with this disease are obese (Wild et al., 2004). Certain racial and cultural groups are at increased risk: Blacks and Hispanics have a twofold to threefold increased risk of developing Type 2 diabetes. Type 2 diabetes also tends to run in families.

Diabetes is one of the leading causes of death by non-communicable diseases worldwide. If not recognized or improperly managed, the high levels of blood glucose can slowly damage both the small and large blood vessels and the imbalance in hormones can impact negatively on the endocrine system. Not only does it result in many serious health complications such as heart disease, it is also a leading cause of adult blindness and kidney disease (Azadbakht et al.,

2003, Pradeepa et al., 2002). At least 50% of all limb amputations, not due to traumatic injury, are due to diabetes. Diabetes is now considered to be a major cause of erectile dysfunction and also recognized to impact severely on reproductive capacity (Azadbakht et al., 2003).

Type 1 and Type 2 diabetes are on the increase throughout the world, with the latter increasingly being described as a "modern disease" caused by lifestyle, diet and obesity. The reason for the increase in Type 1 diabetes is not known, but some scientists are suggesting that genetic factors could be involved, or that viruses could trigger the onset of the disease (Agbaje et al., 2007).

4. Neuroendocrine effects of diabetes mellitus

Diabetes mellitus in humans is often associated with hypofunction of the hypothalamic-pituitary-thyroid axis (HPTA) (Akbar et al., 2006, Hollowell et al., 2002, Papazafiropoulou et al., 2010, Radaideh et al., 2004). Stress, which is associated with diabetes, may also cause changes in the hypothalamus-anterior-pituitary axis in these diabetics. It appears that the presence of sub-clinical hypothyroidism and hyperthyroidism may result from hypothalamus-pituitary-thyroid-axis disorders (Celani et al., 1994). Several investigators have demonstrated that DM affects the function of the hypothalamus. Thyroid hormones affect glucose metabolism via several mechanisms. Hyperthyroidism has long been recognized to promote hyperglycemia (Maxon et al., 1975). During hyperthyroidism, the half-life of insulin is reduced, most likely secondary to an increased rate of degradation and an enhanced release of biologically inactive insulin precursors (Dimitriadis et al., 1985, O'Meara et al., 1993). In addition, untreated hyperthyroidism was associated with a reduced C-peptide to pro-insulin ratio suggesting an underlying defect in pro-insulin processing (Beer et al., 1989). Another mechanism explaining the relationship between hyperthyroidism and hyperglycemia is the increase in the gut glucose absorption mediated by the excess thyroid hormones (Foss et al., 1990). When DM is accompanied by hyperthyroidism, it worsens hyperglycemia through several pathological conditions caused by excessive thyroid hormones, such as increased glucose absorption from the intestine, decreased insulin secretion, decreased peripheral glucose consumption due to insulin resistance, increased hepatic glucose production due to activated glucose metabolism such as gluconeogenesis or glycogenolysis, accelerated breakdown of triglyceride in adipose tissue, and augmented renal clearance of insulin (Bhattacharyya and Wiles, 1999, Foss et al., 1990). As for hypothyroidism, glucose metabolism is affected as well via several mechanisms. A reduced rate of liver glucose production is observed in hypothyroidism (Okajima and Ui, 1979) and accounts for the decrease in insulin requirement in the hypothyroid diabetic patient. Recurrent hypoglycemic episodes are the presenting signs for the development of hypothyroidism in patients with Type 1 diabetes and replacement with thyroid hormones reduces the fluctuations in blood glucose levels (Leong et al., 1999).

Men with Type 2 diabetes mellitus have a higher prevalence of low testosterone levels than age-matched controls. In numerous cross-sectional studies, levels of testosterone in men have been inversely associated with several recognized risk factors for the development of

Type 2 diabetes, such as obesity, central adiposity (belly fat), and an elevated fasting plasma concentration of insulin and glucose. Several prospective studies found that low levels of testosterone and sex hormone–binding globulin predict the subsequent development of Type 2 diabetes among aging men. Low plasma testosterone concentration is associated with other correlates of diabetes, such as cardiovascular disease and hypertension (Khaw et al., 2007).

These neuroendocrine effects may potentiate the adverse effects of diabetes on other organ systems and, in the case of reproductive function, is often of major patient concern.

5. Effects of diabetes mellitus on male fertility

It is estimated that 15% of couples attempting to conceive are not able to do so within one year. Male factor infertility is present in 20%–50% of these couples, either independently or in conjunction with female factor infertility issues (Jarow et al., 2002, Sigman, 1997). Diagnosis of male infertility includes a thorough physical examination, semen analysis, ultrasound, and hormonal tests, if warranted. Male infertility can result from a low sperm count, which means the testes have produced less sperm than normal. The sperm may also have been unable to exit the testes, or they might not be fully functional. Male infertility may also result from a number of factors including: underlying health conditions, retrograde ejaculation, environmental pollutants and lifestyle factors.

Certain diabetic complications can cause issues for men that contribute to infertility (Figure 1). As DM has profound effects on the neuroendocrine axis (Steger and Rabe, 1997), in men, both DM1 and DM2 have long been recognized as major risk factors for sexual and reproductive dysfunction. This primarily includes impotence/erectile dysfunction (ED), ejaculatory (retrograde ejaculation) and orgasmic problems, as well as low desire (reduced libido), but impaired spermatogenesisis is also associated with DM (Bartak et al., 1975, Bhasin et al., 2007, Brown et al., 2005, Fairburn, 1981, Kolodny et al., 1974).

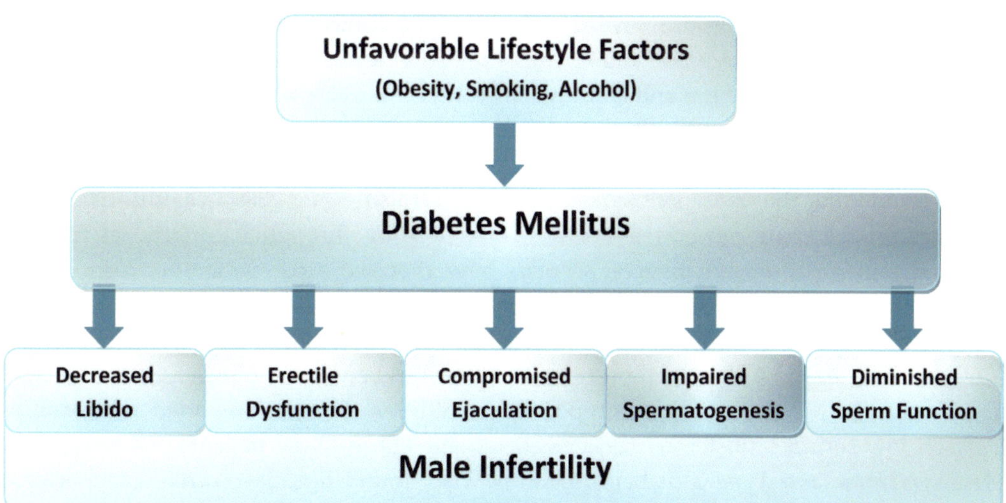

Figure 1. The possible effect of DM and accompanying unfavorable lifestyle choices on male fertility.

Nerve damage or autonomic neuropathy due to diabetes can lead to retrograde ejaculation – where the semen goes into the bladder. Since the semen never reaches the female reproductive system, infertility may be an issue.

The majority of patients with Type 2 diabetes are overweight or obese, which leads to decreased testosterone levels and elevated pro-inflammatory cytokines (substances produced in the cell). This can induce dysfunction in the blood vessel wall through the so-called nitric oxide pathway and further explain the relationship between DM2, obesity and erectile dysfunction(Bhasin et al., 2007, Brown et al., 2005).

Erectile dysfunction, or the inability to achieve an erection, is another diabetes complication that can lead to fertility problems in diabetic men (Brown et al., 2005, Lewis et al., 2004, Rosen et al., 2000). In men with DM, factors including aging, cardiovascular disease, high body mass index (BMI), hypercholesterolemia, smoking, and medication, in combination with DM-specific factors, such as duration and severity of DM and diabetic complications (neuropathy, nephropathy, retinopathy, and vascular damage), there is a strong correlation with ED (Brown et al., 2005, Lewis et al., 2004, Rosen et al., 2000). The mechanisms for ED in men with DM are endothelial dysfunction, dysfunction of the nitric oxide (NO) pathways (down regulation of NO synthase and degeneration of nitrergic nerves), dysfunction of other signal transduction pathways, corporal smooth muscle degeneration, and tissue remodeling (Brown et al., 2005, Saenz de Tejada et al., 1989). Sexual stimulation activates the non-adrenergic, noncholinergic nerve and activates the neural NO synthase/cGMP pathway. The release of NO facilitates the relaxation of penile cavernosal arteries and resistance arterioles, which causes vasodilation, and increases blood flow to the corpus cavernosum. The increased blood flow stimulates the endothelium lining of the lacunar spaces of the corpus cavernosum to release endothelial NO from the endothelium NO synthase. These biochemical and physiological processes result in trabecular smooth muscle relaxation and expansion of the sinusoids within the corpora cavernosa, leading to penile engorgement. This expansion of the corpora cavernosa against the tunica albuginea results in veno-occlusion and trapping of blood under pressure. This process is referred to as the 'veno-occlusive' mechanism. Neural and endothelial NO synthases are regulated by androgens. In addition, the tissue histo-architecture is dependent on androgens. Thus, any perturbations or alterations in the neural, vascular or erectile tissue fibroelastic properties will contribute to ED, by altering the veno-occlusion mechanism (Traish et al., 2009). Obesity essentially impinges on the male reproductive system and fertility through its effects on ED and impaired semen parameters. Several scholars have reported a correlation between obesity and ED. Corona et al. (2006) presented evidence showing that 96.5% of their subjects with metabolic syndrome (MetS), which is characteristic of abdominal obesity, exhibited ED (Corona et al., 2006). A direct proportional relationship between the increasing severity of obesity and the severity of ED was reported. In addition, there are reported relationships between low serum testosterone concentrations and ED in obese patients and those with MetS syndrome and Type 2 diabetes mellitus. They found negative correlations between BMI and self-reported satisfaction with erection as well as between BMI and the percentage of men reporting full erection.

As a consequence of insulin resistance in patients with Type 2 diabetes, high circulating levels of insulin are present in the bloodstream. Hyperinsulinemia, which often occurs in obese men, has an inhibitory effect on normal spermatogenesis and can be linked to decreased male fertility. In a group of diabetic men, apart from semen volume (2.6 vs. 3.3ml), semen parameters (concentration, motility and morphology) did not differ from those of the non-diabetic control group, but the amount of nuclear and mitochondrial DNA damage/fragmentation in the diabetic patients' sperm was significantly higher (52% versus 32%) (Agbaje et al., 2007). There were more deletions in the mitochondrial DNA of diabetic men's sperm cells than those of the non-diabetic men. The mitochondrial DNA deletions in the diabetic men's sperm cells ranged from 3 to 6 and averaged 4, while for the non-diabetic men it ranged from 1 to 4 and averaged 3. Deletions and fragmentation of DNA results in loss of genetic material which, in the case of nuclear DNA, causes infertility as the sperm is not able to deliver its full complement of genetic codes when fusing with the egg in order to create a viable embryo. The researchers concluded that diabetes is associated with increased sperm nuclear and mtDNA damage that may impair the reproductive capability of diabetic men.

In addition to inducing sperm DNA damage, insulin levels have also been shown to influence the levels of sex-hormone-binding globulin (SHBG), a glycoprotein that binds to sex hormones, specifically testosterone and estradiol, thereby inhibiting their biological activity as carriers. High circulating insulin levels inhibit SHBG synthesis in the liver, whereas weight loss has been shown to increase SHBG levels (Lima et al., 2000). In obese males, the decrease in SHBG means that less estrogen will be bound, resulting in more biologically active, free estrogen. In addition to the conversion of testosterone to estrogen in obese patients, the decreased ability of SHBG to sustain homeostatic levels of free testosterone also contributes to abnormal testosterone levels (Jensen et al., 2004). This failure to maintain homeostatic levels might magnify the negative feedback effect of elevated total estrogen levels. Even when the presence of SHBG is accounted for, an independent relationship between insulin resistance and testosterone production can still be demonstrated (Tsai et al., 2004). Therefore, the levels of SHBG might be important only as a marker of altered hormone profiles in obese infertile men. Reductions in semen volume and a higher mean incidence of nuclear DNA fragmentation is seen in diabetic men compared to those without Type 2 diabetes (Agbaje et al., 2007).

Male infertility may represent perturbation in some male patients with MetS,. Obesity is a cardinal feature of MetS. Adverse effects of obesity on male fertility are postulated to occur through several mechanisms. First, peripheral conversion of testosterone to estrogen in excess peripheral adipose tissue may lead to secondary hypogonadism through hypothalamic-pituitary-gonadal axis inhibition Kasturi et al., 2008). Second, oxidative stress at the level of the testicular microenvironment may result in decreased spermatogenesis and sperm damage. Lastly, obesity accompanying DM2 is often associated with decreased physical activity and increased fat deposition. The accumulation of fat in the suprapubic and inner thigh area as well as in the scrotum may result in increased scrotal and testicular temperatures in severely obese men (Kasturi et al., 2008). Increased testicular temperature also adversely affects sperm production Kasturi et al., 2008).

Du Plessis and colleagues (2010) report that an increase in the size or number of adipocytes as a result of obesity can result in both physical changes and hormonal changes. Physical changes can include an increase in scrotal temperature, an increase in the incidence of sleep apnea, and an increase in ED. Hormonal changes might include increases in the levels of leptin, estrogen and insulin, and a decrease in the level of testosterone. These changes, in turn, contribute to oligozoospermia, azoospermia, an increase in the DNA fragmentation index (DFi), and a decrease in semen volume. All three categories of change contribute to obesity-linked male infertility (Azadbakht et al., 2003, Du Plessis et al., 2010).

Du Plessis et al. (2010) propose that the dysregulation of the typical hypothalamic–pituitary–gonadal axis is a consequence of obesity. The increase in estrogen and decrease in testosterone levels negatively affects spermatogenesis as well as regular testicular function. Inhibin B levels are directly related to normal spermatogenesis and thus the low levels of this protein observed in obese males result in abnormal spermatogenesis. The dysregulation of the axis is shown because, despite the low inhibin B levels observed in obese males, there is no compensatory increase in follicle-stimulating hormone (FSH) levels as expected. Increased estrogen levels further contribute to the negative feedback effect on the hypothalamus and lead to decreased gonodoliberin and gonadotropin release (Du Plessis et al., 2010).

It is therefore clear that DM can be associated either directly or indirectly with several disorders of the male reproductive system and sexual functioning (Dinulovic and Radonjic, 1990).

6. Effects of diabetes mellitus on female fertility

Women reach their peak fertility age around their early 20s, but from approximately age 35 to 40, a woman is significantly less likely to fall pregnant. There are many factors that can lead to infertility. In order for a fertilized egg to grow successfully in the womb, it must be released by a woman's ovaries, implanted in the lining of the uterus and survive. Infertility may occur if initially, the ovaries have difficulty producing eggs.. These challenges to fertility can be caused by lifestyle habits or underlying health problems.

Hormonal disorders such as thyroid disease or abnormal hormone levels may also lead to infertility. Chronic diseases including autoimmune disorders, diabetes, cancer and endometriosis also make it more difficult to conceive, as can problems within or around the genital area, such as ovarian cysts or pelvic inflammatory disease. Eating disorders, poor nutrition, obesity and substance abuse may all contribute to infertility in both men and women.

Obesity and insulin resistance are two of the most common factors that lead to infertility, especially female infertility. More patients are diagnosed with Polycystic Ovarian Syndrome (PCOS) and Dysmetabolic Syndrome X, which affects about 25% of the population. A Swedish study, published in 2007, associated Type 1 diabetes with reduced fertility.

PCOS is the most common cause of female infertility (Cupisti et al., 2010). It is related to diabetes because of the strong feature of insulin resistance (inefficient insulin) in this subset of women. Many patients with PCOS have diabetes. PCOS is characterized by irregular or absent menstrual periods, problems with ovulation, increased levels of androgens such as testosterone, and ovaries with multiple cysts (Lobo and Carmina, 2000, Pasquali et al., 2011).

In PCOS, too much testosterone is produced and this affects the ability of the eggs to mature within the ovaries. Because women with PCOS develop insulin resistance, there are often ovulatory problems leading to irregular periods. Because of the irregularity of their cycles, cysts develop, which are fluid-filled cavities within the ovaries. Over time all of these issues make the likelihood of pregnancy begin to seem more and more distant (Lobo and Carmina, 2000).

Anovulation (failure to ovulate) is the causeof about 25% of female infertility cases, with PCOS being the most common cause of anovulation (Cupisti et al., 2010, Goodarzi et al., 2011, Lobo and Carmina, 2000, Walters et al., 2012). This means that PCOS could be a factor in about one-fifth of all infertility cases.

Insulin is said to bind with low affinity to the luteinizing hormone receptor in the theca cells of the ovaries. The hyperinsulinemia or high insulin levels present in obesity, MetS, diabetes, or insulin resistance in general may stimulate ovarian theca cells and thus increase the production of hormones, including androgens. This, in turn, may inhibit normal ovulation because of the hampered development of ovarian follicles. In women with PCOS, immature follicles bunch together to form large clumps. The eggs may mature within the bunched follicles, but the follicles do not break open to release them. Thus, women with PCOS often do not have regular menstrual periods. Also, because the eggs are not released, most women with PCOS have difficulty falling pregnant (Goodarzi et al., 2011, Lobo and Carmina, 2000, Mellembakken et al., 2011, Pasquali et al., 2011, Walters et al., 2012).

There appears to be a higher rate of miscarriage in women with PCOS. Increased levels of luteinizing hormone, which aids in the secretion of progesterone, may play a role. Increased levels of insulin and glucose may cause problems with the development of the embryo. Insulin resistance and late ovulation (after day 16 of the menstrual cycle) also may reduce egg quality, which can lead to miscarriage.

Insulin resistance is found in up to 60% of obese women and 40% of non-obese women. Of the people diagnosed with Type 2 diabetes, 80% to 90% are also diagnosed as obese. This fact provides an interesting clue to the link between diabetes and obesity. The main diabetes complication (including gestational diabetes) related to pregnancy is macrosomia - or a big baby (higher than the 90th percentile in birth weight). Sometimes these babies are not able to pass through the birth canal, so there are higher incidences of caesarean sections, and sometimes it is necessary to induce labor early. Fetal distress can also become an issue. There is also an increased risk of birth defects. This condition is directly related to maternal diabetes problems, especially during the first few weeks when a woman may be unaware she is pregnant. For this reason, women with diabetes are advised to manage their insulin levels under control before attempting to conceive.

Conditions associated with insulin resistance, such as obesity and DM, are often accompanied by increased adiposity or hyperglycemia (Vega et al., 2006). Obesity and diabetes are independently associated with altered female reproductive function (Kjaer et al., 1992, Pettigrew and Hamilton-Fairley, 1997, Zaadstra et al., 1993). Despite the fact that more women suffer from DM than men, and that women share similar risks for diabetic complications with men, less attention has been given to sexual function in women with DM. The prevalence of female sexual dysfunction (FSD) and associated risk factors in diabetic women are less clear than in men (Bhasin et al., 2007). Sexual problems in women with DM may be explained by several possible mechanisms, including biological, social, and psychological factors (Rockliffe-Fidler and Kiemle, 2003): 1.Hyperglycemia may reduce the hydration of mucous membranes in the vagina, leading to decreased lubrication and dyspareunia; 2. Increased risk of vaginal infections increases the risk of vaginal discomfort and dyspareunia; 3. Vascular damage and neuropathy may result in decreased genital blood flow, leading to impaired genital arousal response; and 4. Psychosocial factors such as adjustment to the diagnosis of DM, the burden of living with a chronic disease, and depression may impair sexual function (Giraldi and Kristensen, 2010).

7. Relationship between lifestyle, diabetes mellitus and infertility

Life style habits like smoking, diet, and exercise have an impact on health (Anderson et al., 2010). Obesity is associated with a range of adverse health consequences and this leads to an increased risk of diabetes. Obesity and low weight can impact on reproductive function (Fedorcsak et al., 2004). There is strong evidence of the adverse effects of smoking on fertility. In men, smoking negatively affects sperm production, motility, and morphology, and is associated with an increased risk of DNA damage (Kunzle et al., 2003). There is an increasing body of evidence that shows that life style factors can impact on reproductive performance. Multivariate logistic regression reveals that smoking habits and obesity are significant major contributors for infertility in DM men. Bener et al. (2009) suggest that a lifestyle modification program that includes exercise and improved dietary habits need to be established to lose weight, improve fitness and improve reproductive functioning (Bener et al., 2009). In addition to diabetes, other co-morbid factors for infertility include hypertension, erectile dysfunction, varicocele, and sexually transmitted diseases.

According to a recent review, there are few studies of obesity and male factor infertility amongst couples presenting for infertility treatment (Hammoud et al., 2008). However, the results of the studies that were reviewed generally suggest that there is a relationship between male infertility and an elevated BMI (Hammoud et al., 2008).

Both exercise levels and diet impact upon weight and BMI and may therefore affect fertility. Despite the lack of evidence, given the known health benefits of regular exercise and a balanced, nutritious diet, people trying to conceive are advised to exercise moderately and follow a specific type of diet during the preconception period and beyond (Gardiner et al., 2008, Moore and Davies, 2005). In the general population, female and male fertility is decreased by being both overweight (having a body mass index (BMI) of >25 kg/m^2) and underweight (having a BMI of <20 kg/m^2) (Hassan and Killick, 2004, Ramlau-Hansen et al.,

2007). Fertility treatment is also less successful in overweight or obese women (Fedorcsak et al., 2004, Homan et al., 2007, Lintsen et al., 2005, Maheshwari et al., 2007, Tamer Erel and Senturk, 2009). There are a number of dietary factors that impact upon the human reproductive system.

Heavy alcohol consumption has been shown to affect both female and male fertility (Grodstein et al., 1994, Hakim et al., 1998, Klonoff-Cohen et al., 2003, Windham et al., 1992). In men, alcohol consumption can induce testicular atrophy, impotence, reduced libido and cause a deterioration in sperm count (Donnelly et al., 1999, Muthusami and Chinnaswamy, 2005, Olsen et al., 1997). In women, alcohol can alter estrogen and progesterone levels and it has been associated with anovulation, luteal phase dysfunction and impaired implantation and blastocyst development (Gill, 2000). However, it is unclear from the evidence exactly what level of alcohol consumption has an effect on fertility as a result of the absence of a universal estimation of a 'standard drink' and the fact that self-reported, frequently retrospective data on drinking alcohol are a potential source of bias in located studies (Mukherjee et al., 2005).

Although the precise effect of alcohol use on the risk of diabetes has not been clearly established, evidence suggests that moderate alcohol consumption is associated with a decreased risk of diabetes, while heavy alcohol consumption is associated with an increased risk. Furthermore, the ingestion of moderate amounts of alcohol by diabetics has no acute effect on glycemic control (Howard et al., 2004). A plausible biological mechanism by which moderate alcohol consumption may reduce diabetes risk is less apparent. Alcohol consumption was not found to be associated with changes in fasting insulin levels, a marker of insulin resistance, on longitudinal analysis (Moller and Jespersen, 1995). It is possible that moderate alcohol consumption is a marker for a healthy lifestyle that was not entirely accounted for by adjusting for physical activity and diet (Howard et al., 2004). Moderate alcohol consumption is safe and may be beneficial with regard to cardiovascular risk in diabetics. The effect of alcohol use on the risk of other diabetic complications, including retinopathy, remains uncertain (Howard et al., 2004).

Caffeine, a mild neurostimulant, is the most popular pharmacologically active substance consumed worldwide. Caffeine is found in various food products and beverages, including coffee, tea, chocolate, cocoa products, soft and energy drinks and is also present in certain prescription and non-prescription medications, such as cold and influenza remedies, allergy and headache treatments, diet pills, diuretics and stimulants. A majority of the studies on caffeine and reproductive outcomes present conflicting results and should be interpreted with caution due to numerous methodological shortcomings, such as the following: inaccurate estimation of caffeine consumption; recall bias as result of retrospective assessment of caffeine intake, failure to allow for individual variations in caffeine metabolism; and inadequate control for confounding factors. Evidence suggests that consuming caffeine is associated with an increased time to conception, with a possible dose–response effect (Bolumar et al., 1997, Hatch and Bracken, 1993, Stanton and Gray, 1995). However, when adequately considered alongside other lifestyle factors related to fertility, particularly maternal age, cigarette smoking and alcohol intake, there is little evidence to support the detrimental effect of mild to moderate caffeine consumption on fertility (Leviton and Cowan, 2002, Nawrot et al., 2003).

For reasons of ethical concern and under-reported use of recreational drugs, the evidence about the effect of drug on human reproductive function is sparse and research has been mainly conducted in the form of animal studies (Anderson et al., 2010).

Marijuana is the most commonly used recreational drug worldwide (Battista et al., 2008). Marijuana contains various active components such as cannabinoids that act in both the central and the peripheral nervous system and that interfere with reproductive function at multiple levels. Cannabinoid receptors are located in multiple sites, including reproductive organs such as the ovary, the uterus, the vas deferens and the testis. Acute administration of marijuana in women reduces luteinizing hormone levels, whereas chronic use leads to tolerance and unchanged hormone levels (Park et al., 2004). Cannabinoids can affect fertilisation, oviductal transport and foetal and placental development by dysregulating signalling pathways involved in reproduction and by causing hormonal dysregulation (Battista et al., 2008, Rossato et al., 2008). The existing human data on illicit opiates and reproductive function in women are equivocal and inconclusive (Battista, Pasquariello et al., 2008). Cocaine has been shown to impair ovarian responsiveness to exogenous gonadotrophins in non-human primates and to adversely affect spermatogenesis in rodents (George et al., 1996, Thyer et al., 2001). Abnormal sexual function is common in heroin-addicted men and persists after withdrawal of heroin (Wang et al., 1978). Deterioration of all the sperm parameters, predominantly abnormal motility, have been demonstrated in the majority of heroin-addicted males and to a lesser extent in methadone users (Ragni et al., 1988, Ragni et al., 1985). Normal levels of serum gonadotrophins, with a significant elevation in prolactin and decrease in total and free testosterone levels, were reported in opiate-addicted men (Ragni et al., 1988, Ragni et al., 1985). The effects of cocaine and heroin use during pregnancy include placental disruption, pre-term delivery, low birth weight, neonatal mortality, neonatal withdrawal syndrome and possible long-term neurobehavioral effects, some of which can be associated with poor prenatal care and other substance use rather than purely attributed to cocaine (Hulse et al., 1998, Richardson et al., 1993).

Couple experiencing infertility generally report that is a stressful experience (Anderson et al., 2010). The stress may arise from unfulfilled self-expectations, social pressure, undergoing evaluation and treatment, disappointment with failures and the financial costs associated with the whole process. Infertile women have a significantly higher prevalence of psychiatric disorders relative to fertile women (Chen et al., 2004). Infertile men appear to experience significant distress with transient episodes of impotence and sexual performance anxiety which may contribute to difficulties in achieving natural pregnancy (Peterson et al., 2007, Shindel et al., 2008). Psychological stress has been considered the most common reason for discontinuation of fertility treatment before achieving pregnancy (Olivius et al., 2004, Rajkhowa et al., 2006) and pre-treatment levels of depression have been shown to be highly predictive of patient dropout behavior after only one IVF cycle (Smeenk et al., 2004). Besides stress-related sexual dysfunction and discontinuation of treatment, stress exposure has been directly related to reproductive failure. The pathophysiological rationale behind this assumption is a complex immune-endocrine response to stress that disturbs equilibrium and there is evidence of a stress-associated suppression of reproductive function including the delaying of menarche, hypothalamic amenorrhea, ovarian dysfunction and early-onset perimenopause (Nakamura et al., 2008, Nepomnaschy et al., 2007).

Despite spermatogenesis being a function of only the mature testis, environmental injury during maternal, perinatal and prepubertal phases can indirectly influence eventual sperm production in the adult male. It is believed that exposure during these phases of the developing testis leads to irreversible effects on spermatogenesis, while the accompanying effects of adulthood exposure are in all probability reversible (Dinulovic and Radonjic, 1990).

Evolution has caused our bodies to adapt to their environment. This connection is vital for reproduction as the birth of the young must coincide with plentiful food, and thus increase the chances of survival (Sharpe and Franks, 2002). Although human reproduction is not season specific, sexual behavior and reproduction is notable all year round. Fertility is influenced profoundly by our environment including season and food intake (Sharpe and Franks, 2002).

8. Treatments and solutions for the infertile DM patient: lifestyle changes

Infertility is a global problem. It affects all socioeconomic levels, racial, ethnic and religious groups. Fortunately, in the majority of cases, there is a specific cause for infertility that can be medically resolved. In fact, only about 10% of infertility cases go unexplained.

When a couple seeks medical help, one of the first conditions the doctor will look for is diabetes since the condition can cause fertility complication in both genders. In most instances, simple lifestyle changes like adequate nutrition and weight loss through proper exercise can help reverse the effects of infertility (Figure 2). Fortunately, most cases of infertility, which are related to diabetes, can be treated. In cases where infertility is related to insulin levels, correcting the imbalance is often enough to result in a successful pregnancy. Normal levels of blood sugar are needed to succeed in becoming pregnant. This means insulin, HgbA1c and hemoglobin levels as well as weight need to be monitored. For Type 1 diabetes, insulin replacement therapy is the main treatment regime to be followed as prescribed by the treating physician. Furthermore, when a diabetic subject, exercises properly and ensuring adequate nutrition with a vitamin supplement the chances of conception are improved. Regular exercise helps weight loss and also aids the body in reducing blood glucose levels and in using insulin more efficiently. Newer approaches to treating infertility caused by diabetes and its complications include morbidly obese women undergoing bariatric or gastric bypass surgery (for weight loss). Preliminary successful results have been reported as diabetic women are now able to conceive as they lose weight.

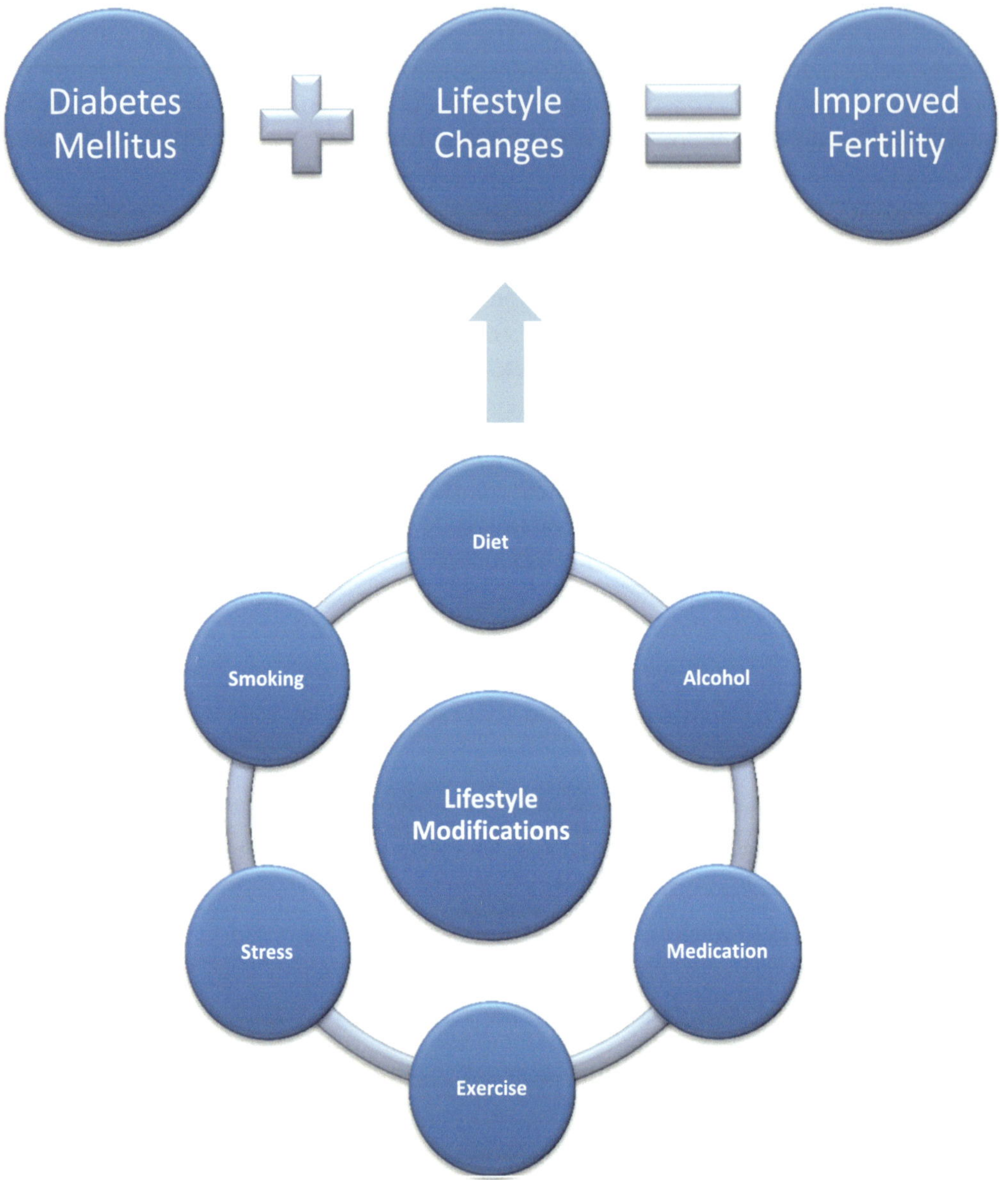

Figure 2. Lifestyle modifications in the DM patient that can help improve fertility

Insulin resistance can be managed with modified diet, exercise, and drugs such as metformin. Exercise programs, vitamin supplements and weight loss alone will better ovulation in one-third of patients. When Clomiphene Citrate, Metformin and Letrozole are used to treat the remainder of infertility patients, more than 80% of infertile couples are able to conceive, as long as there are no other infertility problems reported. This benevolent effect is due to these lifestyle changes and adequate medical intervention in due time (Du

Plessis et al., 2010). Once conception is achieved, the challenge is to control blood sugar levels so that the pregnancy can be carried to full term. The best way to prevent miscarriage in women with PCOS is to normalize hormone levels to improve ovulation, and normalize blood glucose and androgen levels. In recent time, more doctors have been prescribing the drug metformin to help with this problem.

Women who have a body mass index above 35 should lose weight before conception, and this should be an integral part of any fertility program's management of all overweight and obese patients. Weight loss of 5-10 per cent of total body weight can achieve a 30 per cent reduction of visceral adiposity, an improvement in insulin sensitivity, and may help with restoration of ovulation. More often than not, pharmacotherapy for fertility is needed in addition to all these lifestyle changes and thus, the expert management of a fertility specialist is pivotal.

Women with Type 2 diabetes, there have shown a higher incidence of secondary hypogonadotropic amenorrhea (low sex hormones leading to absence of periods), exacerbated by body mass index that is low and glycosylated hemoglobin (HbA1c) that is higher than normal. In women with diabetes mellitus desiring pregnancy, pre-pregnancy counseling is essential before conception is critical to diminish the risk of spontaneous abortion, fetal abnormalities, macrosomia (abnormally big baby), and other pregnancy complications. Diabetic women should aim for a HbA1clevel of below 6 %, or below 7 % if the risk of hypoglycemic episodes is too high, before pregnancy.

Other lifestyle changes or tips for helping fertility in diabetics include: avoiding cigarettes and any drugs that may affect sperm count or may reduce sexual function; getting sufficient rest and reducing stress; males must prevent overheating of the testes and should avoid hot baths, showers, and steam rooms, while avoiding tight underwear; and avoiding use of sexual lubricants, as they may affect sperm motility (Du Plessis et al., 2010).

If fertility issues remain unresolved, intrauterine insemination (also called artificial insemination) and assisted reproductive technologies, such as in vitro fertilization, may be considered.

With careful management of this disorder, people can live long healthy lives and the effects on fertility can be reduced notably.

9. Conclusion

Diabetes mellitus can be either directly or indirectly associated with several disorders of the reproductive system and sexual function. Several studies have demonstrated that diabetes could be prevented by weight loss, regular exercise, modification of diet, abstinence from smoking, and limiting the consumption of alcohol. Weight control would appear to offer the greatest benefit. Education of diabetes is an important first step in order to make healthy lifestyle choices and manage the condition effectively.

Author details

Guillaume Aboua* and Oluwafemi O. Oguntibeju
Department of Biomedical Sciences, Faculty of Health and Wellness, Cape Peninsula University of Technology, Bellville, South Africa

Stefan S. du Plessis
Division of Medical Physiology, Faculty of Health Sciences, Stellenbosch University, Tygerberg, South Africa

10. References

Agbaje, I.M., Rogers, D.A., McVicar, C.M., McClure, N., Atkinson, A.B., Mallidis, C., Lewis, S.E., 2007. Insulin dependant diabetes mellitus: implications for male reproductive function. Hum Reprod 22 (7), 1871-1877.

Akbar, D.H., Ahmed, M.M., Al-Mughales, J., 2006. Thyroid dysfunction and thyroid autoimmunity in Saudi type 2 diabetics. Acta Diabetol 43 (1), 14-18.

Anderson, K., Nisenblat, V., Norman, R., 2010. Lifestyle factors in people seeking infertility treatment - A review. Aust N Z J Obstet Gynaecol 50 (1), 8-20.

Archibong, A.E., Ramesh, A., Niaz, M.S., Brooks, C.M., Roberson, S.I., Lunstra, D.D., 2008. Effects of benzo(a)pyrene on intra-testicular function in F-344 rats. Int J Environ Res Public Health 5 (1), 32-40.

Azadbakht, L., Shakerhosseini, R., Atabak, S., Jamshidian, M., Mehrabi, Y., Esmaill-Zadeh, A., 2003. Beneficiary effect of dietary soy protein on lowering plasma levels of lipid and improving kidney function in type II diabetes with nephropathy. Eur J Clin Nutr 57 (10), 1292-1294.

Bartak, V., Josifko, M., Horackova, M., 1975. Juvenile diabetes and human sperm quality. Int J Fertil 20 (1), 30-32.

Battista, N., Pasquariello, N., Di Tommaso, M., Maccarrone, M., 2008. Interplay between endocannabinoids, steroids and cytokines in the control of human reproduction. J Neuroendocrinol 20 Suppl 1, 82-89.

Beer, S.F., Parr, J.H., Temple, R.C., Hales, C.N., 1989. The effect of thyroid disease on proinsulin and C-peptide levels. Clin Endocrinol (Oxf) 30 (4), 379-383.

Bener, A., Al-Ansari, A.A., Zirie, M., Al-Hamaq, A.O., 2009. Is male fertility associated with type 2 diabetes mellitus? Int Urol Nephrol 41 (4), 777-784.

Bhasin, S., Enzlin, P., Coviello, A., Basson, R., 2007. Sexual dysfunction in men and women with endocrine disorders. Lancet 369 (9561), 597-611.

Bhattacharyya, A., Wiles, P.G., 1999. Diabetic ketoacidosis precipitated by thyrotoxicosis. Postgrad Med J 75 (883), 291-292.

Bolumar, F., Olsen, J., Rebagliato, M., Bisanti, L., 1997. Caffeine intake and delayed conception: a European multicenter study on infertility and subfecundity. European Study Group on Infertility Subfecundity. Am J Epidemiol 145 (4), 324-334.

* Corresponding Author

Brown, J.S., Wessells, H., Chancellor, M.B., Howards, S.S., Stamm, W.E., Stapleton, A.E., Steers, W.D., Van Den Eeden, S.K., McVary, K.T., 2005. Urologic complications of diabetes. Diabetes Care 28 (1), 177-185.

Bruns, C.M., Kemnitz, J.W., 2004. Sex hormones, insulin sensitivity, and diabetes mellitus. Ilar J 45 (2), 160-169.

Celani, M.F., Bonati, M.E., Stucci, N., 1994. Prevalence of abnormal thyrotropin concentrations measured by a sensitive assay in patients with type 2 diabetes mellitus. Diabetes Res 27 (1), 15-25.

Chen, T.H., Chang, S.P., Tsai, C.F., Juang, K.D., 2004. Prevalence of depressive and anxiety disorders in an assisted reproductive technique clinic. Hum Reprod 19 (10), 2313-2318.

Corona, G., Mannucci, E., Schulman, C., Petrone, L., Mansani, R., Cilotti, A., Balercia, G., Chiarini, V., Forti, G., Maggi, M., 2006. Psychobiologic correlates of the metabolic syndrome and associated sexual dysfunction. Eur Urol 50 (3), 595-604; discussion 604.

Cupisti, S., Haberle, L., Dittrich, R., Oppelt, P.G., Reissmann, C., Kronawitter, D., Beckmann, M.W., Mueller, A., 2010. Smoking is associated with increased free testosterone and fasting insulin levels in women with polycystic ovary syndrome, resulting in aggravated insulin resistance. Fertil Steril 94 (2), 673-677.

de Lamirande, E., Gagnon, C., 1992. Reactive oxygen species and human spermatozoa. II. Depletion of adenosine triphosphate plays an important role in the inhibition of sperm motility. J Androl 13 (5), 379-386.

Dimitriadis, G., Baker, B., Marsh, H., Mandarino, L., Rizza, R., Bergman, R., Haymond, M., Gerich, J., 1985. Effect of thyroid hormone excess on action, secretion, and metabolism of insulin in humans. Am J Physiol 248 (5 Pt 1), E593-601.

Dinulovic, D., Radonjic, G., 1990. Diabetes mellitus/male infertility. Arch Androl 25 (3), 277-293.

Donnelly, G.P., McClure, N., Kennedy, M.S., Lewis, S.E., 1999. Direct effect of alcohol on the motility and morphology of human spermatozoa. Andrologia 31 (1), 43-47.

Du Plessis, S.S., Cabler, S., McAlister, D.A., Sabanegh, E., Agarwal, A., 2010. The effect of obesity on sperm disorders and male infertility. Nat Rev Urol 7 (3), 153-161.

Fairburn, C., 1981. The sexual problems of diabetic men. Br J Hosp Med 25 (5), 484, 487, 489-491.

Fedorcsak, P., Dale, P.O., Storeng, R., Ertzeid, G., Bjercke, S., Oldereid, N., Omland, A.K., Abyholm, T., Tanbo, T., 2004. Impact of overweight and underweight on assisted reproduction treatment. Hum Reprod 19 (11), 2523-2528.

Ferrannini, E., 1998. Insulin resistance versus insulin deficiency in non-insulin-dependent diabetes mellitus: problems and prospects. Endocr Rev 19 (4), 477-490.

Foss, M.C., Paccola, G.M., Saad, M.J., Pimenta, W.P., Piccinato, C.E., Iazigi, N., 1990. Peripheral glucose metabolism in human hyperthyroidism. J Clin Endocrinol Metab 70 (4), 1167-1172.

Gardiner, P.M., Nelson, L., Shellhaas, C.S., Dunlop, A.L., Long, R., Andrist, S., Jack, B.W., 2008. The clinical content of preconception care: nutrition and dietary supplements. Am J Obstet Gynecol 199 (6 Suppl 2), S345-356.

George, V.K., Li, H., Teloken, C., Grignon, D.J., Lawrence, W.D., Dhabuwala, C.B., 1996. Effects of long-term cocaine exposure on spermatogenesis and fertility in peripubertal male rats. J Urol 155 (1), 327-331.

Gill, J., 2000. The effects of moderate alcohol consumption on female hormone levels and reproductive function. Alcohol Alcohol 35 (5), 417-423.

Giraldi, A., Kristensen, E., 2010. Sexual dysfunction in women with diabetes mellitus. J Sex Res 47 (2), 199-211.

Glenn, D.R., McClure, N., Lewis, S.E., 2003. The hidden impact of diabetes on male sexual dysfunction and fertility. Hum Fertil (Camb) 6 (4), 174-179.

Goodarzi, M.O., Dumesic, D.A., Chazenbalk, G., Azziz, R., 2011. Polycystic ovary syndrome: etiology, pathogenesis and diagnosis. Nat Rev Endocrinol 7 (4), 219-231.

Grodstein, F., Goldman, M.B., Cramer, D.W., 1994. Infertility in women and moderate alcohol use. Am J Public Health 84 (9), 1429-1432.

Hakim, R.B., Gray, R.H., Zacur, H., 1998. Alcohol and caffeine consumption and decreased fertility. Fertil Steril 70 (4), 632-637.

Hammoud, A.O., Gibson, M., Peterson, C.M., Meikle, A.W., Carrell, D.T., 2008. Impact of male obesity on infertility: a critical review of the current literature. Fertil Steril 90 (4), 897-904.

Hassan, M.A., Killick, S.R., 2004. Negative lifestyle is associated with a significant reduction in fecundity. Fertil Steril 81 (2), 384-392.

Hatch, E.E., Bracken, M.B., 1993. Association of delayed conception with caffeine consumption. Am J Epidemiol 138 (12), 1082-1092.

Hollowell, J.G., Staehling, N.W., Flanders, W.D., Hannon, W.H., Gunter, E.W., Spencer, C.A., Braverman, L.E., 2002. Serum TSH, T(4), and thyroid antibodies in the United States population (1988 to 1994): National Health and Nutrition Examination Survey (NHANES III). J Clin Endocrinol Metab 87 (2), 489-499.

Homan, G.F., Davies, M., Norman, R., 2007. The impact of lifestyle factors on reproductive performance in the general population and those undergoing infertility treatment: a review. Hum Reprod Update 13 (3), 209-223.

Howard, A.A., Arnsten, J.H., Gourevitch, M.N., 2004. Effect of alcohol consumption on diabetes mellitus: a systematic review. Ann Intern Med 140 (3), 211-219.

Hulse, G.K., Milne, E., English, D.R., Holman, C.D., 1998. Assessing the relationship between maternal opiate use and antepartum haemorrhage. Addiction 93 (10), 1553-1558.

Jarow, J.P., Sharlip, I.D., Belker, A.M., Lipshultz, L.I., Sigman, M., Thomas, A.J., Schlegel, P.N., Howards, S.S., Nehra, A., Damewood, M.D., Overstreet, J.W., Sadovsky, R., 2002. Best practice policies for male infertility. J Urol 167 (5), 2138-2144.

Jensen, T.K., Andersson, A.M., Jorgensen, N., Andersen, A.G., Carlsen, E., Petersen, J.H., Skakkebaek, N.E., 2004. Body mass index in relation to semen quality and reproductive hormones among 1,558 Danish men. Fertil Steril 82 (4), 863-870.

Kasturi, S.S., Tannir, J., Brannigan, R.E., 2008. The metabolic syndrome and male infertility. J Androl 29 (3), 251-259.

Khaw, K.T., Dowsett, M., Folkerd, E., Bingham, S., Wareham, N., Luben, R., Welch, A., Day, N., 2007. Endogenous testosterone and mortality due to all causes, cardiovascular disease, and cancer in men: European prospective investigation into cancer in Norfolk (EPIC-Norfolk) Prospective Population Study. Circulation 116 (23), 2694-2701.

Kjaer, K., Hagen, C., Sando, S.H., Eshoj, O., 1992. Epidemiology of menarche and menstrual disturbances in an unselected group of women with insulin-dependent diabetes mellitus compared to controls. J Clin Endocrinol Metab 75 (2), 524-529.

Klonoff-Cohen, H., Lam-Kruglick, P., Gonzalez, C., 2003. Effects of maternal and paternal alcohol consumption on the success rates of in vitro fertilization and gamete intrafallopian transfer. Fertil Steril 79 (2), 330-339.

Kolodny, R.C., Kahn, C.B., Goldstein, H.H., Barnett, D.M., 1974. Sexual dysfunction in diabetic men. Diabetes 23 (4), 306-309.

Kumar, A., Vajpayee, P., Ali, M.B., Tripathi, R.D., Singh, N., Rai, U.N., Singh, S.N., 2002. Biochemical responses of Cassia siamea Lamk. grown on coal combustion residue (fly-ash). Bull Environ Contam Toxicol 68 (5), 675-683.

Kunzle, R., Mueller, M.D., Hanggi, W., Birkhauser, M.H., Drescher, H., Bersinger, N.A., 2003. Semen quality of male smokers and nonsmokers in infertile couples. Fertil Steril 79 (2), 287-291.

Leong, K.S., Wallymahmed, M., Wilding, J., MacFarlane, I., 1999. Clinical presentation of thyroid dysfunction and Addison's disease in young adults with type 1 diabetes. Postgrad Med J 75 (886), 467-470.

Leviton, A., Cowan, L., 2002. A review of the literature relating caffeine consumption by women to their risk of reproductive hazards. Food Chem Toxicol 40 (9), 1271-1310.

Lewis, R.W., Fugl-Meyer, K.S., Bosch, R., Fugl-Meyer, A.R., Laumann, E.O., Lizza, E., Martin-Morales, A., 2004. Epidemiology/risk factors of sexual dysfunction. J Sex Med 1 (1), 35-39.

Lima, N., Cavaliere, H., Knobel, M., Halpern, A., Medeiros-Neto, G., 2000. Decreased androgen levels in massively obese men may be associated with impaired function of the gonadostat. Int J Obes Relat Metab Disord 24 (11), 1433-1437.

Lintsen, A.M., Pasker-de Jong, P.C., de Boer, E.J., Burger, C.W., Jansen, C.A., Braat, D.D., van Leeuwen, F.E., 2005. Effects of subfertility cause, smoking and body weight on the success rate of IVF. Hum Reprod 20 (7), 1867-1875.

Lobo, R.A., Carmina, E., 2000. The importance of diagnosing the polycystic ovary syndrome. Ann Intern Med 132 (12), 989-993.

Maheshwari, A., Stofberg, L., Bhattacharya, S., 2007. Effect of overweight and obesity on assisted reproductive technology--a systematic review. Hum Reprod Update 13 (5), 433-444.

Maxon, H.R., Kreines, K.W., Goldsmith, R.E., Knowles, H.C., Jr., 1975. Long-term observations of glucose tolerance in thyrotoxic patients. Arch Intern Med 135 (11), 1477-1480.

Mellembakken, J.R., Berga, S.L., Kilen, M., Tanbo, T.G., Abyholm, T., Fedorcsak, P., 2011. Sustained fertility from 22 to 41 years of age in women with polycystic ovarian syndrome. Hum Reprod 26 (9), 2499-2504.

Moller, L.F., Jespersen, J., 1995. Elevated insulin levels in men: an 11-year follow-up study. J Cardiovasc Risk 2 (4), 339-343.

Moore, V.M., Davies, M.J., 2005. Diet during pregnancy, neonatal outcomes and later health. Reprod Fertil Dev 17 (3), 341-348.

Mukherjee, R.A., Hollins, S., Abou-Saleh, M.T., Turk, J., 2005. Low level alcohol consumption and the fetus. Bmj 330 (7488), 375-376.

Muthusami, K.R., Chinnaswamy, P., 2005. Effect of chronic alcoholism on male fertility hormones and semen quality. Fertil Steril 84 (4), 919-924.

Nakamura, K., Sheps, S., Arck, P.C., 2008. Stress and reproductive failure: past notions, present insights and future directions. J Assist Reprod Genet 25 (2-3), 47-62.

Nawrot, P., Jordan, S., Eastwood, J., Rotstein, J., Hugenholtz, A., Feeley, M., 2003. Effects of caffeine on human health. Food Addit Contam 20 (1), 1-30.

Nepomnaschy, P.A., Sheiner, E., Mastorakos, G., Arck, P.C., 2007. Stress, immune function, and women's reproduction. Ann N Y Acad Sci 1113, 350-364.

O'Meara, N.M., Blackman, J.D., Sturis, J., Polonsky, K.S., 1993. Alterations in the kinetics of C-peptide and insulin secretion in hyperthyroidism. J Clin Endocrinol Metab 76 (1), 79-84.

Okajima, F., Ui, M., 1979. Metabolism of glucose in hyper- and hypo-thyroid rats in vivo. Relation of catecholamine actions to thyroid activity in controlling glucose turnover. Biochem J 182 (2), 585-592.

Olivius, C., Friden, B., Borg, G., Bergh, C., 2004. Why do couples discontinue in vitro fertilization treatment? A cohort study. Fertil Steril 81 (2), 258-261.

Olsen, J., Bolumar, F., Boldsen, J., Bisanti, L., 1997. Does moderate alcohol intake reduce fecundability? A European multicenter study on infertility and subfecundity. European Study Group on Infertility and Subfecundity. Alcohol Clin Exp Res 21 (2), 206-212.

Papazafiropoulou, A., Sotiropoulos, A., Kokolaki, A., Kardara, M., Stamataki, P., Pappas, S., 2010. Prevalence of thyroid dysfunction among greek type 2 diabetic patients attending an outpatient clinic. J Clin Med Res 2 (2), 75-78.

Park, B., McPartland, J.M., Glass, M., 2004. Cannabis, cannabinoids and reproduction. Prostaglandins Leukot Essent Fatty Acids 70 (2), 189-197.

Pasquali, R., Stener-Victorin, E., Yildiz, B.O., Duleba, A.J., Hoeger, K., Mason, H., Homburg, R., Hickey, T., Franks, S., Tapanainen, J.S., Balen, A., Abbott, D.H., Diamanti-Kandarakis, E., Legro, R.S., 2011. PCOS Forum: research in polycystic ovary syndrome today and tomorrow. Clin Endocrinol (Oxf) 74 (4), 424-433.

Peterson, B.D., Newton, C.R., Feingold, T., 2007. Anxiety and sexual stress in men and women undergoing infertility treatment. Fertil Steril 88 (4), 911-914.

Pettigrew, R., Hamilton-Fairley, D., 1997. Obesity and female reproductive function. Br Med Bull 53 (2), 341-358.

Pradeepa, R., Deepa, R., Mohan, V., 2002. Epidemiology of diabetes in India--current perspective and future projections. J Indian Med Assoc 100 (3), 144-148.

Radaideh, A.R., Nusier, M.K., Amari, F.L., Bateiha, A.E., El-Khateeb, M.S., Naser, A.S., Ajlouni, K.M., 2004. Thyroid dysfunction in patients with type 2 diabetes mellitus in Jordan. Saudi Med J 25 (8), 1046-1050.

Ragni, G., De Lauretis, L., Bestetti, O., Sghedoni, D., Gambaro, V., 1988. Gonadal function in male heroin and methadone addicts. Int J Androl 11 (2), 93-100.

Ragni, G., De Lauretis, L., Gambaro, V., Di Pietro, R., Bestetti, O., Recalcati, F., Papetti, C., 1985. Semen evaluation in heroin and methadone addicts. Acta Eur Fertil 16 (4), 245-249.

Rajkhowa, M., McConnell, A., Thomas, G.E., 2006. Reasons for discontinuation of IVF treatment: a questionnaire study. Hum Reprod 21 (2), 358-363.

Ramlau-Hansen, C.H., Thulstrup, A.M., Nohr, E.A., Bonde, J.P., Sorensen, T.I., Olsen, J., 2007. Subfecundity in overweight and obese couples. Hum Reprod 22 (6), 1634-1637.

Richardson, G.A., Day, N.L., McGauhey, P.J., 1993. The impact of prenatal marijuana and cocaine use on the infant and child. Clin Obstet Gynecol 36 (2), 302-318.

Rockliffe-Fidler, C., Kiemle, G., 2003. Sexual function in diabetic women: A psychological perspective. S. exual and RelationshipTherapy 18, 143-159.

Rosen, R., Brown, C., Heiman, J., Leiblum, S., Meston, C., Shabsigh, R., Ferguson, D., D'Agostino, R., Jr., 2000. The Female Sexual Function Index (FSFI): a multidimensional self-report instrument for the assessment of female sexual function. J Sex Marital Ther 26 (2), 191-208.

Rossato, M., Pagano, C., Vettor, R., 2008. The cannabinoid system and male reproductive functions. J Neuroendocrinol 20 Suppl 1, 90-93.

Roth, L.K., Taylor, H.S., 2001. Risks of smoking to reproductive health: assessment of women's knowledge. Am J Obstet Gynecol 184 (5), 934-939.

Saenz de Tejada, I., Goldstein, I., Azadzoi, K., Krane, R.J., Cohen, R.A., 1989. Impaired neurogenic and endothelium-mediated relaxation of penile smooth muscle from diabetic men with impotence. N Engl J Med 320 (16), 1025-1030.

Saleh, R.A., Agarwal, A., Nelson, D.R., Nada, E.A., El-Tonsy, M.H., Alvarez, J.G., Thomas, A.J., Jr., Sharma, R.K., 2002. Increased sperm nuclear DNA damage in normozoospermic infertile men: a prospective study. Fertil Steril 78 (2), 313-318.

Sexton, W.J., Jarow, J.P., 1997. Effect of diabetes mellitus upon male reproductive function. Urology 49 (4), 508-513.

Sharpe, R.M., Franks, S., 2002. Environment, lifestyle and infertility--an inter-generational issue. Nat Cell Biol 4 Suppl, s33-40.

Shindel, A.W., Nelson, C.J., Naughton, C.K., Ohebshalom, M., Mulhall, J.P., 2008. Sexual function and quality of life in the male partner of infertile couples: prevalence and correlates of dysfunction. J Urol 179 (3), 1056-1059.

Sigman, M., 1997. Male infertility. Med Health R I 80 (12), 406-409.

Smeenk, J.M., Verhaak, C.M., Stolwijk, A.M., Kremer, J.A., Braat, D.D., 2004. Reasons for dropout in an in vitro fertilization/intracytoplasmic sperm injection program. Fertil Steril 81 (2), 262-268.

Stanton, C.K., Gray, R.H., 1995. Effects of caffeine consumption on delayed conception. Am J Epidemiol 142 (12), 1322-1329.

Steger, R.W., Rabe, M.B., 1997. The effect of diabetes mellitus on endocrine and reproductive function. Proc Soc Exp Biol Med 214 (1), 1-11.

Tamer Erel, C., Senturk, L.M., 2009. The impact of body mass index on assisted reproduction. Curr Opin Obstet Gynecol 21 (3), 228-235.

Thorsby, E., Lie, B.A., 2005. HLA associated genetic predisposition to autoimmune diseases: Genes involved and possible mechanisms. Transpl Immunol 14 (3-4), 175-182.

Thyer, A.C., King, T.S., Moreno, A.C., Eddy, C.A., Siler-Khodr, T.M., Schenken, R.S., 2001. Cocaine impairs ovarian response to exogenous gonadotropins in nonhuman primates. J Soc Gynecol Investig 8 (6), 358-362.

Traish, A.M., Feeley, R.J., Guay, A., 2009. Mechanisms of obesity and related pathologies: androgen deficiency and endothelial dysfunction may be the link between obesity and erectile dysfunction. Febs J 276 (20), 5755-5767.

Tsai, E.C., Matsumoto, A.M., Fujimoto, W.Y., Boyko, E.J., 2004. Association of bioavailable, free, and total testosterone with insulin resistance: influence of sex hormone-binding globulin and body fat. Diabetes Care 27 (4), 861-868.

Vega, G.L., Adams-Huet, B., Peshock, R., Willett, D., Shah, B., Grundy, S.M., 2006. Influence of body fat content and distribution on variation in metabolic risk. J Clin Endocrinol Metab 91 (11), 4459-4466.

Walters, K.A., Allan, C.M., Handelsman, D.J., 2012. Rodent Models for Human Polycystic Ovary Syndrome. Biol Reprod.

Wang, C., Chan, V., Yeung, R.T., 1978. The effect of heroin addiction on pituitary-testicular function. Clin Endocrinol (Oxf) 9 (5), 455-461.

Wild, S., Roglic, G., Green, A., Sicree, R., King, H., 2004. Global prevalence of diabetes: estimates for the year 2000 and projections for 2030. Diabetes Care 27 (5), 1047-1053.

Windham, G.C., Fenster, L., Swan, S.H., 1992. Moderate maternal and paternal alcohol consumption and the risk of spontaneous abortion. Epidemiology 3 (4), 364-370.

Zaadstra, B.M., Seidell, J.C., Van Noord, P.A., te Velde, E.R., Habbema, J.D., Vrieswijk, B., Karbaat, J., 1993. Fat and female fecundity: prospective study of effect of body fat distribution on conception rates. Bmj 306 (6876), 484-487.

Chapter 7

The Role of Fruit and Vegetable Consumption in Human Health and Disease Prevention

O. O. Oguntibeju, E. J. Truter and A. J. Esterhuyse

Additional information is available at the end of the chapter

http://dx.doi.org/10.5772/50109

1. Introduction

Several reports have shown that adequate intake of fruits and vegetables form an important part of a healthy diet and low fruit and vegetable intake constitute a risk factor for chronic diseases such as cancer, coronary heart disease (CHD), stroke and cataract formation (Van Duyn & Pivonka, 2000). Scientific evidence indicates that frequent consumption of fruits and vegetables can prevent oesophageal, stomach, pancreatic, bladder and cervical cancers and that a diet high in fruits and vegetables could prevent 20% of most types of cancers (Crawford *et al.*, 1994). According to reports, fruit and vegetable consumption is influenced by gender, age, income, education and family origin (Wardle *et al.*, 2000; Giskes *et al.*, 2002). Other studies suggest that education may influence nutritional knowledge about fruits and vegetables and consequently also influence their intake. Empirical findings also indicate that family origin and socioeconomic status affect the purchasing power of food, food choice, food preparation and food availability which in turn affects consumption. Studies have shown that preferences of fruit and vegetable consumption differ in males and females (Wardle *et al.*, 2000; Wang *et al.*, 2002). A study carried out by Sylvestre *et al* (2006) revealed that mothers consumed 2 1/2 vegetable servings and 2 1/2 fruit servings on average daily and that the reported daily average of fruit and vegetable servings was slightly below the basic recommendation of 5 servings per day (Sylvestre *et al.*, 2006). The same study suggested that children of mothers who consume high fruit and vegetable consumption are more likely to consume fruits and vegetables frequently than children of mothers with low fruit consumption. If the mothers with high fruit and vegetable consumption eat fruits and vegetables at home during meals which are shared with children, then their findings could underpin the importance of fruit and vegetable availability at home. However, it may be important to verify whether the relationship is simply a reflection of the control mothers have over food availability at home or it relates to shared nutritional knowledge about the benefits of fruits and vegetables.

2. Fruits and vegetables as sources of vitamins, minerals and antioxidants

Fruits and vegetables play an important role in human nutrition and health, particularly as sources of vitamin C, thiamine, niacin, pyridoxine, folic acid, minerals and dietary fibre (Wargovich, 2000). In the USA, the consumption of fruits and vegetables as a group is known to contribute to an estimated intake of 91% of vitamin C, 48% of vitamin A, 30% of folate, 27% of vitamin B6, 17% of thiamine and 15% of niacin. It is also known that fruit and vegetable intake supply 16% of magnesium, 19% of iron and 9% of the calories (United States Department of Agriculture, 2000). Other vital nutrients supplied by fruits and vegetables include riboflavin, zinc, calcium, potassium and phosphorus. Some components of fruits and vegetables (phytochemicals) are strong antioxidants and modify the metabolic activation and detoxification/disposition of carcinogens and may even influence processes that may change the course of the tumor cell (Wargovich, 2000). Although antioxidant capacity varies greatly among fruits and vegetables (Kalt, 2002), it is better to consume a variety of them rather than limiting consumption to a few with the highest antioxidant capacity. The United States Department of Agriculture (2000) encourages consumers to take at least two servings of fruits and at least three servings of vegetables per day, choose fresh, frozen, dried or canned forms of a variety of colours, kinds and choose dark-green leafy vegetables, orange fruits, vegetables and cooked dry beans and peas regularly. However, in some countries, consumers are encouraged to eat at least 10 servings of fruits and vegetables per day. There is evidence that consumption of whole foods is better than isolated food components such as dietary supplements and nutraceuticals. For instance, previous reports (Southon, 2000; Seifried *et al.* 2003) showed that increased consumption of carotenoid-rich fruits and vegetables offer a better protective effect than carotenoid dietary supplements by increasing LDL-oxidation resistance, lowering DNA damage and inducing higher repair activity in human volunteers who participated in a study conducted in European countries such as Italy and Spain. High consumption of tomatoes and tomato products have been associated with reduced carcinogenesis, especially of prostate cancer and is thought to be due to the presence of lycopene, which gives red tomatoes their colour (Giovannucci, 2002). Boileau *et al.* (2003) observed that the use of tomato powder significantly reduced prostate carcinogenesis in rats. Examples of fruits and vegetables recommended for daily consumption include spinach, orange, mango, carrot, melon, pineapples red grapefruit etc.

3. Fruit and vegetable consumption: Human health and disease prevention

Childhood and adolescent obesity have reached epidemic proportions especially in the USA and the alarming rate at which this condition continues to increase is of great concern (Muriello *et al.*, 2006). Unfortunately, obesity among children and adolescents is also increasing in South Africa and in other African countries due to western influence, and since behavior-related attitudes to obesity prevention such as physical activity and fruit and vegetable consumption tend to decline with age, it is important that intervention efforts begin early in life (Muriello *et al.*, 2006). Research has shown that the consumption of fruits and vegetables may be associated with a decreased incidence and mortality of a variety of chronic diseases which includes obesity. Fruit and vegetable intake has been shown to have positive effects in terms of weight management and obesity prevention (Tohill *et al.*, 2004). Duncan *et al.* (1983) conducted a study using a diet rich in fruits and vegetables and low in fats versus a diet which was higher in fats but lower in fruits and vegetables. Although both groups were eating to satiety, the group eating the diet rich in fruits and vegetables consumed on average, one half the energy intake when compared to those on high fat, low fruit and vegetable diet. He *et* al. (2006) carried out a study in respect of fruit and vegetable consumption and its relationship to weight management. Their study found that an increase in fruit and vegetable intake was associated with a 24% lower risk of becoming obese.

In a large cohort of pre-adolescents and adolescents living in the USA, body mass index (BMI) changes were relatively consistent during a three year follow-up study. At the beginning of the study, more males than females were overweight and during the follow-up, change in body mass index (BMI) was slightly higher among the boys than in the girls. Among both genders, about 75% of the adolescents did not meet the public health recommendation to consume at least five servings of fruits and vegetables per/day (Field *et al.*, 2003). There are various benefits gained by consuming a diet rich in fruits and vegetables, but it is not clearly understood why a diet rich in fruits and vegetables would prevent obesity or excessive weight gain, suggesting that further studies are needed to elucidate and confirm possible mechanisms involved in the prevention of obesity by fruit and vegetable consumption.

Several cohort studies have examined the relationship between fruit and vegetable intake and coronary heart disease. These studies reported an inverse relationship between intake of fibre from fruits and vegetables and the risk of developing coronary heart disease. Meta-analyses of previous studies showed an inverse association between fruit and vegetable consumption and the occurrence of stroke which supports the concept that fruit and vegetable consumption has the potential to protect against cardiovascular events (Daucher *et al.*, 2005; He *et al.*, 2006). Daucher and co-workers (2006) carried out a meta-analyses of cohort studies and observed that the risk of developing coronary heart disease decreased by 4% for each additional portion per day intake of fruit and vegetables and by 7% for fruit consumption, indicating that fruit offer a more protective effect in reducing the risk of developing coronary heart disease (CHD). It has been observed that clinical and biological investigations support the protective effect offered by the intake of fruit and vegetables against coronary heart disease. Interestingly, the relationship is biologically valid with many clinical and laboratory data showing that the micro- and macro-constituents of fruit and vegetables improve important risk factors of CHD such as hypertension, dyslipidaemia and diabetes (Appel *et al.*, 1997; Van Duyn *et al.*, 2000; Bazzano *et al.*, 2003). In different population studies, adequate fruit and vegetable intake have been shown to correlate with healthy lifestyles which may explain the lower CHD incidence rates among individuals who adequately consume fruits and vegetables. Generally, it is assumed that consumers of fruits and vegetables smoke less, exercise more and are better educated than non-consumers (Joshipura *et al.*, 1999). Although many of the clinical and biological studies adjust for lifestyle factors, basic confounders may still explain part of the favourable association with CHD. High fruit and vegetable intakes are related to a healthy diet pattern (Hu *et al.*, 1999; Hu *et al.*, 2000) and inversely associated with the consumption of saturated fat-rich food (Tucker *et al.*, 2005), which may also contribute to a lower CHD risk (Hu *et al.*, 1999; Hu *et al.*, 2000; Fung *et al.*, 2001). It should be noted however, that most of the clinical and laboratory studies to date have not established a causal relationship between inadequate consumption of fruits and vegetables and the risk of developing CHD. Daucher *et al.* (2006) reported that in different observational studies selected for meta-analyses, the association between vegetable consumption and CHD risk was more pronounced for cardiovascular mortality than for incident CHD. They stated that the reason for the difference is not known but possible explanations may be related to publication bias since mortality studies have fewer outcomes than studies reporting incident CHD or that consumption of vegetables might have specific effects on mortality, a hypothesis that needs confirmation in cohorts with a large number of fatal outcomes. It is also possible that residual confounding factors such as measurement errors affected the association between fruit and /or vegetable intake and risk of developing CHD and differences in study types, including dietary assessment methods, the variety of fruits or vegetables investigated and the definition of the reference group may further explain the difference.

Ness and Powles (1997) reviewed evidence about fruit and vegetable intake and the development of coronary heart disease and found a significant inverse association between the amount of fruits and vegetables consumed and the incidence of coronary heart disease. Alonso *et al.* (2004) also reported a similar association between fruit and vegetable consumption and decreased blood pressure.

A study carried out by He *et al.* (2006) found a significant lower risk of stroke development among those with the highest intake of fruits and vegetables and Lock *et al* (2005) showed that increasing individual fruit and vegetable consumption by 600 grams per day could reduce the global burden of stroke by 19% and decrease the risk of CHD by 31% respectively.

High blood pressure increases the risk of heart disease and stroke (Chobanian *et al.*, 2003). Adding more fruits and vegetables to a healthy diet is one possible pathway to reduce blood pressure. In the Dietary Approaches to Stop Hypertension (DASH) study (Appel *et al.*, 1997), 459 people with and without high blood pressure were randomly assigned to one of three diets: a) a typical American diet that provided about 3 servings per day of fruits and vegetables and one serving per day of a low-fat dairy product, b) a fruit and vegetable diet that provided 8 servings per day of fruits and vegetables and one serving per day of a low-fat dairy product or c) a combination diet (called the DASH diet) that provided 9 servings per day of fruits and vegetables and 3 servings per day of low-fat dairy products. After 8 weeks, the blood pressures of those on the fruit and vegetable diet were significantly lower than those on the typical American diet.

It is believed that the evidence for a beneficial effect of a diet rich in fruits and vegetables on diabetes is not as convincing as it is for heart disease, however the results of a few studies suggest that higher intakes of fruits and vegetables are associated with improved blood glucose control and lower risk of developing type-2 diabetes. In a cohort study of 10, 000 adults in the USA, the risk of developing type-2 diabetes over the next 20 years was about 20% lower in those who reported consumption of at least 5 servings per day of fruits and vegetables as compared to those who did not consume fruits and vegetables (Ford & Mokdad, 2001). In a prospective cohort study that followed over 40 000 USA women for an average of nine years, fruit and vegetable intake was not associated with the risk of developing type-2 diabetes, however higher intakes of green leafy and yellow vegetables were associated with a significant reduction in the risk of developing type-2 diabetes in overweight women (Liu *et al.*, 2004). A cross-sectional study of over 6000 non-diabetic adults in the UK, who consume higher volumes of fruits and vegetables showed to exhibit significantly low levels of glycosylated haemoglobin and it is postulated that potential compounds in fruits and vegetables that may enhance glucose control include fibre and magnesium (Sargeant *et al.*, 2001).

Dietary factors are estimated to account for about 30% of cancers in developed countries, making diet second only to tobacco smoking as a preventable cause of all cancer. This contribution of diet to the incidence of cancer is estimated to be about 20% in developing countries but it may decrease with fruit and vegetable consumption (WHO, 2008). Evidence from case-control and cohort studies has indicated that the intake of fruits and vegetables have a strong protective effect against various types of cancer (oropharynx, oesophagus, stomach, colon and rectum) and that people with a higher intake may have less risk than people with low or very low fruit and vegetable intake (Block *et al.*, 1992; Steinmetz & Jansen, 1996). Van't Veer and co-workers (2000) indicated that people with higher intakes of fruits and vegetables could reduce their risk of developing cancer by 19%. The association between fruit and vegetable intake and the risk of cancer has been said to be relative to the quantities of fruits and vegetables consumed and that there are three potential dose-response associations. It is anticipated that an extra serving of fruit and vegetables might achieve a much greater risk reduction when the total intake is relatively low than when it is high (a vitamin-like minimal requirement) or when the total intake is relatively high (a high threshold effect) and thirdly when intake is at all levels (not higher or lower) (Temple & Gladwin, 2003). With reference to the association between fruit and vegetable consumption, two cohort studies showed contrasting results. A study carried out by Terry *et al.* (2001) reported that fruit and vegetable intake could indicate a protective association only at intakes of about two servings per day whereas Mitchells *et al.* (2000) indicated that fewer than three servings of fruits and vegetables per week are not related to elevated risk of colorectal cancer. However, higher intakes of fruits and vegetables have been associated with a modestly significant reduction in lung cancer risk in a pooled analysis of eight prospective studies (Smith-Warner *et al.*, 2003). Higher intakes of cruciferous vegetables have been linked to a significant reduction in the risk of developing bladder cancer in men (Micaud *et al.*, 1999) and higher intakes of tomato products have been linked to a significant reduction in the risk of developing prostate cancer (Giovannucci *et al.*, 2002). Joseph and coworkers (1999) indicated that supplementation of the diet of rats with fruits or vegetables (blueberry, strawberry or spinach) prevented or reversed age-related changes in neuronal and behavioural function. In our opinion, the finding of Joseph and coworkers is suggestive of a possible association between the mechanisms by which health may be modified by diet in both animal and man by the consumption of fruits and vegetables. A study carried by Galeone *et al.* (2007) showed that a high intake of fruits and vegetables significantly reduced the risk of lung cancer and that the reduced risk was significantly evident in smokers as well as non-smokers.

The incidence of cataracts has been reported to be related to oxidative damage of proteins in the eye's lens which is induced by long-term exposure to ultraviolet light. The cloudiness and discoloration of the lens resulting from such exposure have been known to lead to vision loss that becomes more severe with age. The results of various prospective cohort studies tend to suggest that diets rich in fruits and vegetables, particularly carotenoid and vitamin C-rich fruits and vegetables are associated with decreased incidence and severity of cataracts (Brown *et al.*, 1999; Jacques *et al.*, 2001; Christen *et al.*, 2005). High intakes of broccoli and spinach have been reported to be associated to reduced cataracts among USA males (Brown *et al.*, 1999).

Lutein and zeaxanthin are carotenoids that are found in relatively high concentrations in the retina and could play a role in preventing damage to the retina which is caused by light or oxidants (Mares-Perlman *et al.*, 2002). In two reported case-control studies, high intakes of carotenoid-rich vegetables particularly those rich in lutein and zeaxanthin were said to be associated with a significant reduced risk of developing age-related macular degeneration (Seddon *et al.*, 1994; Shellen *et al.*, 2002). Another study involving more than 118 000 male and female participants found that those who consumed three or more servings of fruits and vegetables daily had their risk of developing age-related macular degeneration reduced by 36% than those participants who consumed less fruits and vegetables (Cho *et al.*, 2004).

A beneficial association between reduced risk of developing chronic obstructive pulmonary disease and fruit and vegetable consumption has been documented (Romieu & Trenga, 2001). Epidemiological studies in Europe and elsewhere showed that higher fruit intake (particularly apple) can be associated with higher forced expiratory volume values, indicating a better lung function (Tabak *et al.*, 2001; Butland *et al.*, 2002). A European study of 2917 participants followed over twenty years with an increase in the daily consumption of fruits has been associated with a 24% decrease in the risk of death from chronic obstructive pulmonary disease. Although the reason for the association between increased fruit consumption and decreased risk of developing chronic obstructive pulmonary disease is not known but it is suggested that antioxidants such as vitamin C or flavonoids found in fruits may be playing a protective role in reducing the risk of developing chronic obstructive pulmonary disease.

Few studies have claimed that antioxidants found in most fruits and vegetable juices could help lower a person's risk of developing Alzheimer's disease. This may be related to the fact that freshly squeezed juices from fruits and vegetables are very good sources of minerals and vitamins which catalyze chemical reactions occurring in the body. Another benefit of fruits and fruit juices is their ability to promote detoxification of the human body. Fruits help to cleanse the body and tomatoes, pineapples and citruses such as oranges, red grapefruits and lemons are well known for their detoxifying properties (Cuthbertson, 2002).

Increased fruit and vegetable consumption of about 3 to 9 servings per day has been shown to decrease urinary calcium loss of about 50 mg/day and lower biochemical markers of bone turnover especially bone resorption (Appel *et al.*, 1997; Lin *et al.*, 2003).

The effects of HIV infection on the nutritional status of persons living with HIV and AIDS have been reported (Oguntibeju *et al.*, 2006; 2007; 2008; 2009). It is known that good nutrition including the consumption of fruits and vegetables can contribute to the wellness and sense of well-being of people living with HIV and AIDS and may even prolong life. Fruits and vegetables are an important part of a healthy food intake and may supply the necessary vitamins, minerals and other substances that could boost the immune system (Department of Health, South Africa, 2001).

4. Possible mechanism of action of fruits and vegetables in human health and disease prevention

It is a common knowledge in biological science that mammalian and plant cells are constantly exposed to a variety of oxidizing agents. These oxidizing agents may be present in air, food, and water, or they may be produced by metabolic activity within the cells, however, it is important to maintain a balance between oxidants and antioxidants to be able to sustain optimal physiological conditions. Overproduction of oxidants can cause an imbalance, leading to oxidative stress (Ames *et al.*, 1993; Adom *et al.*, 2003). Oxidative stress can cause oxidative damage to macromolecules such as lipids, proteins and DNA and consequently lead to increased risk for developing chronic diseases such as cancer and cardiovascular disease (Ames *et al.*, 1993; Liu *et al.*, 1995). In order to prevent or reduce the oxidative stress induced by free radicals, sufficient amounts of antioxidants need to be consumed and fruits and vegetables are known to contain a variety of antioxidant compounds such as phenolics and carotenoids which may help protect cellular systems from oxidative damage and reduce the risk of developing chronic diseases (Wang *et al.*, 1996; Vinson *et al.*, 2001; Adom *et al.*, 2003). It is known that carotenoids demonstrate photoprotection which originate from their ability to quench and inactivate reactive oxygen species (Britton, 1995).

Phenolics provide essential functions in the reproduction and the growth of plants; acting as defense mechanisms against pathogens, parasites, and predators as well as contributing to the colour of plants and may also provide health benefits associated with reduced risk of chronic diseases in humans (Sun *et al.*, 2002).

Different species and varieties of fruits, vegetables, and grains have different phytochemical profiles (Adom & Liu, 2002; Adom *et al.*, 2003) The combination of orange, apple, grape, and blueberry has been shown to display a synergistic effect in antioxidant activity and obtaining antioxidants from dietary intake by consuming a wide variety of foods is of significant importance due to the fact that foods originating from plants contain many diverse types of phytochemicals in various quantities.

Carcinogenesis is a multistep process, and oxidative damage is linked to the formation of tumors through several mechanisms (Ames *et al.*, 1993; Liu *et al.*, 1995). Oxidative stress induced by free radicals causes DNA damage, which, when left unrepaired, can lead to base mutation, single- and double-strand breaks, DNA cross-linking, and chromosomal breakage and rearrangement (Ames *et al.*, 1993). This potentially cancer-inducing oxidative damage might be prevented or limited by the intake of dietary antioxidants which are found in fruits and vegetables. Studies to date have demonstrated that phytochemicals in common fruits and vegetables can have complementary and overlapping mechanisms of action, including antioxidant activity and the scavenging of free radicals, regulation of gene expression in cell proliferation, cell differentiation, oncogenes, and tumour suppressor genes, induction of cell-cycle arrest and apoptosis, modulation of enzyme activities in detoxification, oxidation, reduction, stimulation of the immune system, regulation of hormone metabolism, and antibacterial and antiviral effects (Ames *et al.*, 1993; Liu *et al.*, 1995; Adom & Liu, 2002).

It is believed that fruits and vegetables are rich in precursors to bicarbonate ions which serve to buffer acids in the body, therefore if the concentration of bicarbonate ions is inadequate to maintain normal pH, the body is capable of mobilizing alkaline calcium salts from bone in order to neutralize acids consumed in the diet and those generated by metabolism, thus increased consumption of fruits and vegetables reduces the net acid content of the diet and may preserve calcium in bones which might otherwise be mobilized to maintain normal pH (New, 2002).

The relationship between fruit and vegetable consumption and obesity has also been envisaged. It is not clear how fruit and vegetable consumption prevent obesity or excessive weight gain. However, one possible mechanism could be that fruits and vegetables might serve as healthy substitutes for more calorie-dense foods (Field *et al.*, 2003).

5. Factors affecting the nutritional qualities and consumption of fruits and vegetables

Climatic conditions such as temperature and light intensity have been shown to have a strong effect on the nutritional quality of fruits and vegetables (Mozafar, 1994). Low temperature is believed to favour synthesis of sugar and vitamin C while short duration decreases the rate of ascorbic acid oxidation. Maximum beta-carotene content in tomatoes occurs at a temperature range of 15 to 21°C but beta-carotene content is reduced if temperatures are higher or lower than this range, mainly due to the temperature sensitivity of lycopene, the precursor to beta-carotene and lutein.

The B vitamins are crop specific with reference to temperature sensitivity. Warm season crops (beans, tomatoes, peppers, melons) produce more B vitamins at high (27 to 30 °C versus low (10 to 15 °C) temperatures. In contrast, cool season crops such as broccoli, cabbage, spinach, peas produce more B vitamins at low versus high temperature. It has been reported that light intensity has little effect on the B vitamins but as light intensity increases, vitamin C increases and total carotenoids and chlorophyll decrease (Gross, 1991). Higher light intensities produce more sugars thus favouring the synthesis of vitamins and also increase plant temperatures, inhibiting beta-carotene production which protects chlorophyll from light bleaching. According to Goldman *et al.* (1999), the type of soil, the rootstock used for fruit trees, irrigation, fertilization and other traditional practices influence the water and nutrient supply to the plant and have been shown to affect the composition and quality attributes of fruits and vegetables. Other environmental factors such as altitudes, soil pH, salinity, insects and plant diseases have also been reported to affect composition and quality of fruits and vegetables. Also, processing and cooking methods do affect the nutritional value of fruits and vegetables (Lee & Kader, 2000). For example, water-soluble vitamins such as vitamin C and folic acid are readily lost at high rates when cooking water is discarded.

The level of education has been shown to be related to fruit and vegetable consumption in children and adults. It has been shown that mothers with a higher level of education tend to consume more fruits and vegetables and also influence their children to do so (Gibson, *et al.*, 1998) and that higher income influences the availability of fruits, which in turn affect consumption in both adults and children. Family origin is said to influence food choice and preparation and one study indicated that the frequency of fruit and vegetable consumption in both mothers and children differs according to origin (Shatenstein & Ghadirian, 1998).

6. Recommendations and further studies

For an adequate supply of vitamins, minerals and other compounds from fruits and vegetables, it is important to purchase fresh fruits and vegetables without bruises, soft spots, mold, decay or broken skins. It is very important to wash all fruits and vegetables before cutting, slicing and eating. It is also advisable to store fruit and vegetables in the refrigerator but once cut or sliced, fruits and vegetables should be placed in a refrigerator in tightly sealed plastic bags and consumed within two to three days.

There is a need for more controlled, clinical intervention trials in order to confirm findings that support the view that consumption of fruits and vegetables promotes health and reduces the risk of developing chronic diseases. Accurate assessment of dietary intake remains difficult and cost-efficient methods for estimating fruit and vegetable intake are needed to be able to confirm the relationship between fruit and vegetable consumption. Although research evidence supports the association between fruit and vegetable consumption and decreased incidence and mortality of chronic diseases such as obesity, different cancers and cardiovascular diseases, controversies still exist in the science community with reference to their association, therefore further studies with large population groups over long periods of time is recommended.

Author details

O.O. Oguntibeju, E.J. Truter and A.J. Esterhuyse
Oxidative Stress Research Centre, Department of Biomedical Sciences, Faculty of Health & Wellness Sciences, Cape Peninsula University of Technology, Bellville Campus, South Africa

7. References

Adom KK & Liu RH (2002). Antioxidant activity of grains. J. Agric Food Chem 50: 6182-6187.

Adom KK, Sorrells ME & Liu RH (2003). Phytochemicals and antioxidant activity of wheat varieties. J Agric Food Chem 51: 7825-7834.

Alonso A, de la Fuente C, Martin-Arnau AM, de Irala J, Martinez JA & Gonzalez MA (2004). Fruit and vegetable consumption is inversely associated with blood pressure in a Mediterranean population with a high vegetable-fat intake. Brit J Nutr 92: 311-319.

Ames BN, Shigenaga MK & Gold LS (1993). DNA lesions, inducible DNA repair and cell division: the three key factors in mutagenesis and carcinogenesis. Environ Health Perspect. 101(S5): 35-44.

Appel LJ, Moore TJ & Obarzanek E (1997). A clinical trial of the effects of dietary patterns on blood pressure. DASH Collaborative Research Group. N Engl J Med 336 (16): 117-1124.

Bazzano LA, Serdula MK & Liu S (2003). Dietary intake of fruits and vegetables and risks of cardiovascular disease. Curr Artheroscler Rep 5: 492-499.

Block G, Patterson BH & Subar, AF (1992). Fruit, vegetables and cancer prevention: a review of the epidemiological evidence. Nutr Cancer 18: 1.-4.

Boileau TW, Liao Z, Kim S, Lemeshow S, Erdman JW & Clinton SK (2003). Prostate carcinogenesis in N-methyl-N-nitrosourea (NMU)-testosterone-treated rats fed tomato powder, lycopene or energy-restricted diets. J Natl Cancer Inst 95: 1578-1586.

Britton G (1995). Structure and properties of carotenoids in relation to function. FASEB J 9: 1551-1558.

Brown L, Rimm EB & Seddon JM (1999). A prospective study of carotenoid intake and risk of cataract extraction in USA men. Am J Clin Nutr (70 (4): 517-524.

Butland BK, Fehily AM & Elwood FC (2002). Diet, lung function and lung decline in a cohort of 2512 middle aged men. Thorax 55 (2): 102-108.

Cho E, Seddon JM, Rosner B, Willett WC & Hankinson SE (2004). Propective study of intake of fruits, vegetables, vitamins and carotenoids and the risk of age-related maculopathy. Arch Ophthalmol 122 (6): 883-892.

Chobanian AV, Bakris GL, Black HR (2003). The seventh report of the joint national committee on prevention, detection, evaluation and treatment of high blood pressure. JAMA 289: 2560-2572.

Christen WG, Liu S, Schaumber DA & Buring JE (2005). Fruit and vegetable intake and the risk of cataract in women. Am J Clin Nutr 81 (5): 1417-1422.

Crawford PB, Obarzanek E, Morrison J & Sabry ZI (1994). Comparative advantage of 3-day food records over 24 recall and 5-day food frequency validated by observation of 9-and 10-year girls. J Am Diet Assoc 94 (6): 626-630.

Cuthbertson WFJ (2002). Are the effects of dietary fruits and vegetables on human health related to those of chronic dietary restriction on animal longevity and disease? Brit J Nutr 87 (2): 187-188.

Daucher L, Amouye P & Dallongeville J (2005). Fruit and vegetable consumption and risk of stroke: a meta-analysis of cohort studies. Neurol 65: 1193-1197.

Daucher L, Amouye P, Hercberg S & Dallongeville J (2006). Fruit and vegetable consumption and risk of coronary heart disease: a meta-analysis of cohort studies. J Nutr 136: 2588-2592.

Department of Health, South Africa (2001). South African national guidelines on nutrition for people living with TB, HIV/AIDS and other chronic debilitating conditions.

Duncan KH, Cacon JA, Weinster RI (1983). The effects of high and low energy density diets on satiety, energy intake and eating time of obese and non-obese subjects. Am J Clin Nutr 37: 763-767.

Field AE, Gillman MW, Rosnr B, Rockett HR & Colditz GA (2003). Association between fruit and vegetable intake and change in body mass index among a large sample of children and adolescents in the United States. Int J Obesity 27: 821-826.

Ford ES & Mokdad AH (2001). Fruit and vegetable consumption and diabetes mellitus incidence among USA adults. Prev Med 32 (1): 33-39.

Fung TT, Willett WC, Stampter MJ, Manson JE & Hu FB (2001). Dietary patterns and the risk of coronary heart disease in women. Arch Intern Med 161: 1857-1862.

Galeone C, Negri E & Pelucchi C (2007). Dietary intake of fruits and vegetables and lung cancer risk: a case-control study in Harbin, Northern China. Ann Oncol 18: 388-392.

Gibson EL, Wardle J & Watts CJ (1998). Fruit and vegetable consumption, nutritional knowledge and beliefs in mothers and children. Appet 3 (2): 205-228.

Giovannucci EL, Rimm EB, Liu Y, Stampfer MJ & Willett WC (2002). A prospective study of tomato products, lycopene and prostate cancer risk. J Natl Cancer Inst 94 (5): 391-398.

Giskes K, Turrell G, Patterson C & Newman B (2002). Socio-economic differences in fruit and vegetable consumption among Australian adolescents and adults. Publ Health Nutr 5 (5): 663-669.

Goldman IL, Kader AA & Heintz C (1999). Influence of production, handling and storage on phytonutrient content of foods. Nutr Rev 57: S46-S52.

Gross J (1991). Pigments in vegetables: chlorophylls and carotenoids. AVI Book, Van Nostrand Reinold Pub New York NY.

He FJ, Nowson CA & Macgregor GA (2006). Fruit and vegetable consumption and stroke: meta-analysis of cohort studies. Lancet 367: 320-326.

Hu FB, Rimm EB, Stampter MJ, Ascherio A, Spiegelman D, Willett WC (2000). Prospective study of major dietary patterns and risk of coronary heart disease in men. Am J Clin Nutr 72: 912-921.

Hu FB, Stampter MJ, Manson JE, Ascherio A, Colditz GA & Speizer FE (1999). Dietary saturated fats and their food sources in relation to the risk of coronary heart disease in women. Am J Clin Nutr 70: 1001-1008.

Jacques PF, Chylack LT Jr & Hankinson SE (2001). Long-term nutrient intake and early age-related nuclear lens opacities. Arch Ophthal 119 (7): 1009-1019.

Joseph JA, Denisova NA, Arendash G (1999). Blueberry supplementation enhances signaling and prevents behavioural deficits in an Alzheimer disease model. Nutr Neurosci 6 (3): 153-162.

Joshipura KJ, Ascherio A, Manson JE, Stampter MJ & Rim EB (1999). Fruit and vegetable intake in relation to the risk of ischaemic stroke. JAMA 282: 12331239.

Kalt W (2002). Health functional phytochemicals of fruits. Hort Rev 27: 269-315.

Lee SK & Kader AA (2000). Preharvest and postharvest factors influencing vitamin C content of horticultural crops. Posharv Biol Technol 20: 207-220.

Lin PH, Ginty F & Appel LJ (2003). The DASH diet and sodium reduction improve markers of bone turnover and calcium metabolism in adults. J Nutr 133 (10): 3130-3136.

Liu RH & Hotchkiss JH (1995). Potential genotoxicity of chronically elevated nitric oxide: A review. Mutat Res 339: 73-89.

Liu S, Serdula M & Janket SJ (2004). A prospective study of fruit and vegetable intake and the risk of type-2 diabetes in women. Diab Care 27 (1): 2993-2996.

Lock K, Pomerleau J, Causer L, Altmann DR, McKee M (2005). The global burden of disease attributable to low consumption of fruit and vegetables: implications for the global strategy on diet. World Health Org 83: 100-108.

Mares-Perlman JA, Millen AE, Ficek TL & Hankinson SE (2002). The body of evidence to support a protective role for lutein and zeaxanthin in decaying chronic disease. J Nutr 132 (3): 518S-524S.

Michaud DS, Spiegelman D, Clinton SK, Rimm EB, Willett WC & Giovannucci EL (1999). Fruit and vegetable intake and incidence of bladder cancer in a male prospective cohort. J Natl Cancer Inst 91 (7): 605-613.

Mitchels KB, Giovannucci E & Joshipura KJ (2000). Prospective study of fruit and vegetable consumption and incidence of colon and rectal cancers. J Natl Cancer Inst 92: 1740.

Mozafar A (1994). Plant vitamins: agronomic, physiological and nutritional aspects. CRC Press, Boca Raton FL.

Muriello LM, Driskell MH, Sherman KJ, JohnsonSS, Prochaska JM & Prochaska JO (2006). Acceptability of a school-based intervention for prevention of adolescent obesity. J Sch Nurs 22: 269-277.

Ness AR & Powles JW (1997). Fruit and vegetables and cardiovascular disease: a review. Int J Epidemiol 26 (1): 1-13.

New SA (2002). Nutrition society medal lecture: The role of the skeleton in acid-base homeostasis. Proc Nutr Soc 61 (2): 151-164.

Oguntibeju OO, AJ Esterhuyse & EJ Truter (2009). Possible benefits of micronutrient supplementation in the treatment and management of HIV infection and AIDS. Afri J Pharm & Pharmacol 3 (9): 404-412.

Oguntibeju OO, van den Heever WMJ & Van Schalkwyk FE (2007). Interrelationship between nutrition and immune system in HIV infection: a review. Pak J Biol Sci 10 (24): 4327-4338.

Oguntibeju OO, WMJ van den Heever & FE van Schakwyk (2006). The effect of a liquid nutritional supplement on viral load and haematological parameters of HIV-positive/AIDS patients. Brit J Biomed Sci 63 (3): 134-139.

Oguntibeju OO, WMJ van den Heever & FE van Schalkwyk (2008). Potential effects of nutrient supplement on the anthropometric profiles of HIV-positive patients: complimentary medicine could have a role in the management of HIV/AIDS. Afri J Biomed Res 11: 13-22.

Romieu I & Trenga C (2001). Diet and obstructive lung diseases. Epidemiol Rev 23 (2): 268-287.

Sargeant LA, Khaw KT & Bingham S (2001). Fruit and vegetable intake and population glycosylated haemoglobin levels; the EPIC-Norfolk Study. Eur J Clin Nutr 55: (5): 342-348.

Seddon JM, Ajani UA, Sperduto RD (1994). Dietary carotenoids, vitamins A, C, and E, and advanced age-related macular degeneration. Eye Disease Case-Control Study Group. JAMA; 272(18):1413-1420.

Seifried HE, McDonald SS, Anderson DE, Greenwald P & Milner JA (2003). The antioxidant conundrum in cancer. Cancer Res 63: 4295-4298.

Shatenstein B & Ghadirian P (1998). Influences on diet, health behaviours and their outcome in select ethnocultural and religious groups. Nutr 14 (2): 223-230.

Shellen EL, Verbeek AL, Van Den Hoogen GW, Cruysberg JR & Hoyng CB (2002). Neovascular age-related macular degeneration and its relationship to antioxidant intake. Acta Ophthalmol Scand 80 (4): 368-371.

Smith-Warner SA, Spiegelman D & Yaun SS (2003). Fruits, vegetables and lung cancer: a pooled analysis of cohort studies. Int J Cancer 107 (6): 1001-1011.

Southon S (2000). Increased fruit and vegetable consumption within EU: potential health benefits. Food Res Intl 33: 211-217.

Steinmetz KA & Jansen JD (1996).Vegetables, fruit and cancer prevention: a review. J Am Diet Assoc 96: 1027.

Sun J, Chu, YF, Wu X & Liu RH (2002). Antioxidant and antiproliferative activities of fruits. J Agric Food Chem 50: 7449-7454.

Sylvestre MP, O'Loughlin J, Gray-Donald K, Hanley J & Paradis G (2006). Association between fruit and vegetable consumption in mothers and children in low-income urban neighbourhoods. Health Edu Behav 20: 1-11.

Tabak C, Arts IC, Smit HA, Heederik D & Kromhout D (2001). Chronic obstructive pulmonary disease and intake of catechins, flavonols and flavones: the MORGEN Study. Am J Resp Crit Care Med 164 (1): 61-64.

Temple NJ & Gladwin KK (2003). Fruit, vegetables and the prevention of cancer: research challenges. Nutr 19: 467-470.

Terry P, Giovannucci E & Mitchels KB (2001). Fruit, vegetables, dietary fibre and risk of colorectal cancer. J Natl Cancer Inst 93: 525.

Tohill BC, Seymour J, Serdula M, Kettel-Khan L & Rolls BJ (2004). What epidemiological studies tell us about the relationship between fruit and vegetable consumption and body weight. Nutr Rev 62: 365-374.

Tucker KL, Hallfrisch J, Qiao N, Muller D, Andres R & Fleg JL (2005). The combination of high fruit and vegetable and low saturated fat intakes is more protective against mortality in aging men. J Nutr 135: 556-5561.

United States Department of Agriculture (2000). Nutrition and your health: dietary guidelines for Americans. Home and Garden Bull. 232, USDA, Washington DC (www.usda.gov/cnpp).

Van Duyn MA & Pivonka E (2000). Overview of the health benefits of fruit and vegetable consumption for the dietetics professional. J Am Diet Assoc 99 (10): 1241-1248.

Van't Veer P, Jansen MC, Klerk K & Kok FJ (2000). Fruits and vegetables in the prevention of cancer and cardiovascular disease. Publ Health Nutr 3: 103.

Vinson JA, Hao Y, Su X, Zubik L & Bose P (2001). Phenol antioxidant quantity and quality in foods: fruits. J Agric Food Chem 49: 5315-5321.

Wang H, Cao GH & Prior RL (1996). Total antioxidant capacity of fruits. J Agric Food Chem 44: 701-705.

Wang Y, Bentley ME, Zhai F & Popkin BM (2002). Tracking dietary intake patterns of Chinese from childhood to adolescence over a six-year follow-up period. J Nutr 132 93): 430-438.

Wardle J, Permenter K & Waller J (2000). Nutrition knowledge and food intake. Appet 34 (3): 269-275.

Wargovich MJ (2000). Anticancer properties of fruits and vegetables. Hort Sc 35: 573-575.

WHO (2008). Population nutrient intake goals for preventing diet-related chronic diseases. www.who.int/nutrition.

Chapter 8

Diabetes Mellitus in Developing Countries and Case Series

Omiepirisa Yvonne Buowari

Additional information is available at the end of the chapter

http://dx.doi.org/10.5772/50658

1. Introduction

Diabetes mellitus is a growing public health affecting people worldwide both in developing and developed countries, and poses a major socio-economic challenge [1], [2]. A chronic metabolic disorder of multiple aetiologies is assuming epidemic proportions worldwide [3]. It is also a complex disorder with profound consequences both acute and chronic. Genetic and environmental factors play a role in the development of the disease [4]. The cells of the body cannot metabolise sugar properly due to a total or relative lack of insulin. The body then breaks down its own fat, protein, and glycogen to produce sugar resulting in high sugar levels in the blood with excess by products called ketones being produced by the liver [5]. Diabetes causes disease in many organ systems, the severity of which may be related to how long the disease has been present and how well it has been controlled. The term diabetes mellitus describes a metabolic disorder of multiple aetiology characterised by chronic hyperglycaemia with disturbances of carbohydrate, fat, and protein metabolism resulting from defects in insulin secretion, insulin action or both [6],[7],[8],[9].

Diabetes mellitus may present with characteristic symptoms such as thirst, polyuria, blurring of vision and weight loss [6]. The abnormalities of carbohydrate, fat, and protein metabolism are due to deficient action of insulin on target tissues resulting from insensitivity or lack of insulin [6].

The effects of diabetes mellitus include long-term damage, dysfunction, and failure of various organs [6]. Type 1 diabetes mellitus encompasses the majority of diabetes, which are primarily due to pancreatic islet beta cell destruction and are prone to ketoacidosis [9]. If diabetes is not taken care of, complications such as heart, kidney, and eye diseases, incurable wounds leading to amputations of the extremities and mental disorders follow. Besides this, diabetes related complications inevitably cause high cost of treatment and opportunities for the concerned people and their families especially for poor families the disease and its complications cause severe economical burden. In developing countries, non-communicable diseases are evolving rapidly [8]. Diabetes mellitus places serious constraint on patients' activities [10]. Despite the high prevalence, serious long-term complications, and established evidence based guidelines for management of diabetes mellitus, the quality of care is still deficient in developing countries [11]. Diabetes mellitus is emerging as an epidemic all over the world, represents an important public health problem, and is of clinical concern [12], [13], [14]. Type 1 diabetes has been estimated to affect approximately 19,000 people in the worlds poorest countries but there is lack of good data on the disease prevalence in developing countries and in particular in sub-Saharan Africa[15].

Non-communicable disease such as diabetes mellitus, cardiovascular disease (especially ischaemic heart diseases and hypertension), stroke, cancer and chronic kidney and respiratory diseases have become the leading causes of mortality both in developed and developing nations of the world. The rising prevalence of these diseases is thought to be due to adoption of western lifestyles and urbanization [16]. With the current trend of transition from communicable to non-communicable diseases, it is projected that the later will equal or even exceed the former in developing nations thus culminating in double burden [17]. There is need for health care providers to intensify efforts in educating people living with type 2 diabetes about good personal and environmental hygiene. Emphasis is on early diagnosis of diabetes, good glycaemic and blood control and proper education, programmes for health workers caring for diabetic patients as well as public awareness talks [17]. The prevalence of diabetes mellitus varies between different countries. Diabetes mellitus is defined as a chronic disorder, which is characterised by an elevated level of glucose in the blood due primarily in inadequate secretion or utilization of insulin [18].

Gestational diabetes mellitus is pregnancy induced diagnosed typically in the second half of pregnancy. It occurs when beta cells reserve is unable to counter balance the insulin resistance caused by placental hormone. Systemic hypertension and diabetes mellitus are common chronic conditions that frequently coexist and can significantly affect the health care needs and clinical outcome of affected individuals [19].

The excess global mortality attributable to diabetes in the year 2000 was estimated to be 2.9 million deaths, equivalent to 5.2% of all deaths. Excess mortality attributable to diabetes accounted for 2-3 % of deaths in poorest countries [20]. Diabetes is a serious illness with multiple complications and premature mortality accounting for at least 10 % of total health care expenditure in many countries. Diabetes is often perceived as a disease of affluent countries. A serious chronic disease leads to a substantial reduction in life expectancy, decreased quality of life and increased costs of care [21].

Management of diabetes mellitus is multidisciplinary and this is not readily available in low resource settings. Dietary management is essential in the treatment and it alone may be adequate to achieve and maintain the therapeutic goals to normoglycaemia and normolipidaemia [22]. The care for diabetic patients includes a change in their life style, where the diet plan represents an important pillar of care so they can meet their goals. The management of people with diabetes mellitus is complex and good control significantly reduces the risk of complications yet studies from around the world concisely demonstrate inappropriate variations in care [23].

2. Burden of diabetes mellitus in developing countries

Sub-Saharan Africa will face a double disease burden represented by increased rates of non-communicable diseases added to endemic, pandemic, and emergent infections such as malaria, tuberculosis, and HIV/AIDS. There is dearth of African data concerning the prevalence of type 1 diabetes mellitus [7]. Diabetes mellitus related cardiovascular disease complications are considered rare in Africa but are on the rise and are regularly associated with classic cardiovascular risk factors [24]. A missionary physician stated in 1901 that diabetes was very uncommon in the central region of Africa[25]. There is increased number of people suffering from non communicable diseases and this have been linked to unhealthy ways of living and lifestyle such as consumption of excess calories and reduction in the level of physical activities with the consequent development of obesity and insulin resistance [16].

Obesity, type 2 diabetes mellitus, and their associated long-term complications are emerging as critical, worldwide public health problems. Although few groups have been spared increased in the burden of these conditions, those undergoing rapid westernization, with the transition in diet and activity profiles have been especially affected. Among the most affected groups are those in Africa and the African Diaspora including the Caribbean, Europe, and North America [26]. The probably cause of obesity in developing countries has been attributed to the current lifestyle, where urbanization, better economic development and an increase in income have resulted in diet changes and less physical activity. The care for diabetic patients includes a change in their life style, where the diet plan represents an important pillar of care so they can meet their goals. Obesity increases the risk of developing not only type 2 diabetes, cardiovascular disease, stroke, osteoarthritis and some forms of cancer [27]. Obesity has been clearly linked with diabetic patients from all the major ethnic regions in Nigeria [16]. Over the past century, diabetes was considered a rare medical condition in Africa. However epidemiological studies carried out in the 90's have provided evidence of a different picture[28]. The number of people with diabetes is increasing due to population growth, aging, diet, lifestyle, urbanization, and increased prevalence of obesity and physical activity [12], [28], [29]. Diet and lifestyle are the biggest culprits at least in the case of type 2 diabetes but genetics also have a role to play. Although obesity is an important factor in the diabetes epidemic, it does not alone explain the vast increase in prevalence especially in the developing world [29].

In developing countries, the majority of individuals with diabetes are aged between 45 and 65 years while in developed countries, the majority are older than 64 years. Based on demographic changes by 2030, the number of people older than 64 years with diabetes will be more than 82 million in developing countries and more than 48 million in developed countries. The greatest relative increases are expected to occur in the Middle East crescent, sub-Saharan Africa and India [30]. Some 170 million men and women, who will reside in developing regions of the world in less than 30 years from now, will be suffering from diabetes in their reproductive years of life [31]. In 2003, 194 million people 20 to 79 years of age had diabetes mellitus, almost three quarter of them are living in the developing world. Almost one million people die because of diabetes each year with two-thirds in developing countries. This growing problem will have a significant impact on national and individual economies as well individual health. However, it has proven difficult to determine just what that impact is [32]. Diabetes is an increasing problem in sub-Saharan Africa [33]. It is predicted that the prevalence of diabetes mellitus in adults will increase in the next two decades and much of the increase will occur in developing countries where the majority of patients are aged between 45 and 65 years. The incidence and prevalence of diabetes mellitus has continued to increase globally, despite a great deal of research with the resulting burden resting more heavily on tropical developing countries [17], [34]. Traditional rural communities still have very low prevalence at most 1-2% except in some specific high-risk groups, whereas 1-3% or more adults in urban communities have diabetes. The combination of the rising prevalence of diabetes and the high rate of long-term complications in Africa will lead to a drastic increase of the burden of diabetes on health systems of African countries [34] and may have a devastating human and economic toll if the trends remain unabated [35]. In comparison to previous estimates from sub-Saharan Africa, the prevalence of adult onset diabetes seems to be on the increase[36].

In the last decade, diabetes has become a health problem in developing countries and has been found in a wide variety of atypical forms. Its burden is huge in developing countries due to lack of basic means for reaching diagnosis and a reasonable glycaemic control. The prevalence of type 1 diabetes mellitus varies from country to country in the African sub-region. The low number of health care providers with the requisite knowledge, expertise, and experience in the care of children with diabetes is another major issue. Diabetes care in developing countries needs to address the specific background of the patient population, their needs, medical problems, and social constraints [35]. The region of sub-Saharan Africa contains 33 of the 50 poorest countries in the world and will experience the greatest risk in the prevalence of diabetes over the next 20 years [36].

Most African studies are hospital based and give data on patients that visit the hospital only. Type 1 diabetes has been estimated to affect approximately 19000 people in the world's poorest countries but there is lack of good data on the disease prevalence in developing countries and in particular in sub-Saharan Africa [15]. The present increase in the rate of both type 2 diabetes mellitus and type 1 diabetes mellitus indicate the great and urgent need for more epidemiological surveys in sub-Saharan Africa. Such a need is dictated by the prevalence of undiagnosed diabetes mellitus [7].

The prevalence of diabetes mellitus has significantly increased over recent decades in Tunisia to around 10% [37]. From various African studies in 6299 Africans aged 15 years and above in six Tanzanian villages, 0.87% had diabetes 1.1% males and 0.68% females [38]. In several Nigerian studies a prevalence of 1.6% in two suburban populations in northern Nigeria [39], 1.4% in a rural population in Kwara State [40], 1.6/1000 in children in Sagamu [41], 1.2/1000 in children in Port Harcourt, southern Nigeria [42], case fatality in of 3.4% in Ekiti [43], 17.2% in adults in Port Harcourt [44]. Diabetes was the sixth leading cause of admissions in Enugu, 8.8% admissions into the medical wards at the university of Nigeria teaching hospital with a case fatality of 24% [45] and the leading cause of medical admissions in Nnewi, south east Nigeria [46]. In another Nigerian study in Dakace village about 10 km from Zaria, Zaria 2.0% and all the detected diabetics were males and above 45 years [1]. It was estimated that about 100,000 children less than 15 years developed type 1 diabetes mellitus with wide global variations in incidence rates. There are scanty data on the incidence, aetiology, and outcome of children diabetes mellitus from developing countries like Nigeria [4]. It is also one of the commonest reasons for medical admissions and death in Nigerian hospitals. The disease burden of diabetes mellitus in developing countries is unacceptably high thus necessitating an indebt look at the management techniques and patients' self-care habits due to the burden of diabetes care and the attendant complications, it affects all aspects of the society, and it has become a public health concern globally [47]. The increase in diabetes mellitus in Africa has been attributable in part to urbanization, urban residence, acculturation, abdominal obesity, globalization, westernization, sedentary lifestyle, behavioural habits, systemic arterial hypertension, physical inactivity, low intake of fruits and vegetables, high intake of animal fat and protein, industrialization, health transition, lifestyle changes, and the adoption of western lifestyle [1], [7], [47]. Variations in the type and epidemiology of diabetes between urban and rural areas have also been noted in Africa [47]. For a long-time, Africa was considered safe from many of the diseases that are called "diseases of affluence" which plague the western world. Similarly, there was a time when Africa was thought to be a continent relatively free of diabetes mellitus illness [48]. The disorder was previously thought to be rare or undocumented in rural Africa but over the past few decades, it has emerged as an important non-communicable disease in sub-Saharan Africa [2]. There is increased prevalence of diabetes in developing countries [47]. The high incidence of undiagnosed diabetics poses a major public health challenge in developing countries.

3. Challenges and problems of managing diabetes mellitus in developing and poor resource countries

3.1. Ignorance

There is poor health seeking behaviours in low resource countries because of inaccessible quality health care. Poor health seeking behaviour results in late presentation and is a possible reason why majority of patients in these setting present with complications [14]. For diabetic children, it is possible that some of the affected children succumbed to the illness at home out of parental ignorance and high cost of orthodox medical care. It has been found that some patient sign against medical advice [4]. Some because of finance, others to seek alternative therapy or spiritual help. In a study on childhood diabetes in Kano, northwest Nigeria, three parents/guardians signed against medical advice. They belonged to the lower socioeconomic groups, and their management was largely hindered by lack of funds for investigations and drug procurement [4]. For people with diabetes living at or below the poverty level, the purchase of appropriate footwear may not be feasible or of high priority, (bare foot walking is a common practice in rural communities but may be culturally influenced as well) [49]. Due to this ignorance and poverty, patients present late even with diabetic complications. Patients with diabetic foot continue to insist on medical management to salvage the affected limb until they become surgical emergencies [50]. Such emergency cases come with very little health reserve and clinical information to permit anaesthesia and surgery. The urgent need to save life then becomes the only support to favour surgical intervention. Any delay to allow for more time than necessary for basic investigations, remarkably influences the outcome of the procedures. Diabetics undergoing surgery belong to the high-risk group of patients and the risks are worst in the presence of severe complications such as diabetic foot gangrene [50].

3.2. Economic and cost of management of diabetes mellitus

The cost of management of diabetes mellitus is complex and multidisciplinary therefore expensive in poor resource countries where majority of the population live below a dollar per day. Diabetes mellitus exacts three broad categories of economic costs.

a. **Direct costs on health care:** This includes costs on purchase of medications, and glucometers for those that can afford it. Also the cost on visits to the health care facility and to see the professionals both general and specialist and money spent on hospitalisation both for the diabetes and diabetic complications [29].
b. **Indirect health care costs:** These include care of nursing homes and informal care by relatives and carers. Societal expectations about the appropriate place for professional and informal care certainly have important economic consequences [29]. Relatives and friends who care for the patient, may loose productive hours at their work or business.
c. **Productivity costs**: This includes the loss of earnings from mortality and morbidity that is time taken by otherwise economic individuals with diabetes to treat their condition and disability associated with diabetes and its complications [29]. In developing countries with scarce resources, it is still possible to put in place effective programs to combat diabetes. Some patients in developing countries travel great distances to medical care facilities, which meant that greater earnings needed to be sacrificed in order to attend to medical visits and check-up. This discourages individuals from seeking an early diagnosis and is loss lost to follow up [29].

This growing problem of diabetes mellitus will have significant impact on national and individual economies as well as on individual health. The indirect costs of diabetes such as lost productivity are at least as high and increased as more economically productive people are affected [32]. Good data on the direct medical costs of diabetes are not available for most developing countries [32].

3.3. Poverty

Health conditions in most African countries are poor and a large percentage of families live below the poverty line of one United States dollar per month [35]. Access to health services is limited and living conditions are poor. The low number of health care providers with the requisite knowledge, expertise, and experience in the care of children with diabetes is another major issue where the facilities are available; there is lack of basic diagnostic and monitoring tools as well as irregular supply of insulin. Insulin is still not available on an uninterrupted basis in many parts of the developing world [15]. The prognosis is likely to be poor for patients with type 1 diabetes in sub-Saharan Africa and only wealthy patients own their own glucose meter. Some patients have their glucose concentrations monitored without charge in public health facilities. Patients with comorbidity with diabetes is associated with considerable consequences for health care and related costs and comorbidity has been shown to intensify utilization of health care facilities and to increase medical care costs on patients with diabetes [51].

3.4. Use of alternative and complementary therapy

There are many forms of treatment in the African region. Most of the time, the patients visits the local traditional healers before coming to the hospital [4]. Traditional healers are an integral part of the health care system [37]. Many traditional healers had heard of diabetes and knew at least the disease was characterised by excessive thirst and urination[37]. Traditional medicine or complementary and / or alternative medicine (CAM) refers to health practices, approaches, knowledge and beliefs incorporating plant, animal and mineral based medicines, spiritual therapies, manual techniques and exercises applied singularly or in combination to treat, diagnose and prevent illness or maintain well being [52], [53]. It describes a diverse group of medical and health care system practices and products not currently considered an integral part of conventional medicine [3], [54], [55] and are consequently not taught as part of the medical curriculum [56]. Traditional medicine is often referred to as complementary therapy when used in combination with orthodox medicine and alternative therapy when used in place of orthodox medicine [54], [57]. CAM is also referred to as holistic or integrative and describes a heterogeneous collection of non-traditional therapies from chemical substances to prayer [58]. The frequency of utilization of CAM is increasing worldwide and is well documented in both African and global populations to be between 20 to 80%[56]. In chronic conditions in which health outcomes are closely linked to adherence to treatment in which diabetes mellitus is one of them, the use of CAM may potentially adversely affect outcome. Multiple therapy practices involving combined use of CAM particularly herbal medicines and prescription medications has also been identified as being prevalent in some populations. Many herbal remedies have not undergone careful scientific assessment and some have the potential to cause serious toxic effects and major drug-to-drug interactions. Cultural and economic reasons are largely responsible for use of CAM [56]. Researchers have given several reasons for the increased prevalence of CAM utilization. These include failure of modern medicine to cure the underlying problem and the perception that CAM is cheaper than conventional medicine. In countries like Nigeria, possible reasons for the use of CAM include the strong advertisement by alternative practitioners that CAM is a panacea to all diseases thus encouraging patients to try them. Another possible explanation is the cultural beliefs of Africans that illnesses have a spiritual origin. Patients are thus interested in finding an explanation for their symptoms or the root cause of their problems and therefore consult with alternative practitioners. In Nigeria, the use of herbal remedies are perceived to be cheaper, may be on the increase due to the poor economic state and the increasing costs of orthodox medicines also cultural and economic reasons are largely responsible for the use of CAM [56]. The use of alternative therapy has become more popular in both developed and developing countries in recent times [56]. There advertising strategies on the media and especially using vehicles with megaphone from one neighbourhood to another, which do not necessarily inform but persuade customers, have also made the use more popular [57]. CAM is increasingly used in adults and children [59]. Over 80% of the populations in some African and Asian countries depend on traditional medicine for primary health care [60]. The use of CAM among diabetics is common [53], [55]. Although some of those therapies may be effective, others can be ineffective or even harmful. Patients who use CAM should keep their health care providers informed [55]. West Indians Africans, Indians, Latin Americans, and Asians mostly use CAM [54]. Prayer, acupunction, massage, hot tub therapy, biofeedback, and yoga have been used as well as various plant remedies for treating diabetes [54]. Several CAM practices and herbal remedies are promising for diabetes treatment but further vigorous study is needed in order to establish safety, efficacy, and mechanism of action because many patients with diabetes may be using CAM and to consider potential interactions with conventional medicines being used [54]. The increasing cost and distrust of modern western medical care in recent years has promoted the use of alternative and traditional therapies and has attracted the interest of health professionals, researchers, government, and policy makers. The use of CAM has not been limited to resource poor settings alone but also among the elites. Claims and refutations by various individuals and professional groups of cure for chronic ailments with alternative therapy have been reported. Furthermore, inadequate access to modern health care services and a trend towards naturalness have strengthened the shift to alternative therapy. The unregulated or inappropriate use of alternative therapy has also been documented to have negative effects on its users. Alternative therapy medications are not so regulated in most countries. There is increased acceptance and use of traditional medicines in recent times [57].

Globally, people developed unique indigenous healing traditions adapted and defined by their culture, beliefs and environmental which dissatisfied the health needs of their communities over centuries. Over 80% of the population in some Asian and African countries depend on traditional medicine for primary health care [2]. Herbal medicine is an integral part of traditional medicine and traditional medicine has a broad range of characteristic and elements, which earned it the working definition from the World Health Organization. Traditional medicines are diverse health practices, approaches, knowledge an beliefs that incorporated plant, animal and/ or mineral based medicines, spiritual therapies, manual techniques, and exercise, which applied singularly or in combination to maintain wellbeing as well as treatment, diagnosis or prevent illness. In a study in Lagos, Nigeria, 16.2% of respondents' use herbal medicine to decrease blood sugar [52]. Some other attractions to alternative therapies may be related to the power of the underlying philosophies they share, which involve closeness to nature, spirituality and the fact that these therapies often go along with the cultural beliefs of the people [61], [62]. In another Nigerian study, 46% of diabetics used herbal medicine [63]. CAM is an emerging aspect of the management of chronic disease worldwide. The main forms of CAM usage in diabetes mellitus include bitter leaf *vernonia amygdalina,* aloe Vera, garlic, ginger and local herbs. There is an increasing use of CAM in diabetes mellitus and this cut across the two main types of diabetes mellitus as CAM usage has been reported in type 1 and 2 diabetes mellitus. In the African setting for most chronic ailment there are often underlying explanations, which are founded on cultural and spiritual beliefs thus, necessitating the use of traditional medicines, which are of herbal nature. Of increasing importance in the Nigerian scenario is the use and claim of the glucose lowering effects of bitter leaf *vernonia amygdalina*. This is a small shrub with a dark green stem that grows widely in tropical and subtropical Africa and is widely used for its medicinal properties. One reason commonly adduced for its usage stems from the fact that it is bitter tasting and thus is able to neutralize the sweetness present in the blood of people with diabetes mellitus. Use of CAM is suggested by well meaning family members or neighbours or other people that had diabetes mellitus and used.

4. Case series

4.1. Case 1

A 42-year-old woman a known diabetic of three years went to seek spiritual help for her ailment at a spiritual healing home in Nigeria. She was told to observe a seven days fasting with some herbal concoction. On the fifth day of the fasting programme, she went comatose and was rushed to the hospital. Her blood sugar was 42 mmol/l with ketones in urinalysis, foul smelling breath. The electrolytes, urea, and creatinine were deranged. Respiratory rate was 40 breaths/minute, pulse rate 120 beats/minutes, pale, anicteric, afebrile, and dehydrated. Blood pressure was 90/40 mmhg. A diagnosis of diabetic ketoacidosis was made. She was placed on intravenous ampiclox, metronidazole, intravenous access was established, and normal saline set up and Insulin therapy commenced, the blood pressure, pulse rate and respiratory rate was measured every 30 minutes. She was managed and recovered consciousness two days later.

Case discussion: Use of alternative therapy is common in Nigeria and other African countries. Most of the components of these herbal remedies are not known therefore if it contains dangerous toxic substances that can have negative effects on the patient as seen in case 1.

4.2. Case 2

A 64-year-old man not a known diabetic presented with two weeks history of pains, swelling and sore on the right leg. At the onset of the illness, the patient applied several herbs on the leg, which started with severe pains and swellings, burst and gave rise to the swelling. On presentation he was ill looking, conscious, and alert, blood pressure 120/70 mmhg, pulse rate 100 beats /minute, pale, dehydrated with a sore on the right shin, which was discharging foul smelling substance. The leg was gangrenous. Haemoglobin concentration was 7%, electrolytes, urea, and creatinine where within normal ranges, random blood sugar was 36 mmol/l. On urinalysis there was glucose +++ in urine. A diagnosis of diabetic foot was made. The patient was placed on subcutaneous soluble insulin, haematinics, intravenous antibiotics, and analgesics. Wound swab microscopy, culture, and sensitivity were done. He was counselled for below knee amputation and to provide two units of blood as blood products where not available at the centre. He said he should be given time to think about the amputation. In the evening, he attempted suicide when his wife who raised alarm stopped him. He became depressed but later gave consent and the amputation was done.

Case 2 discussion: Diabetic foot results in a large increase in the use of general practice care and in the use of medical specialist care and hospital care [51]. This is the case in developing countries where most of the populace are poor and do not have assess to quality medical care. There are also limited specialist doctors. Patients with diabetes do not only have diabetes related co-morbidity but also have non-diabetes related co-morbidity such as depression and musculoskeletal diseases [51]. Depression can progress to attempted and actual suicide especially when an arm or limb needs to be amputated. Individuals with type 2 diabetes mellitus are known to have a higher prevalence of depression [63]. Depression is common in patients with diabetes mellitus [64]. Diabetes may increase risk of depression because of the sense of threat and loss associated with receiving this diagnosis and the substantial lifestyle changes necessary to avoid developing debilitating complications [65]. Patients with diabetes are more likely to experience depression than the general population and the presence of depression is associated with poor quality of life, increase in hyperglycaemia, health care utilization, risk of complications, functional impairment, and risk of mortality. The relationship between depression and worst outcomes in diabetes could be explained in part through depression relationship to poorer self-care and treatment adherence [66]. The patient was not depressed or attempted suicide until he was counselled for amputation. Amputation is the removal of a body extremity by trauma or surgery. As a surgical measure, it is used to control pain or a disease process in the affected limb such as malignancy or gangrene. The prevalence of depression is roughly twice as high among diabetic patients as among the general population. Depressed patients with diabetes have poorer glycaemic control, more severe diabetes symptoms and disability, added complications and higher health care use relative to patients with diabetes but on depression [67]. Psychological problems from limb amputation persistently retard rapid rehabilitation. Some diabetic foot ulcer patients shy away from attending the hospital for fear of amputation and eventually some of them die due to infections [68].

4.3. Case 3

A 49-year-old man known diabetic for more than two years with poor drug compliance on oral hypoglycaemic agents presented with complaints of fever, vomiting, polydipsia, weakness, and anorexia. A thorn pierced the big toe at the farm of two weeks prior to presentation. There was no feeling of pain at the time of impact and an ulcer developed after one week, which was worsening and not healing. The ulcer started discharging purulent fluid. He is a known hypertensive of five years duration not compliant with medications. On examination the patient was febrile temperature 38 [0] C, dehydrated, ill looking with periorbital oedema. There was right foot swelling with hypopigmentation, the right big toe was gangrenous and tied with a dirty bandage. Haemoglobin estimation was 10%. Electrolytes, urea, and creatinine were deranged. A diagnosis of diabetic nephropathy with diabetic foot was made. The patient was counselled for disarticulation of the big toe and was referred to a tertiary centre for possible dialysis and expert management.

Case 3 discussion: Diabetes mellitus is a chronic disease with a long-term macrovascular and microvascular complications including diabetic nephropathy, neuropathy and retinopathy [1]. Macrovascular complications such as stroke, heart disease, peripheral vascular disease and foot problems. Miocrovascular complications are diabetic eye diseases (retinopathy and cataracts), renal disease, erectile dysfunction, and peripheral neuropathy [68]. From various African studies, clinical diabetic nephropathy in Sudan 11.6% [69], 19% in 1971 in Nigeria [70], 46% in Kenya [71] and 6% in Ethiopia [72]. The exact cause of diabetic induced complications are not fully understood, the underlying factor that appears to make those with diabetes more prone to many health problems is prolonged and frequently elevation of blood sugar [14]. Diabetes mellitus is a complex metabolic disease that can have devastating effects on multiple organs in the body. It is the leading cause of end stage renal disease in the United States of America and is a common cause of vision loss, neuropathy, and cardiovascular diseases [73]. One of the most potentially serious complications regards neuropathy is when it is most severe can lead to amputation [74]. The effects of diabetes mellitus include long-term damage, dysfunction, and failure of various organs including the kidneys [69]. The prevalence of clinical nephropathy has been reported to be between 15 % and 40% generally in the developed countries [72].

4.4. Case 4

A 62-year-old woman known diabetic of eight years duration presented with injury to her left big toe after placing it over a hot object, which she did not know she stepped on a hot object. The toe was already gangrenous at the time of presentation. She had a right above knee amputation two years prior to presentation for gangrenous diabetic foot. She was counselled for disarticulation of the left toe. She refused and signed against medical advice.

Case 4 Discussion: Diabetes is an important cause of amputation of the lower limb resulting from of non-traumatic origin as well as blindness and kidney failure. Problems of the foot are the most frequent reason for hospitalization amongst patients who have diabetes. Many hospital visits due to diabetes related foot problems are preventable through simple foot care routine. Amongst people who have diabetes, amputations are reported to be 15 times more common than amongst other people. 50% of all amputations occur in people who have diabetes [74]. Diabetic ulcers are the most common foot lesions leading to lower extremity amputation [68]. Management of the diabetic foot requires a thorough knowledge of the major risk factors for amputation, frequent routine evaluation, and preventive maintenance. The aetiology of lower extremity diabetic ulcer includes injury complicated by underlying neuropathy, ischemia, or both [68]. Lower limb amputation remains one of the commonest surgical procedures. In a ten-year review from 1997-2006 of lower limb amputation at a Nigerian private tertiary hospital, 64 amputations were done due to gangrenous diabetic foot [75]. Foot lesions cause pain, morbidity, have substantial economic consequences beside the direct costs relating to loss of productivity, individual patients and family costs and loss of health related quality of life. The lifetime risk of a person with diabetes developing a foot ulcer could be as high as 25% and it is believed that every 30 seconds a lower limb is lost somewhere in the world because of diabetes. People with diabetes are prone to developing foot ulcer amputation and other lower extremity. Diabetic foot problems are a common occurrence throughout the world, resulting in major economic consequences for patients, their families, and society. Because foot ulcer are most likely to be of neuropathic origin they are eminently preventable in the developing countries that will experience the greatest increase in the prevalence of type 2 diabetes in the next 20 years [76]. People at the greatest risk of the ulceration can easily be identified by careful examination of the feet, education and frequent follow up is indicated in these patients [76]. Diabetic foot complications constitute an increased public health problem and are a leading cause of admission, amputation, and mortality in diabetic patients and yet since neuropathy is the major cause, they should be in many cases preventable. Early diagnosis, education, and treatment are crucial. Diabetic foot problem are common all over the globe and have major economic consequences to society, diabetic patients and their families [76]. The recurrence rates of foot ulcers are > 50% after 3 years, an important thing to remember when assessing the economic impact of diabetic foot disease. Cost of diabetic foot diseases therefore includes not only the immediate episode but also social services home care and subsequent ulcers [76]. Diabetic foot ulcers are associated with significant morbidity and mortality in individuals with diabetes mellitus. Diabetic foot ulcer is the leading cause of non-traumatic lower extremity amputations worldwide. Preceding events of diabetic foot ulcers include trauma, wearing ill-fitting shoes and burns [77]. When foot ulceration presents late and is most frequently associated with neuropathy and infections. The region of sub-Saharan Africa contains 33 of the 50 poorest countries in the world and will experience the greatest risk in the prevalence of diabetes over the next 20 years. Diabetic foot complications constitute an increasing public health problem and are a leading cause of admission, amputation and mortality in diabetic patients and yet since neuropathy is the major cause, they should been many cases preventable. Early diagnosis, education, and treatment are crucial. Educational programs must meet the specific needs of the patient, understanding their social background. An integrated approach to foot care can improve patients' outcomes even in rural areas. A review of the epidemiology of diabetic foot problems in Africa highlighted not only the frequency of neuropathy but also the increasing frequency of peripheral vascular disease, presumably in result of increasing urbanization. Diabetic foot is the most frequent cause of prolonged hospital admission in diabetic patients and is significantly a contributor to the considerable morbidity associated with the diabetic foot. Foot complications in Africa are mainly because of infection in the neuropathic foot rather than due to peripheral vascular disease. Although neuropathy is often the initiating factor for foot ulceration, ischemia is critically important in determining healing despite a relative low prevalence rate of peripheral vascular disease in diabetic patients with foot ulcers in Africa; amputation is a frequent outcome mainly due to uncontrolled infection. Several factors have been identified as greatly increasing the risk factors of neuropathy. Poverty and barefoot walking, inappropriate footwear, poor foot hygiene and delay in seeking medical attention [78].

Diabetic foot ulcers are estimated to affect 15% of all diabetics during their lifetime and precede almost 85% of all amputations. Diabetes by virtues of its complications like neuropathy and vasculopathy and other factors affect the musculoskeletal and soft tissue mechanics in a manner that elevates planter pressure and makes tissue damage more likely, causing non-resolving neuroischeamic ulcers at the weight bearing sites [79]. There is rising incidence of diabetic foot in Nigeria, which has recently become an important indication for lower limb amputation in Nigeria [80]. In a 15-year review in Nigeria, amputation following diabetic foot was the third indication of amputation 12.3% of diabetic gangrene [81]. Diabetics undergoing surgery belong to the high-risk group of patients. The risks are worst in the presence of severe complications such as diabetic foot gangrene. Foot problems are a major cause of hospital bed occupancy by diabetic patients. Early counselling and psychotherapy are necessary to avoid delayed consent for amputation [50]. Factors associated with poor outcomes include delays in seeking medical attention and ulcers that have progressed to gangrene at the time of presentation. In Africa, foot complications are the main cause of prolonged hospital stays for people with diabetes and are associated with substantial mortality, constituting a major public health problem[49]. In Tanzania, the highest mortality rates are observed in people with severe gangrenous ulcers not treated with aggressive surgery. Diabetic foot infection is a limb threatening complications and several studies have shown it to be the immediate cause of amputation in 25-50% of people with diabetes [49]. In sub-Saharan Africa, peripheral neuropathy is the principal underlying risk factor in the pathogenesis of foot ulcers in people with diabetes [49]. Foot infections usually begin in foot ulcers that are sequalae of existing neuropathy, macrovascular diseases, or certain metabolic disturbances. Risks of infection are exacerbated by the decrease in cellular immunity caused by acute hyperglycaemia and circulatory deficits caused by chronic hyperglycaemia. Diabetic foot infection is a limb threatening complication and several studies have shown it to be the immediate cause of amputation in 25-50% of people with diabetes [49]. In developing countries, increasing prevalence of diabetes and emergence of resistant strains of bacteria are among several factors related complications to the burden of infection related complications. Infection complications are noted among the commonest surgical presentations in diabetes foot. The diabetic patient has a greater susceptibility to infections that arise from several aspects of an altered immunity foot infections are a common problem in developing countries where diabetes mellitus is an emerging problem. The high incidence of undiagnosed diabetics poses a major public health challenge in developing countries. Amputations remain one of the key indications of severe diabetic foot disease.

5. Conclusion

Diabetes mellitus is a public health problem in developing countries and education should be a high priority intervention for all developing regions. Proper education regarding footwear and foot care is necessary in diabetics.

Author details

Omiepirisa Yvonne Buowari
Medical Women Association of Nigeria, Rivers State Branch, Nigeria

6. References

[1] Dahiru T, Jibo A, Hassan AA, Mande AT. Prevalence of diabetes in a semi-urban community in northern Nigeria. Nig J Med. 2008. 17 (4): 414-416.

[2] Mbanya JCN, Motala AA, Sobngwi E, Assah FK Enora ST. Diabetes in sub-Saharan Africa. Lancet 375. 2010.: 2254-2266. www.lancet.com

[3] Ogbera AO, Dada O, Adeleye F, Jewo PI. Complementary and alternative medicine use in diabetes mellitus. West Afr J Med. 2010. 29(3): 158-162.

[4] Adeleke SI, Asani MO, Belonwu RO, Gwarzo GD, Farouk ZL. Childhood diabetes mellitus in Kano, North West Nigeria. NIG J Med. 2010. 19(2): 145-147.

[5] French G. Clinical management of diabetes during anaesthesia and surgery. Update Anaesth. 2000. 11(13): 1-3.

[6] Definition, diagnosis, and classification of diabetes mellitus and its complications. Report of a World Health Organization consultation. Part 1: Diagnosis and classification of diabetes mellitus. WHO department of non-communicable disease surveillance. Geneva. 1999. www.who.int

[7] Kasiam LO, Long-Mbenza B, Nge OA, Kangola KN, Mbungu FS, Milongo DG. Classification and dramatic epidemic of diabetes mellitus in Kinshasa hinterland: the prominent role of type 2 diabetes and lifestyles changes among Africans. Nig J Med. 2009. 18(3): 311-320.

[8] Gohl D. Subjectively perceived barriers and resources for diabetes self-management by participants of a peer education project in Cambodia. Master Thesis. 2008. retrieved www.charite.de

[9] Alebiosu CO. Clinical diabetic nephropathy in a tropical African population. West Afr J Med. 2003. 22(2): 152-155.

[10] Issa BA, Baiyewu O. Quality of life of patients with diabetes mellitus in a Nigerian teaching hospital. Hong Kong J Psych. 2006. 16: 27-33.

[11] Balaji A. Quality of care among type 2 diabetes mellitus patients residing in an urban slum of Chennai Corporation: a community based cross sectional study. J Indian Med Assoc. 2011. 109(7): 462-4.

[12] Zafar J, Bhatti F, Aktar N, Rasheed U, Humayun S, Waheed A, Younus F et al. Prevalence and risk factor for diabetes mellitus in a selected urban population of a city Punjab. J Pakistan Med Assoc. 2011. 61(1): 40-7.
[13] Grover S, Avasthi A, Bhansali A, Chakrabartis S, Kulhura P. Cost of ambulatory care of diabetes mellitus: a study from north India. Postgrad Med J. 2005. 81(956): 391-395
[14] Nwafor A, Owhoji A. Prevalence of diabetes mellitus among Nigerians in Port Harcourt correlates with socio-economic status. J Appl Sci Environ Manag. 2001. 5(1): 75-77.
[15] Beran D, Yudkin JS, de Courten M. Access to care for patients with insulin requiring diabetes in developing countries: case studies of Mozambique and Zambia. Diabetes Care. 2005. 28(9): 2136-2140.
[16] Okafor CI, Ofoegbu EN. Indications and outcome of admissions of diabetic patients into the medical wards in a Nigerian tertiary hospital. Nig Med J. 2011. 52(2): 86-89.
[17] Chijioke A, Adamu AN, Makusidi AM. Mortality pattern among type 2 diabetes patients in Ilorin, Nigeria. JEMDSA. 2010. 15(2): 1-4.
[18] Wirth DP, Mitchell BJ. Complementary healing therapy for patients with type 1 diabetes mellitus. J Sci Explo. 1994. 8(3): 367-377.
[19] Omotoso ABO, Opadijo OG, Araoye MA. Hypertension and diabetes mellitus in Nigerians: a review of 572 patients. Nig J Med. 1999. 8(3): 108-111.
[20] Roglic G, Unwin N, Bennett PH, Mathers C, Tuomilehto J, Nag S, Cannolly V, King H. The burden of mortality attributable to diabetes: realistic estimates for the year 2000. Diabetes Care. 2005. 28(9): 2130-2135.
[21] O'Connor PJ, Crain AL, Rush WA, Hanson AM, Fisher LR, Kluznik JC. Does diabetes double the risk of depression? Ann Fam Med. 2009. 7(4): 328-335.
[22] Edo AE, Adediran OS. Carbohydrates in diabetic diet in Nigeria: is it evidence based? Nig J Gen Pract. 2006. 7(9): 19-23.
[23] Alberti H, Boudriga N, Nabli M. Primary care management of diabetes in a low /middle income country: a multi-method, qualitative study of barriers and facilitators to care. BMC Family Practice. 2007. 8:63. www.biomedcentral.com/1471-2296/8/63
[24] Kengne AP, Amoah AGB, Mbanya J. Cardiovascular complications of diabetes mellitus in sub-Saharan Africa. Circulation. 2005. 112(23): 3592-601.
[25] Cook AR. Notes on the diseases met with in Uganda, central Africa. J Trop Med. 1901. 4: 175-178.
[26] Gucciardi E, Wang SC, Demelo M, Amaral L, Stewart DE. Characteristics of men and women with diabetes: observations during patients' initial visit to an education centre. Can Fam Physician. 2008. 54 (2): 219-227.
[27] Evaristo-Neto AD, Foss-Freitas MC, Foss MC. Prevalence of diabetes mellitus and impaired glucose tolerance in a rural community of Angola. Diabetol Metab Synd. 2010. 2:63. www.dmsjournal.com/content/2/1/63
[28] Jeffrey S, Freeman DO. The increasing epidemiology of diabetes and review of current treatment algorithms. J Am Osteopathic Assoc. 2010. 110. 7(Suppl 7). Retrieved www.jaoa.org
[29] 1998 press release. Global burden of diabetes. Press release WHO/63.1998 in www.who.int

[30] Narayan KMV, Zhang P, Ramachandran A, Kanaya A, Imperatore G, Williams D, Engelgau M. How should developing countries manage diabetes: CMAJ. 2006. 175(7): 733-736.
[31] Levitt NS. Diabetes in Africa: epidemiology, management, and health care challenges. Heart. 2008. 94(11):1376-1382.
[32] Sobngwi E, Mauvais-Javis F, Vexiau F, Mbanya JC, Gautier JF. Diabetes in Africans. Part 1: Epidemiology and clinical specificities. Diabetes Metab. 2001. 27(6): 628-34.
[33] Majaliwa ES, Elusiyan BE, Adesiyun OO, Laigong P, Adeniran AK, Kandi CM et al. Type 1 diabetes mellitus in the African population: epidemiology, and management challenges. Acta Biomed. 2008. 79(3): 255-259.
[34] Owoaje EE, Rotimi CN, Kaufman JS, Tracy J, Cooper RS. Prevalence of adult diabetes in Ibadan, Nigeria. East Afr Med J. 1997. 74(5): 299-302.
[35] Bouguerra R, Alberti H, Salem LB, Rayana CB, Atti JE, Gaigi S et al. The global diabetes pandemic: The Tunisian experience. Eur J Clin Nutr. 2007. 61(2): 160-165.
[36] McLarty DG, Kitange HM, Mtinangi BL, Makane WJ, Swai AB, Masuki G et al. Prevalence of diabetes and imparted glucose tolerance in rural Tanzania. Lancet. 1989. 1 (8643): 871-875.
[37] Bakari AG, Onyemelukwe GC, Sani BG, Hassan SS, Aliyu TM. Prevalence of diabetes in suburban northern Nigeria, results of a public screening survey. Diabetes Int. 1999. 9:59-60.
[38] Erasmus RT, Ebonyi E, Fakeye C. Prevalence of diabetes mellitus in a rural Nigerian population. Nig Med Parct. 1988. 15:128-38.
[39] Fetugua M, Ogunlesi TA, Adekanbi AF, Olanrewaju DM. Clinical presentation of childhood diabetes mellitus in Olabisi Onabanjo University Hospital, Sagamu. Nig Hosp Pract. 2007. 1(3): 70-3.
[40] Anochie IC, Nkanginieme KEO. Childhood diabetes in Port Harcourt, southern Nigeria. Diabetes Int. 2002. 12: 20-21.
[41] Ajayi EA, Ajayi AO. Pattern and outcome of diabetic admission at a federal medical centre: a five-year review. Ann Afr Med. 2009. 8(4): 271-275.
[42] Unachukwu CN, Uchenna DI, Young E. Mortality among diabetes In-patients in Port Harcourt, Nigeria. Afr J Endo Metab. 2008. 7(1): 1-5.
[43] Ike SO. The pattern of admissions into the medical wards of the university of Nigeria teaching hospital, Enugu. Nig J Clin Pract. 2008. 11(3): 185-192.
[44] Osuafor TO, Ele PU. The pattern of admissions in the medical wards of Nnamdi Azikiwe University Teaching Hospital (NAUTH). Orient J Med. 2004. 16(1): 11-15.
[45] Asumanu E, Ametepi R, Koney CT. Audit of diabetic soft tissue and foot disease in Africa. West Afr J Med. 2010. 29(2): 86-90.
[46] Azevedo M, Alla S. Diabetes in sub-Saharan Africa: Kenya, Mali, Mozambique, Nigeria, South Africa, and Zambia. Int J Diabetes Dev Countries. 2008. 28(4): 101-108.
[47] The diabetic foot in sub-Saharan Africa: a new management paradigm. Wounds International. www.woundsinternational.com
[48] Ezike HA. Anaesthetic challenges in the surgical management of diabetic foot disease in Enugu. Niger Med J. 2008. 49(3): 59-62.

[49] Struijs JN, Baan CA, Schellevis FG, Westert GP, Geertrudis AM. Comorbidity in patients with diabetes mellitus: impart on medical health care utilization. BMC Health Serv Res. 2006. 6:84. doi 10.1186/1472-6963-6-84.

[50] Oreagba IA, Oshikoya KA, Amachree M. Herbal medicine use among urban residents in Lagos, Nigeria. BMC Complementary Alternative Med. 2011. 11:17 www.biomedcentral.com/1472-6882/11/117

[51] Al-Kindi RM, Al-Mushrafi M, Al-Rabaani M, Al-Zakwani I. Complementary, and alternative medicine use among adults with diabetes in Muscat region, Oman. Sultan Qaboos Uni Med J. 2011. 11(1): 62-68.

[52] Dham S, Shah V, Hirsch S, Banerji MA. The role of complementary and alternative medicine in diabetes. Current Diab Rep. 2006. 6(3): 251-8.

[53] Complementary and alternative medical therapies for diabetes. www.nccam.nih.gov

[54] Amira CO, Okubadejo NU. Frequency of complementary and alternative medicine utilization in hypertensive patients attending an urban tertiary care centre in Nigeria. BMC Complementary and alternative medicine. 2007. 7: 30 www.biomedcentral.com/1472-6882/7/30

[55] Abodunrin OL, Omojasola TP, Rojugboka OO. Utilization of alternative medical services in an urban centre of north central Nigeria. Nig Health J. 2011. 11(2): 51-55.

[56] Shapiro S, Rapaport R. The role of complementary and alterative therapies in paediatric diabetes. Endocrinol Metab Clin North Am. 2009. 38(4): 791-810.

[57] Dannemann K, Hecker W, Haberland H, Herbst A, Galler A, Schafer T, Brahler E at al. Use of complementary and alternative medicine in children with type 1 diabetes mellitus-prevalence, pattern of use and costs. Pediatr Diabetes. 2008. 9(3): 228-350.

[58] WHO media centre. Traditional medicine. 2008. Fact sheet N° 134. www.who.int/mediacentre/factsheets/fs/34/en

[59] Kaptchuk TJ, Eisenberg DM. The persuasive appeal of alternative medicine. Ann Intern Med. 1998. 129 (12):1061-1065.

[60] Astin JA. Why patients use alternative medicines: results of a national study. JAMA. 1998. 279(19): 1548-1553.

[61] Nguyen TT, Wong TY, Islam FM, Hubbard L, Miller J, Haroon E et al. Is depression associated with microvascular disease? Depress anxiety. 2008. 25(11): E158-62.

[62] Abrahamian H, Hofmann P, Prager R, Toplak H. Diabetes mellitus and co-morbid depression treatment with milnacipran results in significant improvement of both diseases (results from the Austrian MDDM study group). Neuropsychiatr Dis Treat. 2009. 5: 261-266.

[63] Mezuk B, Eaton WW, Albrecht S, Golden SH. Depression and type 2 diabetes over the lifespan: A meta-Analysis. Diabetes Care. 2008. 3(12): 2383-2390.

[64] Gonzalez JS, Peyrot M, McCart LA, Collins EM, Serpa L, Miniaga MJ, Safren S. Depression and diabetes treatment nonadherence: A meta-Analysis. Diabetes Care. 2008. 13(12): 2398-2403.

[65] Lin EHB, Katon W, Rutter C, Simon GE, Ludman EJ, Korff MV et al. Effects of enhanced depression treatment on diabetes self care. Ann Fam Med. 2006. 4(1): 46-53.

[66] Ikeh EI, Puepet F, Nwadiaro C. Studies on diabetic foot ulcers in patients at Jos University Teaching Hospital, Nigeria. Afr J Clin Experimental Microbiol. 2003. 4(2): 52-61.
[67] El Mahdi EM. Pattern of diabetes mellitus in the Sudan. Trop Geog Med. 1989. 41(4): 353-357.
[68] Osuntokun BO, Akinkugbe FM, Francis TI, Osuntokun O, Taylor GO. Diabetes mellitus in Nigerians: a study of 832 patients. West Afr Med J Niger Pract. 1971. 20(5):295-312.
[69] Abdullah MS. Diabetic nephropathy in Kenya. East Afr Med J. 1978. 55(11): 512-8.
[70] Lester FT. Clinical features complications and mortality in type 2 (non-insulin dependent) diabetic patients in Addis Abeba (1976-1990). Ethiopia Med J. 1993. 31(2): 109-126.
[71] Harper W. Diabetes Mellitus. www.drharper.ca
[72] Diabetes and amputation. www.diabetes.co.uk
[73] Obalum DC, Okeke GC. Lower limb amputation at a Nigerian private tertiary hospital. West Afr J Med. 2009. 28(1): 24-7.
[74] Boulton AJM. An Integrated Health Care Approach Is Needed: The Global Burden of Diabetic Foot Disease. Diabetic Microvascular Complications Today. 2006. 23-25.
[75] Edo AE, Eregie A, Ezeani UI. Diabetic foot ulcers following rat bites. Afr J Diabetes Med. 2010. 18(2): 19.
[76] Tesfaye S, Gill G. Chronic diabetic complications in Africa. Afr J diabetes Med. 2011.9(1): 37-40 www.africanjournalofdiabetesmedicine.com
[77] Gaur DS, Varma A, Gupta P. Diabetic foot in Uttaranchal. JK Sci. 2007. 9(1): 18-20.
[78] Solagberu BA. Diabetic foot in Nigeria-a review article. Afr J Med Med Sci. 2003. 32(2): 111-8.
[79] Thianni LO, Tade AO. Extremity amputation in Nigeria-a review of indications and mortality. Surgeon. 2007. 5(4): 213-7.

Chapter 9

Principles of Exercise and Its Role in the Management of Diabetes Mellitus

Yıldırım Çınar, Hakan Demirci and Ilhan Satman

Additional information is available at the end of the chapter

http://dx.doi.org/10.5772/50503

1. Introduction

It is known that a sedentary life style diminishes life expectancy and worsens existing chronic illnesses. Exercise not only promotes health but also prevents illness and can be used in the treatment of most of the well-known metabolic and chronic diseases. It reduces insulin resistance, helps regulate blood glucose, lowers uric acid and triglycerides and leads to an increase in the HDL/LDL cholesterol ratio [Banfi et al., 2012].

For a healthy beginner the intensity of the exercise should be at a specific percentage of their age-predicted maximum heart rate (calculated as 220 - age). A practical method to determine the appropriate exercise intensity is to use the "talk test" [Quinn, 2011]. This refers to an intensity of exercise that allows individuals to still talk to a partner exercising with them without any dyspnea. Individuals should slow down if they cannot speak to their partner comfortably.

Exercise is recommended for all patients with diabetes mellitus (DM) if there is no contraindication. However, it is important that they are educated regarding the impact of exercise on their blood glucose levels. Insulin dose adjustments are required when individuals with DM exercise to ensure that their plasma glucose levels are regulated. Exercise facilitates injected insulin absorption via increased blood flow to muscles and this may result in hypoglycemia. Therefore, the site of the insulin injection should not be the extremities or muscles contracting during exercise. The insulin response to exercise and hypoglycemia risk differs from one patient to the other and therefore individual evaluation and education is mandatory. Duration and intensity of exercise, injection placement, previous insulin dose and timing determines patients' insulin requirements when they exercise.

Patients with diabetes mellitus are advised to carry an identity card or a bracelet indicating that they are diabetic, especially when they are exercising alone.

2. Healthy life

A healthy life can be maintained by following all the recommendations that help protect against the development of metabolic and non-communicable diseases (NCD) (chronic diseases). There are a number of studies advising exercise and dietary interventions to maintain wellness [ADA, 2008 & Scott, 2005]. It is known that a sedentary life style worsens cardiopulmonary capacity and existing chronic illnesses and diminishes life expectancy. A number of studies have investigated the optimal exercise model for preventing or reducing NCDs, including the type, duration, intensity and mode of exercise [Jeon et al., 2006 & Kruger et al., 2009]. It is important that exercise programming is individualized.

3. Definitions of physical activity exercise and sports

Examples of physical activity are occupational activities and walking slowly (lower than 80 steps per minute) for short periods [Ogilvie et al., 2007]. Although physical activity refers to body movements that require active muscle contraction and energy expenditure, the effects of regular daily activity on metabolism and physiological capacity are different and less than those of exercise.

Exercise is defined as body movements that are planned and organized. These are whole body or selected muscle group movements that are performed regularly with the aim of achieving a specific level of fitness. When investigating the effects of exercise on an individual it is important to consider their physiological capacity, eating habits and life style. Regular exercise helps regulate blood glucose levels independently from its weight-loss effect [Boule et al., 2001]. The exercise-induced increase in lean muscle mass may be responsible for the reduced weight-loss. The duration of exercise is regulated based on the intensity of exercise and how it impacts on thermoregulation, cardiopulmonary capacity and fatigue. A short exercise period can be performed as part of a warm up to enhance sports performance.

Currently, the words exercise and sports are incorrectly used interchangeably. Exercise refers to planned and provoked body movements that can be modified according to personal daily conditions and medical aims. Sport refers to a specific sport ritual with its accompanying rules and mandatory time and may be performed at a recreational or competitive level. Swimming is an exercise however it is also a sport and may be performed competitively according to time or distance. The energy expenditure and intensity of movement is not regulated for individual wellness during sports, unlike exercise where there is usually a "prescription". Sports may become a cultural subject and have intellectual benefits in addition to positive effects on physical and moral capacities.

In medicine, exercise is considered to be all the activities that are measurable; where gains and losses can be calculated; and where intensity, duration and mode can be planned according to needs of the person.

4. Physiological and metabolic effects of exercise

It is well known that exercise affects both physiological and metabolic mechanisms of humans. Through these mechanisms, exercise not only promotes health but can be used as "medicine" to prevent and treat various diseases including NCDs.

4.1. Cardiac and pulmonary diseases

In relation to cardiac and pulmonary diseases; exercise results in physiological myocardial hypertrophy that is accompanied by an increase in stroke volume, slower heart rate and improved collateral circulation [Burton et al., 2004]. It also promotes an increase in respiratory capacity that is accompanied by increased O_2 transport, a considerable decrease in peripheral vascular resistance and diastolic blood pressure, increased fibrinolytic activity, and increased sarcolemma and myoglobin in muscles. In addition, exercise may strengthen the rectus abdominus muscle that helps to increase endurance capacity and protect against postural hypotension. Patients suffering from respiratory distress have demonstrated a considerable recovery with the help of respiratory muscle exercises [Cinar et al., 2011].

4.2. Endocrinology and metabolism

Most diseases, especially malignancies, have catabolic effects on the body. Exercise has an anabolic effect and the positive effect of exercise on appetite has been suggested as an explanation for its anabolic effect. However, exercise does not always result in an increased appetite. Exercise has been shown to normalize the appetite as well as reduce the excess drive for feeding. Therefore, exercise has regulator effect on abnormal appetites [Hopkins et al., 2010]. Exercise reduces insulin resistance, helps regulate blood glucose, lowers uric acid and triglycerides and leads to an increase in the HDL/LDL cholesterol ratio, glycogen stores, cortisol and growth hormone secretion [Banfi et al., 2012]. Although exercise facilitates glycolysis and increases the transport of glucose into the muscle cell, hypoglycemia is rarely seen in non-diabetics. Blood glucose level is regulated hormonally during prolonged exercise or when blood glucose levels are low. Specifically, glucagon and catecholamines increase while insulin secretion diminishes and the liver continues to release glucose.

4.3. Obesity and weight control

Health professionals recommend a combination of exercise, diet and lifestyle changes for weight-loss. Weight loss obtained solely from exercise is negligible. Energy expenditure during a single, acute, 60 minute bout of exercise does not result in significant weight-loss. For example, a person with a mass of 70 kg and a height of 170 cm, walking at 80 steps per minute, will expend approximately 100 kcal in an hour, the amount of kcals found in three average sized apples or 25 grams of carbohydrate or 11 grams of butter. A reduction in body-weight after exercise typically reflects water loss because of sweating and urination. A fat loss of 700 kcal (1 gram fat equal to 9kcal) due to aerobic exercise is preferable to a 700 kcal food restriction, although this kind of heavy exercise is not suitable for most individuals. Therefore, in most situations, the exercise, dietary and lifestyle habits of individuals need to be planned to optimize weight and weight-loss. It is important that weight-loss reflecting a reduction in fat mass should be monitored over time, for example monthly, rather than over a few hours or days.

4.4. Metabolic syndrome

Increased and inappropriate eating behavior and a lack of physical activity is associated with the metabolic syndrome. Insulin resistance, obesity, hypertension, dyslipidemia and stroke are associated with this syndrome. Exercise has been shown to protect individuals from developing metabolic syndrome that could be result in DM [Onat, 2011].

4.5. Musculoskeletal diseases

Exercise is important for musculoskeletal strength maintenance and the prevention of postural abnormalities. Growing children should be advised to exercise. The majority of the postural abnormalities in adulthood are related to muscular weakness.

4.6. Osteoporosis

Sedentary behavior is one of the leading causes of osteoporosis. Physicians recommend exercise, dietary and supplement alterations as well as sunlight exposure to prevent and treat osteoporosis. Exercise has been shown to increase or maintain bone density [Iwamoto, 2011].

4.7. Mental health

Exercise reduces depression, increases optimism and regulates biorhythms. Research has suggested that group exercise and physical activity have benefits on psychological wellness [Tordeurs et al., 2011].

5. Medical evaluation as a part of exercise planning

Cardiac output increases in parallel to exercise intensity. During exercise, there is a redistribution of the cardiac output, with an increased blood flow to the contracting, exercising muscles and a reduction in flow to other organs, for example the gastrointestinal system. Performing exercise while experiencing increased blood flow to the gastrointestinal system due to a heavy meal, results in a circulatory burden. The energy expenditure of food digestion depends on the nature of the meal. The process of protein and carbohydrate digestion increases energy expenditure. Therefore, eating, particular protein and fried food, just before exercise should be avoided. Dietary consultation is recommended prior to participation in exercise of different modalities and intensities.

Exercise is influenced negatively by the following factors; an acute increased circulatory burden when performing resistance exercise, unsuitable durations and intensity of endurance exercise, inappropriate clothing and shoes, poor environmental conditions, inadequate healing of existing injuries, inadequate warm-up, heavy meals before exercise, and fatigue (Table 1).

1.	Acute circulatory burden
2.	Unsuitable exercise planning
3.	Inappropriate wearing
4.	Environmental conditions
5.	Inadequate warm-up
6.	Heavy meals before exercise
7.	Fatigue

Table 1. Factors negatively affecting exercise

The present and past health status of individuals, together with their exercise history, should be determined before they participate in exercise. Individuals with a history of hypertension, DM and coronary artery disease should undergo a more in-depth examination. American College of Cardiology (ACC) and American Heart Association (AHA) guidelines recommends that men ≥40 years and women ≥50 years who would like to perform heavy exercise must undergo an exercise stress test that is supervised by a physician [ACC/AHA, 1997]. Individuals who did not participate in exercise until the age of 20 years should be advised not to perform heavy exercise, but rather light aerobic exercise, at the start of an exercise program. In such individuals, there will be an improvement in physical capacity, including metabolic adaptations, although the degree of cardiovascular adaptations is unclear. In more experienced individuals, such as marathon runners, they may have hypertrophied myocardial muscles with the diameter of their coronary arteries being larger than that of normal. However, these changes may be because of heavy training. Exercise performed at a mild to moderate intensity may result in these beneficial, physiological adaptations.

For individuals at risk, ECG and blood pressure evaluations should be performed by a physician before the individual participates in an exercise program. A treadmill stress test is recommended for these individuals. Pre-participation medical evaluations are required for pregnant women, women with history of gestational diabetes mellitus (GDM), diagnosis of DM before the age of 40 years, myocardial infarction (MI) and stroke, hypertension, dyslipidemia, smoking, and family history of premature death. Persons who experience palpitations, tachycardia, sweating and dyspnea at the beginning of exercise may be at risk need to be examined.

The American Heart Association (AHA) and the American College of Sports Medicine (ACSM) has a pre-participation screening questionnaire that should be used to determine whether individuals can start exercising or should have a medical examination prior to starting an exercise program. It is called the **AHA/ACSM Health/Fitness Facility Preparticipation Screening Questionnaire** (http://www.wm.edu./offices/recsports/documents/fitnessquestionnaire.pdf).

5.1. Recommendations for medical evaluations

If there are no contraindications, for example arterial insufficiency, then exercise should be encouraged as long as a diabetic is educated regarding the effects of exercise on blood glucose levels and how to regulate their glucose levels when exercising. Patients that have severe arterial problems like angina pectoris, claudication or proliferative retinopathy should not perform heavy exercise. Exercise-induced pain, early fatigue, difficulty in breathing, tachycardia, excessive sweating, patients prone to hypoglycemia, prolonged tiredness after exercise are all signs that require evaluation and a decision should be made as to whether the individual should continue exercising. In these cases, physicians should check if there is a severe underlying medical illness (Table 2).

1. Angina pectoris
2. Retinopathy
3. Hypoglycemia attacks
4. Respiratory problems
5. Early fatigue
6. Tachycardia

Table 2. Whom to evaluate?

Individuals should be encouraged to start an exercise program and improve their wellness as this will enhance their quality of life. Physicians should ensure that they have an understanding of the effect of exercise that they "prescribe" for medically ill patients. Consideration of the disease and medical history will reduce the risk of harm, and enhance the benefits of the exercise.

5.2. Contraindications for exercise

Patients using insulin and who are at risk for hypoglycemia should avoid solitary sports like mountain climbing or diving. In addition, if the hypoglycemia is uncontrolled, this is also a contraindication for exercise. High intensity exercise is not recommended for individuals with proliferative retinopathy as the risk of hemorrhage increases [Sigal et al., 2006]. For patients with a history of coronary artery disease or if there is suspicion of coronary artery disease, a consultation with a specialist is required prior to starting an exercise program. To estimate coronary artery disease risk, calculation instruments are present and there is one available on the American Diabetes Association web site: (American Diabetes Association's Diabetes PHD (Personal Health Decisions) (http://diabetes.org/diabetesPHD).

Individuals suffering from severe peripheral neuropathy should be advised about their risk of injury during exercise. For example, they may have balance problems or difficulty in walking that places them at risk for falling. Patients that experience postural hypotension, induced by autonomic neuropathy or dehydration (related to severe sweating) must be evaluated medically prior to exercise participation. Although high intensity exercise does not cause microalbuminuria, it is not usually recommended as it may cause slight but transient proteinuria. There is currently no consensus regarding whether exercise-induced proteinuria causes renal impairment. Albumin is typically not found in urine after exercise unless there is a glomerular damage.

6. Exercise prescription

Before beginning an exercise program, balance, flexibility, joint pathology, muscle strength and stability should be examined, with precautions taken to prevent the occurrence of injuries. If possible, it is recommended that light strengthening exercises should be performed prior to the start of the exercise program. Without examining the above parameters it is possible that individuals will not cope with a structured exercise program and may become de-motivated and drop-out.

For the elderly and other individuals who struggle with ambulation, non-weight bearing exercises are recommended initially, for example riding a bicycle, swimming or light exercise in the water. These activities will enhance their exercise capacity. For other individuals, weight-bearing exercises such as walking, jogging, or rhythmic group dancing are recommended.

Walking is the preferred exercise modality as it is cheap and easy to perform. When starting an exercise program, this may be the exercise of choice. However, as individuals increase their fitness, and as their compliance to the exercise improves, different exercises may be introduced to strengthen weak muscles. For example, if the individual walks at work, their lower limbs may receive enough exercise and a physician may recommend exercises aimed at strengthening the rectus abdominus and diaphragm muscles to improve pulmonary capacity. Improving exercise capacity through walking and strengthening the rectus abdominus reduces fatigue and improves recovery time after exercise. Patients suffering from neuropathic pain and who have problems with their lower extremities may prefer swimming, cycling at home or exercises performed while sitting (Figure 1).

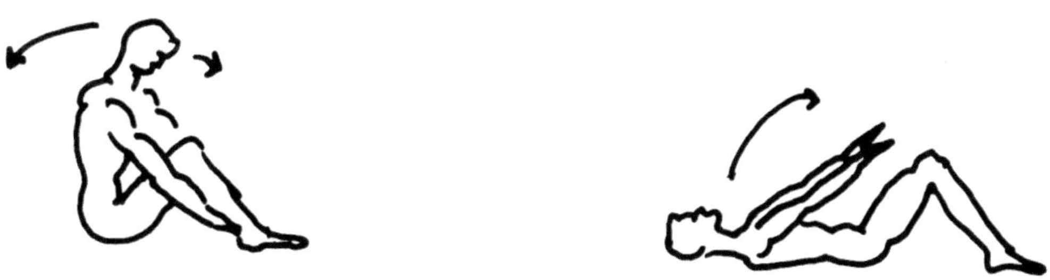

Figure 1. Twist sit-up can easily be performed by anyone.

In healthy individuals, an approximately 25% increase in exercise capacity is possible by the end of three months of training. To ensure improvements in capacity, the exercise program must include the principle of progressive overload. Intensity and duration of the exercise should be altered and other muscle groups may be included in the program at the appropriate time to ensure progression. Patients should be advised how and when to change their programs. The introduction of more intense, longer duration or new exercises will ensure continued adaptations and will improve program compliance.

7. Loading, progression and frequency of exercise

The exercise program must take into account personal preferences in terms of the mode of exercise, the venue and the capacity of the individual.

7.1. Phases of an exercise program

The first 5-10 minutes of an exercise session is the warm-up phase that prepares individuals for the main conditioning phase of the session. The second conditioning phase includes 20-40 minutes of continuous exercise that is performed at a specific intensity. The final third phase is the cool down period that lasts for 5-10 minutes (Table 3). It is crucial that an individual performs the warm-up and cool-down phases to ensure adequate preparation and recovery from exercise, respectively. The cool-down ensures adequate recovery of metabolic, cardiovascular, and neuroendocrine responses to within a normal range. If the individual cannot perform the exercise continuously it can be broken-up into intervals of exercise separated by rest periods or a reduced intensity.

1. **Warm-up**: 5-10 minutes
2. **Conditioning:** 20-40 minutes
3. **Cool-down:** 5-10 minutes

Table 3. Three phases of an average exercise

7.2. Intensity, duration and frequency of exercise

Exercise plays an important role in health promotion and the maintenance of health. The intensity of exercise is regulated according to age, environmental conditions, physical capacity, the general health of the patient, as well as the aims of the program. The aims may include increasing endurance capacity, muscle strengthening, targeting of specific organ systems like the respiratory system, decreasing insulin resistance and weight-loss or weight maintenance.

For novice exercisers the program should promote health and ensure that the individuals remain motivated. The movements required during the initial phases of the program should be easy to perform and evoke a sensation of wellness and success. It is recommended that patients with diabetes perform life-long exercise if they have no contraindications and therefore they should find it easy to adapt to the exercise and the movements and goals should be achievable. Difficult exercise programs that are difficult to adapt should be avoided.

There are various opinions regarding the most appropriate exercise recommendations for healthy subjects. In general, aerobic exercise performed 3-5 times per week for no more than 20-40 minutes is advised. Up to 150 minutes of exercise (30 minutes/day) per week has been suggested to play a role in developing fitness and promoting health. As mentioned in the previous section, each exercise session that aims to improve cardiovascular adaptations, starts with light movements during the warm-up phase that aims to prepare the body for exercise. This is then followed by 20-40 minutes of the main conditioning phase followed by a short period of cooling down. It is generally accepted that exercise time less than 20 minutes is not adequate for muscle (increased sarcolemma) or vascular adaptations (including coronary arteries) that include the stimulation of angiogenesis. The AHA recommends daily, moderate intensity exercise that lasts for 30 minutes or more. It takes time to achieve this recommendation, and therefore each exercise program should be individualized.

Generally, the method used to prescribe exercise intensity is to base each session on a specific percentage of an individual's age-predicted maximum heart rate. However, the use of this prediction may be dangerous for some people. For a healthy beginner, prediction of their maximum heart rate can be determined using 220 - age. In addition, a safe low to moderate intensity exercise target heart rate could be calculated using 160 - age. To improve endurance capacity the target heart rate could be calculated as 180 - age. It is difficult to measure heart rate during exercise if one is not using a portable heart rate monitor. A simple method of monitoring heart rate during exercise is to use the "talk test" [Quinn, 2011]. This refers to an intensity of exercise that allows an individual to talk (without dyspnea) to a partner exercising with them. The individual should slow down if they cannot speak comfortably to their partner. This simple method is recommended to regulate heart rate during exercise and to reduce the stress of worrying about heart rate in novice exercisers. Generally, if it is difficult to talk during exercise, this suggests that there is either a cardiovascular problem or in most cases hyperventilation due to lactic acid increase in circulation and metabolic acidosis related to anaerobic exercise. This "talk test" is especially important for individuals that have any kind of disease as well as elderly individuals in order to ensure that they perform exercise at a low to moderate intensity to minimize cardiac risks.

The metabolic equivalent (MET) unit is used to represent exercise intensity. One MET represents 3.5 mL O_2 uptake (oxygen consumption) per kg of muscle mass and is considered to be the metabolic rate of an individual at rest. Playing golf or walking at 4.5-6 km/hr is equal to 3-5 METs. A person weighting 70 kg, with a step length of 75 cm, walking 80 steps per minute (3.6 km/hr) will expend an additional 100 kcal/hr of energy [Porter et al., 2011]. Energy consumption will increase when walking speed increases. Playing tennis against a partner is equal to about 5-7 METs. Heavy occupational activity or walking/running at 9-10 km/hr is the equivalent of 9 METs. Moderate intensity exercise is considered to be 3-6 METs with the equivalent heart rate being 50-60% of maximal heart rate. High intensity or vigorous exercise is considered to be greater than 6 METs with the equivalent heart rate being ≥70% of maximum.

To ensure that the recommended caloric equivalents for healthy individuals are achieved, daily 20 minutes efforts (for 150 kcal energy consumption) excluding warming or 60 minutes efforts (for 300 kcal energy consumption) including warm-up are recommended. Personal health conditions, training experience, physiological and metabolic capacity, age, level of fatigue experienced, aims of the program should all be taken into account when planning the exercise program. With time, alterations will be made in the program to ensure appropriate adaptations. It is important that education is provided to individuals regarding the planning and application of exercise.

A primary benefit of exercise training is the reduction of insulin resistance. A break from exercise that is longer than two days is not recommended in these patients because the exercise-induced insulin sensitization lasts for no longer than 72 hours after an exercise bout. If exercise is stopped for longer than 1-2 weeks then a new exercise program should be developed that takes into account that a level of detraining may have occurred. Therefore, the first week of exercise should be of a light to moderate intensity and shorter in duration to ensure that the individual does not start exercising too hard.

7.3. Exercise progression

Intensity, duration, and frequency of an exercise are increased slowly over a number of months to ensure that individuals continue to benefit from the program. The planning of the exercise progression should have the aim of ensuring that the individual does not experience excessive fatigue but experiences an increase in aerobic exercise capacity.

8. Exercise associated physiological and environmental conditions

8.1. Diabetes mellitus and food supplementation

Conditions differ for patients with type 1 and type 2 DM as well as for insulin using type 2 DM patients. Insulin dose adjustments are required when individuals with DM exercise to ensure that their plasma glucose levels are regulated. For example, a plasma glucose level of 200 mg/dL may decrease by 40-60 mg/dL after an hour of walking. This effect of exercise places patients with DM in a vulnerable situation if their glucose levels are not regulated suitably. A decrease in plasma glucose triggers counter mechanisms to increase plasma glucose and therefore exercise can only drop plasma glucose if there is hyperglycemia. However, individuals who have a tendency towards developing hypoglycemia are advised to perform exercise after eating appropriate food so that they can perform exercise without the risk of developing hypoglycemia.

8.2. Water supplementation and exercise

As water loss may cause fatigue and a decreased motivation to exercise, hydration practices before and during exercise must be taught. During exercise individuals should not drink more than one glass of water. Drinking a large amount of water may cause a full stomach. This in turn causes a redistribution of blood flow to the stomach that induces cardiac burden and a sensation of fatigue. It is recommended that appropriate amounts of water and food are consumed 30 minutes before exercise. If the individual gets thirsty during exercise, small amounts (100-200 mL/15 minutes) of water can be drunk at intervals. This will also help prevent an excessive rise in core temperature during the exercise. The amount of water lost in sweat is difficult to estimate during exercise due to the associations between climate, clothing and individual characteristics. However, individuals are advised to check their weight-loss as a measure of fluid-loss and restore the lost water by drinking after exercise. A marathon runner may experience core temperatures of 38.5°C, similar to that of a fever, and may lose one liter of water per hour through sweating [Cheuvront, 2001]. After competitive exercise, it takes 2-4 days to replace lost water. One reason for this delay is the time it takes to distribute water to the intracellular and extracellular compartments. For these reasons, the amount of water lost during exercise should be monitored and precautions should be taken to maintain a healthy hydration status during exercise. Weighing individuals before and after exercise may help determine whether fatigue is related to water loss or because of anaerobic metabolism due to the exercise being too strenuous. Sweating also results in a loss of salts (NaCl) leading to a sensation of fatigue and discomfort. During summer and in hot climates excessive sweating should be avoided and unsuitable clothing that prevents heat loss should be avoided. Exercising individuals should replace the salt that is lost. Another problem is that the recommendation for restriction of salt intake is sometimes misunderstood and patients unfortunately stop salt intake. Salt intake must be in equilibrium and if salt intake is largely changed, it takes two months for the kidneys to adapt via tubular re-absorption. Salt depletion may result in fatigue and an increased consumption of sodium rich products like cola, salty biscuits, and adding extra salt to meals.

8.3. Environmental conditions

Hot, cold, windy or rainy conditions result in an extra circulatory burden and are not suitable for walking and sports performed outdoors. Exercise performed in the morning is more beneficial. Heavy exercise performed late in the evening increases metabolism and possibly disturbs sleeping patterns. Walking on level ground is preferred. Patients with DM should also avoid sudden increases in running speed to avoid sudden stress being placed on the cardiovascular system. Therefore, football is not a recommended sport for patients with DM. However, there are well-known insulin using professional football players with DM. Activities such as walking, swimming and tennis requiring whole body movements are preferable. The exercise area must also be clean, private and comfortable. Group sports may add to the enjoyment and improve group dynamics as well as have beneficial psychological effects.

8.4. Clothing

Clothing must be light, allowing the skin to breathe and to help sweat transfer away from the body and preferably be made from cotton. Socks made from cotton may keep the sweat inside the shoe and therefore are not appropriate. Thin wool socks transfer sweat and keep the foot dry thereby preventing injuries. Shoes that allow the foot to breathe and have a hard base, preventing unnecessary horizontal flexion but allowing slight vertical compression at the heel are recommended. Patients with neuropathy as well as the elderly should wear boots that support the ankles. This is because these individuals are more prone to early fatigue and they have difficulty in maintaining appropriate foot control. Using slightly compressible red soil tracks diminishes joint injury risk. However, it is not always possible to use such tracks, where it is advised to wear suitable shoes that have compressible heels. Persons with diabetes should not exercise wearing clothing such as nylon wind jackets because these prevent the skin from "breathing" and may cause excessive sweating during the exercise. Exercising in hot environments places an extra stress on the body, and it is recommended that when exercising on hot sunny days that sunglasses and a hat are worn.

9. What kind of exercise to prescribe?

9.1. Aerobic exercise

Aerobic exercise promotes health and wellbeing. Aerobic exercise conditions the aerobic energy system to ensure that enough energy can be produced for movement by oxidative metabolism. During aerobic exercise, glucose, amino acid and fatty acid oxidation take place within the mitochondria. Fatty acid is transported into mitochondria via carnitine and degradation to acetyl-CoA occurs via beta oxidation. Glycolysis converts glucose into pyruvate and with the presence of oxygen in cells pyruvate is oxidized to acetyl-CoA. Fatty acids and glucose converted into acetyl-CoA that enters the citric acid cycle and oxidized to CO_2. Amino acid degradation also results in the formation of acetyl-CoA that also enters in the citric acid cycle. The chemical energy that is produced during these reactions is used for production of adenosine triphosphate (ATP). However, under anaerobic conditions (during high intensity exercise), glucose is converted into pyruvate in the cytoplasm, in the absence of oxidative metabolism. ATP synthesis in mitochondria is not available in the absence of oxygen and pyruvate does not enter the mitochondria. The result is that there is an increase in Nicotinamide adenine dinucleotide (NADH) in the cytoplasm, with the accumulated pyruvate in the cytoplasm being converted to lactic acid. Under anaerobic conditions the energy system works without oxygen and there is an increase in lactic acid that causes metabolic acidosis, fatigue, tachypnea and possibly sensation of dyspnea.

Studies on cardiopulmonary exercise test have shown that anaerobic metabolism increases, together with an accumulation of blood lactate, at an oxygen consumption of approximately 40-60% of maximal aerobic capacity (VO_{2max}) or a heart rate of 50-70% of maximal heart rate [Quinn, 2011]. To compensate for the increase in lactate and consequently increased CO_2 resulting in metabolic acidosis, hyperventilation occurs to release the excess CO_2. Hyperventilation and dyspnea can be used in a practical setting to guide exercise intensity. When dyspnea occurs, this may suggest that there is an increase in anaerobic metabolism and individuals should reduce their exercise intensity. The intensity of exercise that anaerobic metabolism occurs can be determined through an exercise test with gas analysis.

Overtraining, including exercising frequently at high intensities should be avoided by individuals who are not training for competition as well as individuals seeking health, fitness or weight-loss. Examples of aerobic exercise include walking and cycling. These exercises can be performed comfortably for long durations to improve fitness. Aerobic exercise enhances heart health and prevents the development of osteoporosis. When an individual experiences hyperventilation and a loss of concentration during exercise this may suggests an increase in anaerobic metabolism. High intensity or vigorous exercise causes an increase in the production of energy from anaerobic metabolism because energy production from the aerobic energy system is insufficient. The anaerobic energy system is most active during high intensity, short duration exercise. For comfortable and healthy exercise, individuals should avoid intensive exercise that activates the anaerobic energy system. Sprinting, weightlifting and heavy physical activities all require anaerobic metabolism.

9.2. Flexibility exercise

Keeping joints flexible and improving flexibility are important for the rehabilitation of bed-ridden patients as well as the elderly. Warm-up and flexibility exercises help decrease the risk of injury during exercise. Following a suitable warm-up, soft and slow movements have a beneficial effect on muscle length and result in an improvement in joint range-of-motion. This in turn may correct body posture.

Flexion movements are recommended only when the body has undergone a warm-up condition. The warm-up will reduce muscle viscosity and increase flexibility and therefore reduce the risk of injury from flexion movements. This is the reason why experienced sportsmen continue to move and try to keep warm when a game is interrupted for a short period at any stage.

9.3. Resistance exercise for strength

Isometric contractions: These are contractions where force is generated in the muscle but there is no lengthening or shortening of the muscle. In addition, the object that the force is being applied to does not move. This type of contraction enables a better muscle contraction compared with weightlifting. Pushing the head against the stable hands is an isometric contraction and strengthens the neck muscles. These contractions are recommended in cases where joints movements are not indicated. Advantages include a low risk for injury as well as no equipment required (Figure 2).

Isotonic contractions: These are the typical weight-lifting movement where the mass of the object being lifted remains constant. This contraction is produced by lengthening and shortening of muscles (Figure3).

Isokinetic contractions: Measured using an isokinetic dynamometer. The speed of the contraction is regulated and kept constant however there is accommodating resistance (Figure 4). Isotonic and isokinetic exercises are preferred for elderly people. Isometric exercises increase blood pressure and cardiac burden.

During resistance exercise, the anaerobic energy system is dominant and there is an increase in both muscle mass and strength. Muscle and liver glycogen stores are also increased. If the exercise includes resistance or strength training, then the session should include 1-3 sets of 10-20 repetitions, with 20- 60 second rests between sets without allowing the individual to "cool-down". The rest periods between the sets should be adequate to ensure recovery (gaining power again) prior to the start of the next set. By the end of the exercise session the individual should feel a slight tiredness and must be satisfied with the exercise. Excessive tiredness should be avoided to ensure adherence to the exercise program. Well-known contraindications for exercise are listed in Table 4.

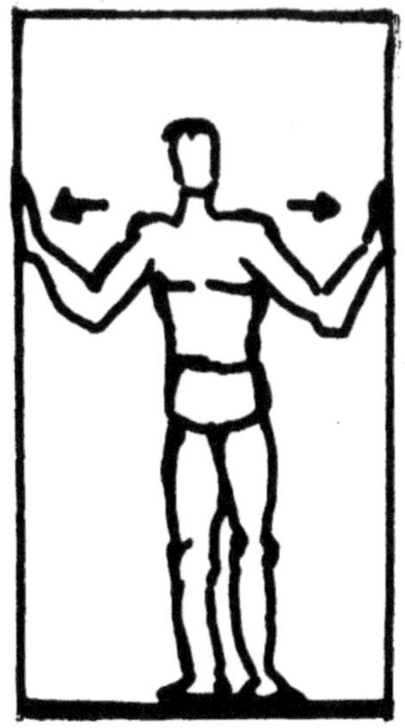

Figure 2. Isometric exercise (wall press)

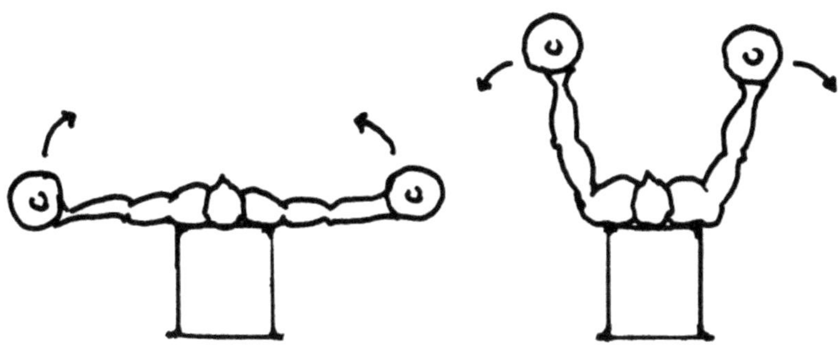

Figure 3. Isotonic exercise (pectoral strengthening)

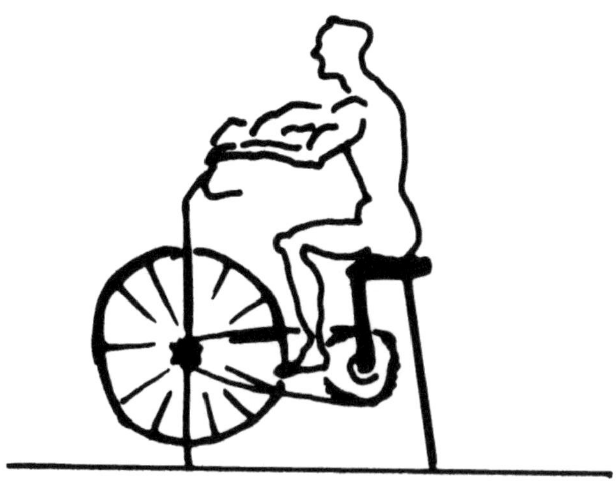

Figure 4. Isokinetic exercise (stationary bicycle)

For beginners a strength training program that includes of 1-3 sets of 8-12 repetitions of all the major muscle groups is recommended. The program may then be adjusted according to how the individual adapts. To prevent early fatigue it is important that the muscle group being exercised is considered. For example, to prevent fatigue in one muscle group, the exercise prescription recommended is 3 sets of 3 types of exercise, rather than 9 sets of one type of exercise.

1.	Excessive tiredness
2.	Hunger
3.	Cold sweating
4.	Tachycardia
5.	Dizziness
6.	Nausea and vomiting
7.	Respiration difficulty
8.	Chest pain or heaviness on the chest
9.	Impaired consciousness
10.	Excessive sweating and feeling of excessive mouth dryness.
11.	Pain at any location or sensation of cramping
12.	Balance impairment
13.	Blurred vision
14.	Low back pain or bleeding during pregnancy
15.	Fatigue
16.	Hypoglycemia
17.	Dehydration
18.	Uncontrolled hypertension
19.	Arrhythmia with syncope
20.	Unhealed injuries

Table 4. Contraindications for exercise

10. Diabetes and exercise

Exercise is recommended for all patients with DM if there is no contraindication however, it is important that they are educated regarding the impact of the exercise on their blood glucose levels. An exercise program consisting of at least 30 minutes of exercise 5 days per week (150 minutes/week) is recommended. As mentioned previously, each session would start with a 5-10 minute warm-up, followed by a conditioning period of 20-40 minutes of aerobic exercise, and then ending with 5-10 minutes of cool-down. All patients should be encouraged to be more physically active during the day. Walking is advised, rather than driving, for individual who live close to work. In addition, spending more time in the garden should be recommended. Sudden effort loading movements like climbing may activate anaerobic metabolism and ischemia and should be avoided.

Depending on the type of diabetes as well as the exercise session planned, consideration must be given to appropriate caloric intake before exercise. At the beginning of an exercise session, energy is obtained from glycogen stores. A normal liver stores about 200 grams of glycogen. During prolonged exercise, glucose and fatty acids produced by the liver are used. However, exercise that lasts for 2-3 hours results in a reduction in glycogen stores and hypoglycemia may occur. If the depletion is treated by consuming glucose containing food like honey or jam then hyperinsulinemia may be experienced within 30 minutes resulting in a second hypoglycemic response. Walking at an average speed of 80 feet/min will only result in 100 kcal being expended per hour, while vigorous exercise results in an energy expenditure of 700 kcal in an hour. During comfortable walking, consumption of 20-40 grams of carbohydrate can maintain blood glucose levels. Prolonged exercises may cause an inhibition of insulin secretion and may stimulate counter regulatory hormones. Glucose transport into muscle cells is facilitated by muscle contraction. Hypoglycemia may occur at any time during exercise. After vigorous exercise, while the muscle and liver are replacing their glycogen and energy stores, hypoglycemia may occur in the periphery up to 24 hours after the exercise. Therefore, appropriate caloric intake should be maintained after vigorous exercise and insulin dose adjustments may be required.

10.1. Exercise for patients with type 2 diabetes mellitus

Exercise is recommended for patients with diabetes to decrease hyperglycemia. The increased prevalence of diabetes has been linked to sedentary behavior. Resistance exercise has been shown to be moderately beneficial as it delays mortality and reduce the risk of becoming a diabetic in populations where diabetes may be common. In addition, resistance exercise has been associated with reduced cardiovascular complications and mortality. Research demonstrated that the HbA1c values of elderly individuals (mean age 66 years) were decreased by 1-2 % after performing resistance exercise. Type 2 diabetes patients have hepatic and peripheral insulin resistance. Therefore, they can have hyperinsulinemia when they are hungry. However, during exercise, glucose uptake exceeds its production. Because exercise regulates plasma glucose there can be a decrease in insulin. The American Diabetes Association (ADA) recommends that if plasma glucose regulation is obtained through the intake of oral antidiabetic drugs then extra caloric intake is not required.

Patients with diabetes who plan to exercise should know how to check their plasma glucose levels before and after the exercise. They should also learn about the possible blood glucose changes that may occur during exercise and how to manage if anything goes wrong. Diuretic treatment modifications need to be provided to patients that sweat excessively during exercise. Patients using beta-blockers may experience a hidden hypoglycemia. Multi drug users must consult with their doctors regarding continued use of the drugs, as well as possible changes in their exercise regimen and caloric intake. Precautions must be adhered to at all times when they are exercising. For example, they may be required to carry small amounts of food with them. Patients with DM are advised to carry an identity card that includes an emergency contact telephone number as well as information that the person has diabetes. They could also wear a bracelet identifying that they have DM.

10.2. Exercise in insulin user patients with type 2 diabetes mellitus

Because exercise augments the insulin effect, the insulin doses that normally regulate plasma glucose may easily cause hypoglycemia. ADA recommends carbohydrate supplementation before exercise for individuals who use insulin or drugs that cause insulin secretion and in those individuals whose plasma glucose is less than 100 mg/dL (5.6 mmol/L). Insulin dose may be reduced in type 2 DM patients who exercise. In addition, 20-40 grams carbohydrate supplementation before exercise should also be considered. Over time the insulin requirements and response to insulin may change and therefore the patient must be monitored closely. Insulin users should determine blood glucose when the insulin effect is at its maximum level and when he/she should have to eat food. They should also be aware of the relationship between exercise and plasma glucose. Sulfonylurea- or insulin-using patients are more prone to experiencing hypoglycemia during exercise. However, hypoglycemia is not as frequent as in type 1 diabetes.

Exercise facilitates insulin absorption via increased blood flow to muscles and this may result in hypoglycemia. Insulin is preferably injected into sites away from the moving extremities/contracting muscle groups. Insulin user type 2 DM patients who exercise may use approximately 30-50% less insulin than usual although they should be aware of their glucose levels at all times. Before and after the exercise, plasma glucose measurements should be taken and it should be remembered that hypoglycemia may occur up to 24 hours after the exercise session.

10.3. Exercise in patients with type 1 diabetes mellitus

The insulin response and hypoglycemia risk differs from one patient to the other and therefore individual evaluation and education is mandatory. For patients with type 1 DM, plasma glucose measurements must be performed before and after the exercise. Insulin must be injected at the appropriate time to avoid hypoglycemia and 20-40 grams of carbohydrate is recommended before exercise. If the exercise will last more than an hour, and intake of 20-40 grams of carbohydrate per hour is recommended. Before exercise, food that is hard to digest should be avoided.

If the insulin dose is adjusted, patients with type 1 DM can perform most sports. The duration of exercise, loading level, injection placement, previous insulin dose and timing determines patients' insulin requirements when they exercise. Long acting insulin may result in a higher level of insulin than expected at the periphery. If insulin is injected into the actively contracting muscle this may cause a rapid absorption of the insulin and hypoglycemia may occur. Injuries and infections may increase insulin requirements. However, healing may decrease the amount of insulin requirements and this may result in hypoglycemia.

The hormone responses during exercise are inappropriate in type 1 DM. In these patients, even though insulin is deficient, exercise causes an activation of the counter insulin system leading to ketoacidosis. Acute and vigorous exercise stimulates the counter insulin responses, with catecholamines, growth hormone, glucagon and cortisol to increase blood glucose and may cause hyperglycemia. However, hypoglycemia may occur 4-48 hours following the exercise.

When peripheral glucose use is restricted, lipid mobilization increases and ketogenesis is stimulated. In type 1 DM measuring ketones in the blood or urine is recommended if hyperglycemia exists. Hypoglycemia means excessive insulin or insufficient carbohydrate intake and ketonemia means insufficient insulin and carbohydrate. In type 1 DM exercise worsens the clinical situation if ketosis is present. Before exercise, if plasma glucose is under 100 mg/dL (5.6 mmol/L), it is advised that an individual consumes food containing carbohydrate such as fruit. Type 1 DM patients with plasma glucose ranging 100-250 mg/dL (5.6-14 mmol/L) do not need extra food prior to moderate exercise. Plasma glucose levels over 250 mg/dL (>14 mmol/L) and ketosis then require insulin and should receive extra attention [ADA, 2003]. Ketonuria should be checked before exercise. It may indicate that there is not enough insulin in the body. If there is a ketoacidosis risk then it is better to avoid exercising.

10.4. Exercise in pregnant women with diabetes mellitus

Exercise is important and is recommended for pregnant women with DM. Fitness and appropriate muscle tone reduces back pain related to muscle problems arising from the fetus weight. These exercises may also be beneficial during labor. The rectus abdominus, diaphragm and respiratory muscles are required to be strong to produce pressure during labor. In some countries there are group exercise programs to prepare pregnant women for labor. Before participating in an exercise program a gynecologic examination is mandatory. Exercise programs can be followed throughout pregnancy. Women who start exercising once they are pregnant and pregnant women with advanced age must be under the supervision of a physician.

Pregnant women should stop exercise when specific symptoms occur. These include lower back pain and vaginal bleeding. To prevent dehydration, drinking water before, during and after exercise is recommended.

Recommendations of The American College of Obstetricians and Gynecologists (ACOG) can be found at 'Gestational Diabetes (FAQ177)' and 'Exercise during treatment (FAQ 119)' (http://www.acog.org/For_Patients.aspx).

Author details

Yıldırım Çınar
Department of Internal Medicine, Faculty of Medicine, Trakya University, Edirne, Turkey

Hakan Demirci
Department of Family Medicine, Sevket Yilmaz Training and Research Hospital, Bursa, Turkey

Ilhan Satman
Division of Endocrinology and Metabolism, Department of Internal Medicine,
Istanbul Faculty of Medicine, Istanbul University, Istanbul, Turkey

11. References

American Diabetes Association (ADA). (2003). Physical activity/exercise and diabetes mellitus (Position Statement). Diabetes Care, Vol. 26, pp. (73-77).

American Diabetes Association (ADA). (2008). Nutrition recommendations and interventions for diabetes. Diabetes Care, Vol. 31, pp. (61-78).

American Heart Association (AHA). (1997). ACC/AHA guidelines for exercise testing: executive summary. Circulation, Vol. 96, pp. (345-354).

Banfi G, Colombi A, Lombardini G, Lubkowska A. (2012). Metabolic markers in sports medicine. Adv Clin Chem, Vol. 56, pp. (1-54).

Boule NG, Haddad E, Kenny GP. et al. (2001). Effects of exercise on glycemic control and body mass in type 2 diabetes mellitus. JAMA, Vol. 286, pp. (1218-1227).

Burton DA, Stokes K, Hall GM. (2004). Physiological effects of exercise. Conti Educ Anaesth Crit Care Pain, Vol. 4, No.6, pp. (185-188).

Cheuvront SN, Haymes EM. (2001). Thermoregulation and marathon running: biological and environmental influences. Sports Med, Vol. 31, No. 10, pp. (743-762).

Cinar Y, Kosku N. (2011). The role of inspiratory muscle exercises in patients with respiratory distress: increase in respiratory capacity. International conference on life science and technology IPCBEE, Vol. 3, IACSIT press, Singapore.

Hopkins M, King NA, Blundell JE. (2010). Acute and long-term effects of exercise on appetite control: is there any benefit for weight control? Curr Opin Clin Nutr Metab Care, Vol. 13, No.6, pp. (635-640).

Iwamoto J. (2011). Effect of exercise on developing bone mass and cortical bone geometry. Clin Calcium, Vol. 21, No.9, pp. (1323-1328).

Jeon CY, Lokken RP, Hu FB, van Dam RM. (2007). Physical activity of moderate intensity and risk of type 2 diabetes. Diabetes Care, Vol. 30, pp. (744-752).

Kruger J, Buchner DM, Prohaska TR. (2009). A prescribed amount of physical activity in randomized clinical trials in older adults. The Gerontologist, Vol. 49, pp. (100-107).

Ogilvie D, Foster CE, Rotnie H. et al. (2007). Interventions to promote walking: systematic review. BMJ, pp. (1-10).

Onat A. (2011). Metabolic syndrome: nature, therapeutic solutions and options. Expert Opin Pharmacother, Vol. 12, No.12, pp. (1887-1900).

Porter RS, Kaplan JL. (2011). Endurance exercise and metabolic requirements. The Merck Manuel of diagnosis and therapy (19th Edition). Merck Sharp and Dohme Corp. Whitehouse company New Jersey, pp. (3461-3462).

Quinn TJ, Coons BA. (2011). The talk test and its relationship with the ventilator and lactate thresholds. J Sports Sci, Vol. 29, No.11, pp. (1175-1182).

Scott CB. (2005). Contribution of anaerobic energy expenditure to whole body thermogenesis. Nutrition and metabolism, Vol. 2, pp. (1-9).

Sigal RJ, Kenny GP, Wasserman DH, et al. (2006). Physical activity/ exercise and type 2 diabetes. Diabetes Care, Vol. 29, pp. (1433-1438).

Tordeurs D, Janne P, Appart A, Zdanowicz N, Reynaert C. (2011). Effectiveness of physical exercise in phychiatry: a therapeutic approach? Encephale, Vol. 37, No.5, pp. (345-352).

Chapter 10

Hyperglycemia and Diabetes in Myocardial Infarction

Marco A. López Hernández

Additional information is available at the end of the chapter

http://dx.doi.org/10.5772/48091

1. Introduction

The proposal of this chapter is explain the importance and relevance of the understanding of the role that play the level in the serum glucose during the acute myocardial infarction (AMI). Since many years the investigation in this area has showed that the hyperglycemia is a strong predictor of mortality in acute myocardial infarction, as representation of the response of the myocardial cell to the ischemic injury, related mainly to acute catecholamine release.

Cardiovascular disease (CVD) is the leading cause of morbidity and mortality in individuals with diabetes, for which 65% of deaths are attributable to heart disease or stroke. Hyperglycemia is encountered in up to 50% of all ST elevation myocardial infarcted (STEMI) patients, whereas previously diagnosed DM is present in only 20% to 25% of STEMI patients.[1] When admission glucose level exceeds 200 mg/dL, mortality is similar in non-DM and DM subjects with MI. Admission glucose has been identified as a major independent predictor of both in-hospital congestive heart failure and mortality in STEMI.[2]

In the HEART2D Study treating diabetic survivors of AMI with prandial versus basal strategies achieved differences in fasting blood glucose, less-than-expected differences in postprandial blood glucose, similar levels of A1C, and no difference in risk for future cardiovascular event.[3]

Recently the glucose variability has been highlighted. In the results in a re analysis of HEART2D study results, the intraday glucose variability as target compared with the basal glucose, in diabetic type 2 patients after myocardial infarction, showed similar overall glycemic control but did not result in a reduction in cardiovascular outcomes[4]. Treating diabetic survivors of AMI with prandial versus basal strategies achieved differences in fasting blood glucose, less-than-expected differences in postprandial blood glucose, similar levels of A1C, and no difference in risk for future cardiovascular event.

2. Diabetes mellitus and risk for myocardial infarction

The main cause of death in the industrialized countries is the coronary artery disease (CAD). The risk of myocardial infarction is high in patients with diabetes mellitus. In United States, diabetes is the most prevalent risk factor for cardiovascular events[5] The patient with diabetes mellitus have increased risk for cardiovascular disease, a risk that contributes to a significant decrease in life expectancy. The patients with diabetes have a risk for myocardial infarction (MI) comparable to that of the risk of recurrent myocardial infarction in a patient without diabetes. The association between diabetes and cardiovascular disease has been well identified, and the increased of risk for acute coronary syndromes and the poor outcome linked to raised blood glucose levels has been studied in many trials.

A Finnish population-based study has shown that patients with diabetes without a previous MI have as great a risk for infarction as individuals without diabetes with a previous myocardial infarction (Figure 1).11 The 7-year incidence rates of MI (fatal and nonfatal) in subjects without diabetes were 18.8% in those with a previous MI and 3.5% in those without a history of infarction; the corresponding rates in individuals with diabetes were 45.0% and 20.2%, respectively[6]

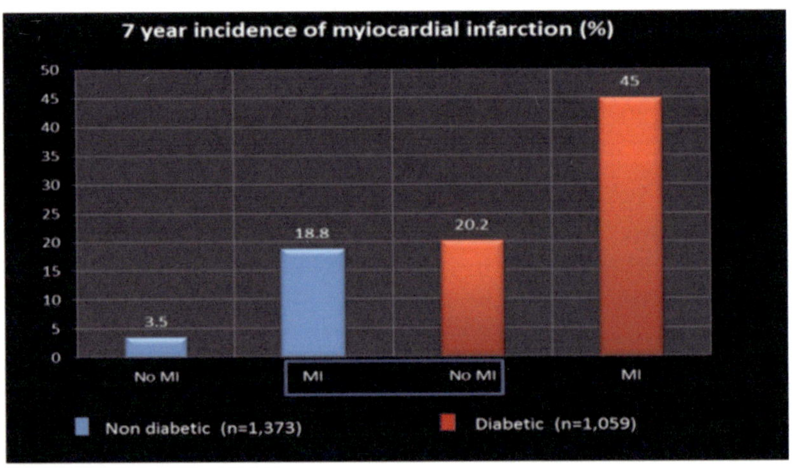

Figure 1. Diabetes mellitus as a risk equivalent of coronary artery disease.
(Adapted from Hafner S M,N Engl J Med.1998;339:229.342)

Diabetes mellitus is associated with a 2 to 4 fold increase of the risk for cardiovascular disease.[7,8] 75 to 80% of the deaths in patients with diabetes mellitus are conditioned by a thrombotic event[5] This increased risk is the main factor underlying the excess mortality and reduced life expectancy of people with type 2 diabetes; the life expectancy of people with type 2 diabetes at the age of 40 is reduced by an estimated 8 years in comparison with individuals without diabetes[9]

The prognosis is poorer in patients with diabetes mellitus type 2 that suffers a myocardial infarction compared with people without diabetes mellitus. In patients with acute myocardial infarction the underlying mechanism in the increase of mortality associated to glucose levels are poor understood. In a study by Nicolau JC and cols, with 52 patients with acute myocardial infarction with ST segment elevation and hyperglycemia, in the first 24 hours compared radionuclide ventriculography at day 4 and six months, finding that basal glucose level like independent and powerful predictor of left ventricular growth after an acute myocardial infarction[10]

Hyperglycemia increases the morbility and mortality in hospitalized patients in Intensive Care Units with acute myocardial infarction, stroke and those with aortocoronary bypass. The treatment with infusion of insulin has showed a better outcome in these patients[11]

A1c hemoglobin (A1cHb) or glycosilated hemoglobin is a marker of the glucose level in two previous months, and that is affected in minimal mode by the levels of glucose associated to acute coronary syndromes. In the OPTIMAAL study, in Danish population with acute myocardial infarction complicated with heart failure, was concluded that A1cHb levels showed to be a predictor of mortality in patients without diabetes previously known.[12]

In a Japanese study was evaluated the impact of elevated level of glucose in patients with acute myocardial infarction with percutaneous coronary intervention, concluding that the hyperglycemia at time of admission was associated with a increased mortality a short term (30 days), and that the presence de diabetes mellitus was associated a poor outcome at long term (3 years), considering that both, the acute hyperglycemia in myocardial infarction and diabetes mellitus must be treated as two different problems[13]

3. Mechanisms induced by hyperglycemia than increased risk in acute myocardial infarction

Acute phase hyperglycaemia and diabetes are both associated with adverse outcomes in acute myocardial infarction, with higher reported incidences of congestive heart failure, cardiogenic shock, and death. However, the association between hyperglycaemia and adverse outcomes is not confined to patients with diabetes. The mechanism is not clear, but it is commonly regarded as a response to stress resulting from catecholamine induced glycogenolysis. Hyperglycemia, therefore, is seen as an epiphenomenon that is associated with poor outcomes only because adrenergic stress is closely related to the extent of myocardial injury.

The possible mechanisms that influence the increased risk in diabetes for cardiovascular events include, insulin resistance, changes in endothelial function, dyslipidemia, chronic inflammation and release of mediators of inflammation, procoagulability and impaired fibrinolysis.

3.1. Insulin resistance

Insulin resistance is a hallmark in diabetes mellitus type 2 and obesity, the resistance to action of insulin in skeletal muscle, leads to a decrease in the glucose disposal and the use of fatty acids and compensatory hyperinsulinemia.[14] With relative insulinopenia, however, the ischemic myocardium is forced to use free fatty acids instead of glucose as an energy source because myocardial glucose uptake is acutely impaired. Thus, a metabolic crisis may ensue as the hypoxic myocardium becomes less energy efficient in the setting of hyperglycemia and insulin resistance.

The SMART study group published a prospective cohort study in 2611 patients with manifest arterial disease without known diabetes. Homeostasis model of insulin resistance (HOMA-IR) was used to quantify insulin resistance. The relation of HOMA-IR with cardiovascular events (vascular death, myocardial infarction or stroke) and all causes of mortality were assessed. In patients with manifest arterial disease without known diabetes, the results of this trials concludes than insulin resistance increases with the number of metabolic syndrome components, and elevated insulin resistance increases the risk of new cardiovascular events[15]

Diabetes mellitus type 2 is result of two developments, a chronic overnutrition with resultant insulin resistance and least a relative failure of pancreatic ß-cells to release sufficient insulin to maintain glucose homeostasis. Insulin resistance is the basic mechanism, but its diagnosis is not straightforward. Commonly, attempts are made using the homeostasis model of insulin resistance[16]

Intact pro insulin is a precursor molecule of the insulin that is released into circulation. Proinsulin is associated with increased resistance to insulin, and have a similar adipogenetic activity than insulin, but only the 10% to 20% of the glucose-lowering effect. Recently, determination of proinsulin has been used as a diagnostic tool because an increasing proinsulin to insulin ratio predicts insulin resistance and deterioration of glucose tolerance.[17] Hyperglycemia is a reflection of relative insulinopenia, which is associated with increased lipolysis and free fatty acid generation, as well as diminished myocardial glucose uptake and a decrease in glycolytic substrate for myocardial energy needs in STEMI. Myocardial ischemia results in an increased rate of glycogenolysis and glucose uptake via translocation of GLUT-4 receptors to the sarcolemma.[18]

Finally, in the setting of acute MI and revascularization, blood glucose control in patients with diabetes should routinely involve fasting and post meal glucose measurements (such as hyperglycemic peaks with the associated sequelae of hyperinsulinemia, reactive oxygen species generation, and endothelial dysfunction) because only the latter reflects the amount and type of ingested carbohydrates.[19-20]

3.2. Endothelial dysfunction

A single layer of endothelial cells lines the inner surface of all blood vessels, providing a metabolically active interface between blood and tissue that modulates blood flow, nutrient delivery, coagulation and thrombosis, and leukocyte diapedesis. It synthesizes important bioactive substances, including nitric oxide and other reactive oxygen species, prostaglandins, endothelin, and angiotensin II, that regulate blood vessel function and structure. Nitric oxide potently dilates vessels and mediates much of the endothelium's control of vascular relaxation. A number of fundamental mechanisms contribute to the decreased bioavailability of endothelium-derived nitric oxide in diabetes:

1. Hyperglycemia inhibits production of nitric oxide by blocking eNOS synthase activation and increasing the production of reactive oxygen species, especially superoxide anion (O2–), in endothelial and vascular smooth muscle cells. Superoxide anion directly quenches nitric oxide by forming the toxic peroxynitrite ion, which uncouples eNOS by oxidizing its cofactor, tetrahydrobiopterin, and causes eNOS to produce O2
2. Insulin resistance leads to excess liberation of free fatty acids from adipose tissue, which activate the signaling enzyme protein kinase C, inhibit phosphatidylinositol-3 (PI-3) kinase (an eNOS agonist pathway), and increase the production of reactive oxygen species—mechanisms that directly impair nitric oxide production or decrease its bioavailability once produced.
3. Production of peroxynitrite decreases synthesis of the vasodilatory and antiplatelet prostanoid prostacyclin.

In addition to reducing ambient concentrations of nitric oxide, diabetes increases the production of vasoconstrictors, most important, endothelin-1, which activates endothelin-A receptors on vascular smooth muscle cell to induce vasoconstriction.

Acute coronary syndromes are associated to unestable atheromatous plaques in which inflammation and endothelial dysfunction play key roles, as well as in subsequent occlusive coronary thrombosis a global flow abnormality affecting the entire coronary tree is associated with adverse clinical outcomes in patients with ACS and might be caused by a combination of global inflammation and vasoconstriction.[21-22]

Endothelial dysfunction is caused by acute hyperglycemia. Williams et al assessed endothelium-dependent vasodilation through brachial artery infusion of methacholine chloride in non-diabetic subjects. They showed that hyperglycemia significantly attenuated the forearm blood flow response to methacholine, but did not reduce endothelium-independent vasodilation to verapamil.[23]

3.3. Dyslipidemia

Characteristic abnormalities in the lipid profile in type 2 diabetes include elevated triglyceride levels, decreased atheroprotective high-density lipoprotein (HDL) levels, and increased levels of small dense LDL. Increased efflux of free fatty acids from adipose tissue and impaired insulin-mediated skeletal muscle uptake of free fatty acids increase hepatic free fatty acid concentrations.[24] In response, the liver increases VLDL production and cholesteryl ester synthesis.[25]

Free fatty acids combine with a cholesterol molecule to form a cholesteryl ester. Cholesteryl ester concentrations may regulate VLDL production, with increased concentrations resulting in elevated VLDL synthesis. Overproduction of triglyceride-rich lipoproteins and impaired clearance by lipoprotein lipase lead to the hypertriglyceridemia common in diabetes. Low levels of HDL represent the second common abnormality in type 2 diabetes. Elevated levels of triglyceride rich lipoproteins lower HDL levels by promoting exchanges of cholesterol from HDL to VLDL via cholesteryl ester transfer protein. Diabetic patients with CAD more commonly have the combination of elevated triglycerides and low HDL than elevated total and LDL cholesterol levels.

Strongly related to insulin resistance, obesity is a known risk factor for heart failure. Animal studies suggest that the underlying mechanisms are overstorage of lipids and lipotoxic injury to myocytes associated with high serum levels of free fatty acid and triglycerides that involve increased free fatty acid uptake, diminished mitochondrial oxidative capacity, generation of ROS, and increased apoptosis.

3.4. Inflammation

In a study Esposito et al[26] measured circulating levels of cytokines, including interleukin (IL)-6, IL- 18 and tumor necrosis factor-α in subjects with normal or IGT during 3 consecutive pulses of intravenous glucose separated by a 2-h interval. The plasma cytokine levels increased as the blood glucose level increased but immediately returned to normal as glucose returned to normal levels. Interestingly, when the first elevation in the blood glucose level was maintained by subsequent continuous intravenous glucose infusion, plasma cytokine concentrations gradually returned to normal levels.

The exact mechanism by which glucose stimulates pro inflammatory events is not clear, although indirect evidence suggests that it does so possibly by stimulating production of tumor necrosis factor (TNF)-α (a pro inflammatory cytokine). A diet with a high glycemic load and hyperglycemia induced production of acute-phase reactants. Similar to glucose, TNF-α also enhances free radical generation by augmenting polymorphonuclear leukocyte NADPH oxidase activity, activates NF-κB, and increases intercellular adhesion molecule-1 expression in endothelial cells. This similarity in the actions of glucose and TNF-α, and the ability of former to enhance acute phase reactants suggests, but does not prove, that glucose may enhance TNF-α production and brings about its pro inflammatory actions.

TNF-α is secreted by adipose tissue, macrophages and cardiac tissue, and plays roles in the pathogeneses of insulin resistance, type 2 diabetes mellitus, inflammation, and septic shock. Release of TNF-α occurs early in the course of AMI and reduces myocardial contractility in a dose dependent manner.[27-28]

It has been suggested that four key biochemical changes induced by hyperglycemia: increased flux through the polyol pathway (in which glucose is reduced to sorbitol, reducing levels of both NADPH and reduced glutathione), increased formation of advanced glycation end products, activation of protein kinase C (with effects ranging from vascular occlusion to expression of pro-inflammatory genes), and increased shunting of excess glucose through the hexosamine pathway (mediating increased transcription of genes for inflammatory cytokines and plasminogen activator inhibitor-1 [PAI-1]) – are all activated by a common mechanism: overproduction of superoxide radicals. Excess plasma glucose drives excess production of electron donors (mainly NADH/H+) from the tricarboxylic acid cycle; in turn, this surfeit results in the transfer of single electrons (instead of the usual electron pairs) to oxygen, producing superoxide radicals and other reactive oxygen species (instead of the usual end product, H2O). The superoxide anion itself inhibits the key glycolytic enzyme glyceraldehyde-3-phosphate dehydrogenase (GADPH), and in consequence, glucose and glycolytic intermediates spill into the polyol and hexosamine pathways, as well as additional pathways that culminate in protein kinase C activation and intracellular AGE formation.[29] (Figure 2)

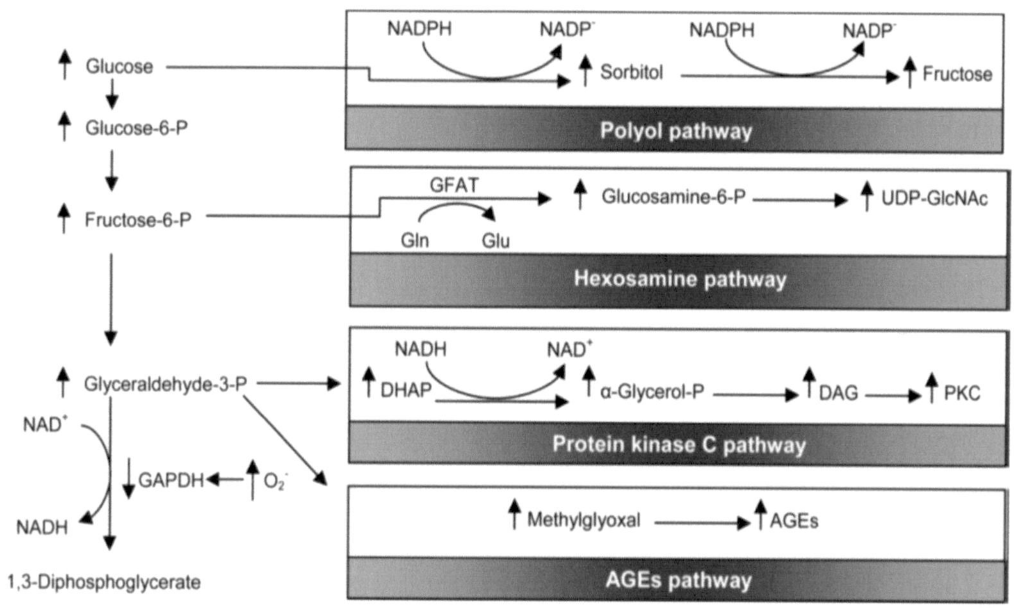

Figure 2. Potential mechanism by which hyperglycemia-induced mitochondrial superoxide overproduction activates four pathways of hyperglycemic damage. Excess superoxide partially inhibits the glycolytic enzyme glyceraldehyde-3-phosphate dehydrogenase (GAPDH), thereby diverting upstream metabolites from glycolysis into pathways of glucose overutilization. This results in increased flux of dihydroxyacetone phosphate (DHAP) to diacylglycerol (DAG), an activator of protein kinase C (PKC), and of triose phosphates to methylglyoxal, the main intracellular AGE precursor. Increased flux of fructose-6-phosphate (Fructose-6-P) to UDP-N-acetylglucosamine increases modification of proteins by O-linked N-acetylglucosamine(GlcNAc), and increased glucose flux through the polyol pathway consumes NADPH and depletes glutathione. GFAT, glutamine: fructose-6-phosphate aminotransferase; Gln, glutamine; Glu, glutamate; NAD, nicotinamide dinucleotide; UDP, uridine diphosphate. Adapted from Ceriello A. Diabetes care 2009 Nov;32 Suppl 2:S232-6

3.5. Procoagulability

Hyperglycemia also stimulates coagulation and platelet aggregation. It has been reported that hyperglycemia elevates coagulant activation markers, including thrombin antithrombin complexes and soluble tissue factor, whereas hyperinsulinemia inhibits fibrinolysis.

Platelets can modulate vascular function and participate significantly in thrombus formation. Abnormalities in platelet function may exacerbate the progression of atherosclerosis and the consequences of plaque rupture. Intraplatelet glucose concentration mirrors the extracellular concentration, since glucose entry into the platelet does not depend on insulin. In the platelet, as in endothelial cells, elevated glucose levels lead to activation of protein kinase C, decreased production of platelet-derived nitric oxide, and increased formation of O2−

Patients with diabetes have increased platelet-surface expression of glycoprotein Ib (GpIb), which mediates binding to von Willebrand factor, and GpIIb/IIIa, which mediates platelet fibrin interaction. These abnormalities may result from decreased endothelial production of the anti aggregants nitric oxide and prostacyclin, increased production of fibrinogen, and increased production of platelet activators, such as thrombin and von Willebrand factor. Thus, diabetic abnormalities increase intrinsic platelet activation and decrease endogenous inhibitors of platelet activity

3.6. Impaired fibrinolysis

Patients with type 2 diabetes have impaired fibrinolytic capacity because of elevated levels of plasminogen activator inhibitor type 1 in atherosclerotic lesions and in non atheromatous arteries.[30] Diabetes increases the expression of tissue factor, a potent procoagulant, and plasma coagulation factors such as factor VII and decreases levels of endogenous anticoagulants such antithrombin III and protein C.[31-32]

Impaired fibrinolysis, due to elevated levels of plasminogen activator inhibitor type 1 (PAI-1), further contributes to a hypercoagulable state in patients with diabetes. PAI-1 inhibits the conversion of plasminogen into plasmin and consequently reduces fibrinolytic activity. An in vivo study in healthy volunteers using a hyperinsulinemic euglycemic clamp, demonstrated a 2.5-fold increase in levels of PAI-1 relative to baseline. This study suggested that impaired fibrinolysis in patients with diabetes is mediated by hyperinsulinemia rather than hyperglycemia.[33]

Hyperinsulinemia increases PAI-1 levels by stabilization of the PAI-1 messenger RNA transcript through the actions of insulin and insulin-like growth factor type 1. Adipocytes have been found to be a major source of PAI-1, providing a direct link between obesity and a suppressed fibrinolytic system. Finally, inflammatory cytokines such as transforming growth factor-beta and tumor necrosis factor-alpha both of which are believed to have important roles in the metabolic syndrome increase the release of PAI-1 from adipose tissue

4. The hyperglycemic effect in the outcomes in acute coronary syndromes

Acute hyperglycemia is associated with multiple biological effects that contribute to a poor outcome of the acute coronary syndromes, [34] this effects are listed in the table number 1 Admission hyperglycemia is associated with long-term risk for ACS mortality[35] ,but this association is not homogeneous in different ACS presentations,[36] unstable angina, NSTEMI, or STEMI. Besides, mortality up to 1 year can be predicted both by admission glucose and fasting blood glucose, but the better predictor of mortality for longer periods is fasting glucose.[37]

In the OASIS registry, a 6-nation study of unstable angina and non–Q-wave MI, diabetes independently increased the risk of death by 57%.[38] Elevated plasma glucose and glycated hemoglobin levels on admission are independent prognosticators of both in-hospital and long-term outcome regardless of diabetic status.[39-40] For every 18 mg/dL increase in glucose level, there is a 4% increase in mortality in nondiabetic subjects.[41]

Hyperglycemia also interferes with ischemic preconditioning. Ischemic preconditioning is a potent endogenous cardioprotective mechanism that is promoted by the brief transient ischemia proceeding subsequent prolonged ischemia and reperfusion. In the clinical setting, it has been demonstrated that prodromal angina occurring shortly before the onset of AMI is associated with smaller infarct size, preserved LV function and lower mortality after reperfusion therapy.[42]

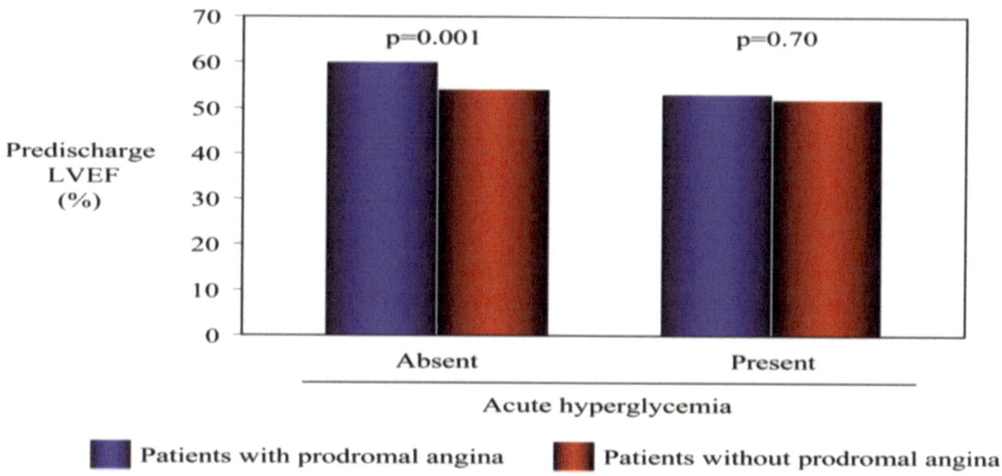

Figure 3. In the absence of acute hyperglycemia, prodromal angina was associated with preserved predischarge in left ventricular ejection fraction (LVEF). Among patients with acute hyperglycemia, there was no significant difference in predischarge LVEF between patients with (blue bars) and without prodromal angina (red bars). Adapted from Ishihara et al Ischemic preconditioning delays infarct progression during the early hours after the onset of AMI and extends the window of time for reperfusion therapy[43]

Endothelial dysfunction
Platelet hyperreactivity
Increased cytokine activation
Increased lipolysis and free fatty acid levels
Reduced glycolysis and glucose oxidation
Increased oxidative stress (Increased myocardial apoptosis)
Impaired microcirculatory function ("no-reflow" phenomenon)
Impaired ischemic preconditioning
Impaired insulin secretion and insulin stimulated glucose uptake

Table 1. Acute Cardiovascular Effects of Hyperglycemia

5. Importance of glucose levels in diabetic and nondiabetic patients in acute myocardial infarction.

Elevation of blood glucose on admission is a common feature during the early phase after acute myocardial infarction, even in the absence of a history of diabetes mellitus.[44] However the optimal plasma glucose level may be different between diabetic and nondiabetic patients. Many studies have shown that an elevated plasma glucose level on admission is a major independent predictor of in-hospital and long-term outcome in patients with acute myocardial infarction, regardless of diabetes status.

Acute hyperglycemia is common in patients with STEMI even in the absence of a history of diabetes. Hyperglycemia is encountered in up to 50% of all STEMI patients, whereas previously diagnosed diabetes mellitus is present in only 20% to 25% of STEMI patients. The prevalence of type 2 diabetes mellitus or impaired glucose tolerance may be as high as 65% in myocardial infarction patients without prior diabetes when oral glucose tolerance testing is performed.

High blood glucose concentration may increase risk of death and poor outcome after acute myocardial infarction. Capes SE et al did a systematic review and meta-analysis to assess the risk of in-hospital mortality or congestive heart failure after myocardial infarction in patients with and without diabetes who had stress hyperglycemia on admission. Concluding that acute hyperglycemia with myocardial infarction is associated with an increased risk of in-hospital mortality in patients with and without diabetes; the risk of congestive heart failure or cardiogenic shock is also increased in patients without diabetes (Figure 4)

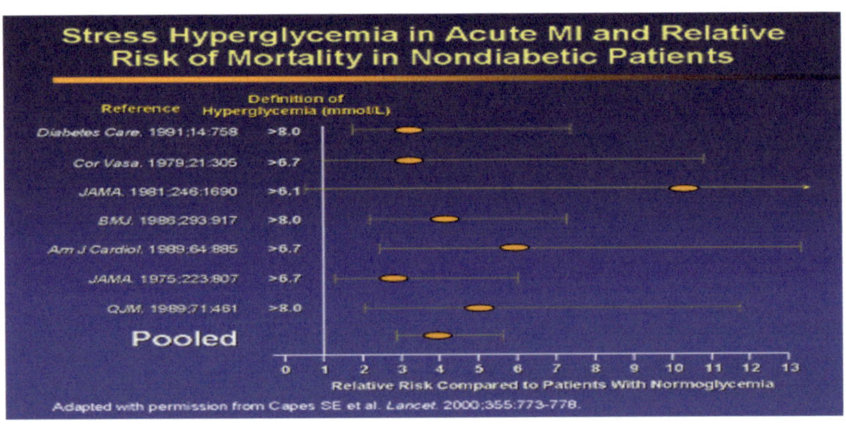

Figure 4. Stress hyperglycemia in acute MI and relative risk of mortality in nondiabetic patients

Acute hyperglycemia is common among patients with acute myocardial infarction. The prevalence of acute hyperglycemia in prior studies varies from <10% to >80%.[45-46] It mostly depends on the definition of acute hyperglycemia, which is differs from study to study. Threshold glucose concentration used to define acute hyperglycemia has ranged from 6.1 mmol/L (1 mmol/L=18 mg/dl) to 11.0 mmol/L. There is a linear correlation between the blood glucose level on admission and mortality after acute myocardial infarction. Therefore, there is no clear cut-off value of blood glucose to predict mortality and no consensus about the appropriate definition of acute hyperglycemia for patients with myocardial infarction. In most of the recent studies, 10.0 mmol/L or 11.0 mmol/L of blood glucose on admission is used to define acute hyperglycemia.

Diabetes has been a consistently powerful risk factor for development of post infarction heart failure, accounting for 66% of mortality during the first year. The combination of diabetes and HF after MI requires preventive action because it is usually not associated with the characteristic left ventricular remodeling. If left ventricular remodeling does develop, it requires appropriate treatment that includes revascularization and metabolically and hemodynamically effective treatment strategies that limit infarct size, cardiac dysfunction, and left ventricle remodeling

In patients without a history of diabetes, there was a linear relation between admission blood glucose level and in-hospital mortality (Figure 5)

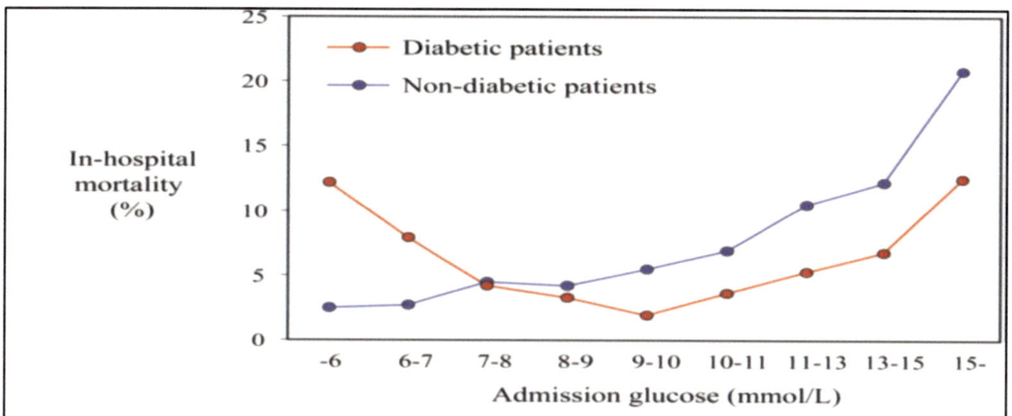

Diabetic patients (n)	41	76	96	92	104	112	187	161	321
Non-diabetic patients (n)	394	490	532	384	238	173	171	82	96

Figure 5. Relationship between admission blood glucose level and in-hospital mortality. It is near-linear in patients without diabetes (blue) but U-shaped in patients with diabetes (red). Adapted from Ishihara M, et al. Am J Cardiol 2009; 104: 769-74

In the presence of hyperglycemia, proteins and lipids are irreversibly glycated by non-enzymatic mechanisms, and these advanced glycated end products accumulate in the cells and extracellular space of blood vessels, enhancing atherogenic processes. A cell surface receptor for this glycated end products (a "RAGE") has been isolated; binding of AGEs and other pro inflammatory ligands to this signal-transducing receptor has a multitude of effects, including increased smooth muscle cell proliferation, migration and activation of mononuclear phagocytes, induction of cytokines such as TNF-α, and in endothelial cells, increased vascular permeability, oxidative stress, vasoconstriction and expression of adhesion molecules. Glucotoxic effects involve three additional mechanisms for dysfunction in the diabetic heart. These involve:

1. Reactive oxygen species that amplify hyperglycemia induced activation of protein kinase C isoforms.
2. Increased formation of glucose derived advanced glycation end products
3. Increased glucose flux through the aldose reductase pathways

Admission glucose levels have a prognostic role in patients with acute myocardial infarction and in patients with heart failure.[47-48]

In a Spanish study, the findings highlight a 2-fold increase in mortality risk with hyperglycemia after STEMI, as an additive to clinical parameters. Moreover, it is of interest to note that the probability of mortality was not modified when DM was added in the model, indicating that the predictive influence of DM was marginal.[49] Similar results were found by Pinto et al.[50] in a subgroup of patients in CLARITY-TIMI 28 study trial. In 1027 patients with STEMI treated with PCI, with 26% incidence of DM.

6. The effect of hyperglycemia and diabetes in outcomes for thrombolysis, arrhythmias and left ventricle function

In patients with acute STEMI, thrombolysis in myocardial infarction (TIMI) frame counts may show significant variability despite presence of grade 3 TIMI flow after successful reperfusion and lower TIMI frame counts after reperfusion are associated with more favorable prognosis. No data are present regarding TIMI frame counts and admission glucose values in non-diabetic patients with acute ST elevation MI who undergo successful primary percutaneous coronary intervention. In STEMI subjects, acute hyperglycemia is associated with reduced TIMI grade 3 flow before intervention compared with normal glucose blood levels and is the most important predictor of the absence of coronary perfusion.[51] Similarly, diabetic subjects have reduced myocardial blush grades and diminished ST-segment resolution after successful coronary intervention in STEMI, consistent with diminished microvascular perfusion.[52] Acute hyperglycemia also is associated with impaired microcirculatory function as manifest by "no reflow" phenomenon on myocardial contrast echocardiography after percutaneous coronary intervention.[53]

Elevated admission glucose levels are associated with increased risk of life-threatening complications, especially arrhythmias in diabetic and non-diabetic AMI patients. This increased risk of complications is one of the possible explanations for the elevated in-hospital mortality in AMI patients presenting with hyperglycemia. In a clinical study by Dziewierz et al[54] admission hyperglycemia was associated with increased risk of ventricular tachycardia/ventricular fibrillation, atrial fibrillation, second to third atriventricular block, pulmonary edema. A analysis from the Krakow Registry of Acute Coronary Syndromes database, found that diabetes mellitus and presence of chest pain on admission, as well as heart rate and systolic blood pressure on admission, were independent predictors of new onset of atrial fibrillation[55]

In a Spanish study with the aim to evaluate the impact of glucose levels on admission and high risk ventricular tachyarrhythmia in hospital mortality in patients with acute myocardial infarction, the admission glucose levels >180 mg/dL had a significantly increased risk in in-hospital only high risk ventricular tachyarrhythmia only in patients without diabetes[56]

Several mechanisms promote metabolic consequences that lead to cardiac dysfunction and heart failure in diabetes. An important mechanism deduced mainly from experimental work is myocardial energy demand/supply mismatch from increased oxygen demand in the diabetic myocardium related to increased vascular stiffness; and decreased energy supply from myocardial underperfusion.

The CARISMA study enrolled patients with a recent MI and LV systolic dysfunction. The patients were implanted with an implantable loop recorder and followed for 2 years allowing continuous monitoring and diagnosis of asymptomatic and symptomatic arrhythmias.[57] Diastolic dysfunction in post myocardium infarcted patients with moderate-to-severe left ventricle systolic dysfunction predisposes to cardiovascular ischemic events such as re-infarction and stroke. New-onset atrial fibrillation also occurs more frequently in patients with diastolic dysfunction. Re-infarction and stroke were more frequent in patients with new onset atrial fibrillation, but the increased risk of ischemic events was independent of development of atrial fibrillation, suggesting that diastolic dysfunction in infarcted patients by itself is an important risk factor for ischemic events.[58]

Diabetes is associated with a higher risk of death or heart failure hospitalization across the spectrum of left ventricle ejected fraction (LVEF) in high-risk post-myocardial infarction patients. The magnitude of reduction in risk of death or heart failure hospitalization associated with increasing LVEF is significantly attenuated among patients with diabetes when compared to patients without diabetes[59]

VALIANT was a randomized, double-blind trial of the efficacy and safety of Valsartan versus Captopril versus combination therapy following MI complicated by clinical or radiological signs of heart failure, evidence of left ventricle systolic dysfunction (LVEF ≤ 35% by echocardiography or ≤40% by radionuclide ventriculography), or both[60]

7. Glucose variability in acute myocardial infarction

Hyperglycemia is a strong predictor of mortality in patients hospitalized with acute myocardial infarction. Professional society guidelines have accordingly advised glucose control in hyperglycemic patients. These same guidelines also recommend avoiding hypoglycemia, even though the association between hypoglycemia and adverse outcomes in acute myocardial infarction patients is controversial. In a meta-analysis of OASIS-6 and CREATE-ECLA studies Goyal A. et al conclude that both admission and post admission hyperglycemia predict 30-day death in acute myocardial infarction patients. In contrast, only hypoglycemia on admission predicted death, and this relationship dissipated after admission. These data suggest hypoglycemia may not be a direct mediator of adverse outcomes in myocardial infarction[61]

Short-term variation in blood glucose levels is a daily challenge for patients with diabetes. It confers a possible increased risk for hypoglycemia, and it has been suggested that glucose variability is related to cardiovascular risk [62–64]. However, reanalysis of the Diabetes Control and Complications Trial (DCCT) and DCCT/Epidemiology of Diabetes Interventions and Complications (EDIC) dataset examining the predictive value of glucose variability on microvascular and neurologic complications did not show an effect of glucose variability independent from mean glucose and HbA1c, and randomized controlled trials specifically targeting glucose variability are lacking

Oscillating hyperglycemia also induces apoptosis of cells. Risso et al reported that intermittent high glucose enhanced apoptosis of human endothelial cells that were incubated in media containing different glucose concentrations.[65] Apoptosis, which was studied by viability assay, cell cycle analysis, DNA fragmentation, and morphological analysis, was enhanced in human umbilical vein endothelial cells exposed to intermittent, rather than constant, high glucose concentrations.

They are secondary to deterioration in microvascular function causing a decrease in myocardial blood flow. In diabetic patients without microvascular or macrovascular complications, postprandial myocardial perfusion defects may represent an early marker of the atherogenic process in the coronary circulation; hence, its reversal constitutes a potential goal of treatment[66]. (Figure 6)

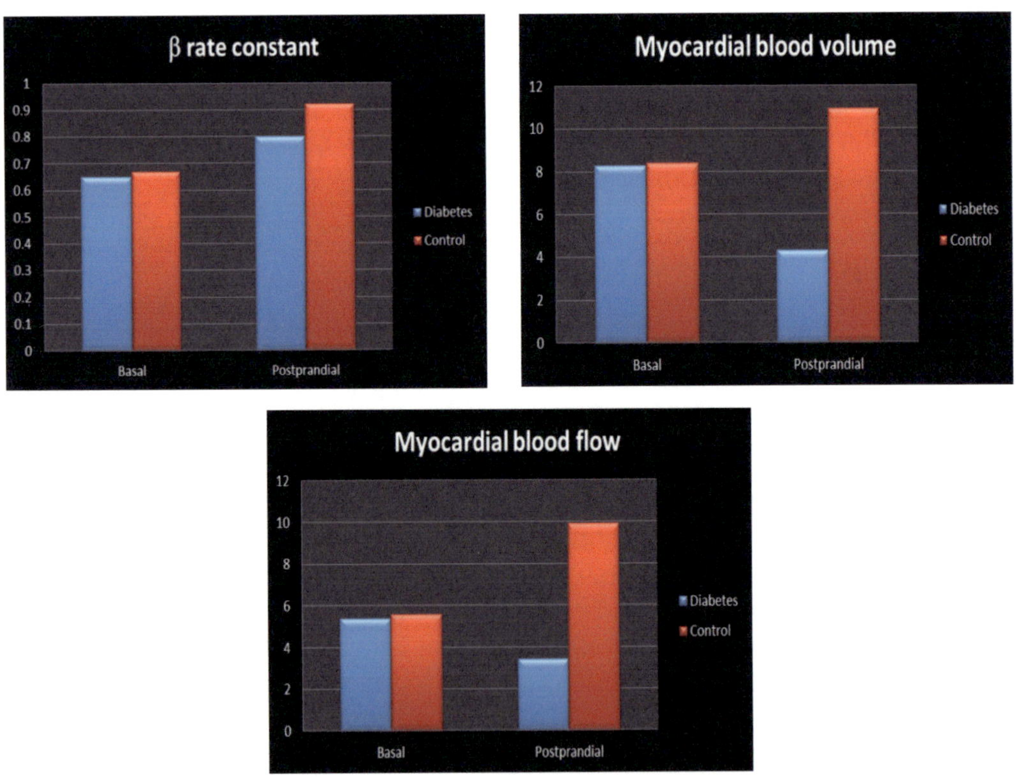

Figure 6. Changes in myocardial perfusion indexes after overnight fasting (baseline) and 120 minutes after standard mixed meal ingestion (postprandial) in type 2 diabetic patients (blue bars) and control subjects (red bars). Adapted from Scognamiglio R et al. Circulation 2005;112:179-84.

The American Heart Association Diabetes Committee of the Council on Nutrition, Physical Activity, and Metabolism prepared a scientific statement summarizing the current understanding of the association between elevated glucose and patient outcomes in acute coronary syndromes and identifying major knowledge gaps that remain for further investigation efforts.

The committee assessed data from the Diabetes Mellitus Insulin-Glucose Infusion in Acute Myocardial Infarction (DIGAMI), Hyperglycemia: Intensive Insulin Infusion In Infarction (HI-5), Clinical Trial of Reviparin and Metabolic Modulation in Acute Myocardial Infarction Treatment and Evaluation-Estudios Clinicos Latino America (CREATE-ECLA), and other clinical trials in ACS patients with hyperglycemia.

Most cardiovascular disease risk factors make similar contributions to risk among patients with and without diabetes, and the relationship between fasting plasma glucose or HbA1C levels and macrovascular complications among diabetic patients is not strong. For example, the United Kingdom Prospective Diabetes Study Group (UKPDS) study found that "intensive" control of fasting blood glucose among diabetic patients reduced the relative risk for myocardial infarction by only 16% as compared to conventional, diet-based therapy ($p=0.052$).[67] What, then, accounts for the greatly increased cardiovascular risk among patients with diabetes? Postprandial hyperglycemia, which captures "spikes" in blood glucose levels that may not be fully reflected in fasting blood glucose or glycosylated hemoglobin levels[67], has historically been overlooked as a CV risk factor among diabetic patients, those with isolated impaired glucose tolerance and those in the general population.

8. Treatment of acute hyperglycemia in acute myocardial infarction

Many clinicians caring for diabetic patients have a "fasting glucocentric" outlook: they focus on fasting blood glucose and HbA1C levels as the main measures of glycemic status when evaluating a diabetic patient's cardiovascular risk. However, there is broad epidemiological evidence that just as acute hyperglycemia portends a poorer clinical outcome among critically ill patients, postprandial hyperglycemia predicts cardiovascular disease and mortality not only among patients already identified as diabetic, but also among subjects in the general population. Mounting mechanistic evidence suggests that acute hyperglycemia has myriad adverse effects that are mediated through oxidative stress. Moreover, some available interventional studies suggest that strategies directed toward decreasing postprandial glucose in outpatients and acute hyperglycemia during hospitalizations for cardiovascular events may improve clinical outcomes. Postprandial hyperglycemia determines myocardial perfusion defects in type 2 diabetic patients.

The concept of a metabolic cocktail (GIK) to stabilize cell membranes through potassium influx, promote glucose oxidation, and reduce free fatty acid accumulation to protect the ischemic myocardium dates back to the work of Sodi-Pallares et al.[68] However, the CREATE-ECLA study showed no benefit of GIK in a large number of STEMI subjects, dampening the enthusiasm for aggressive use of a metabolic cocktail in STEMI[69]

The Normoglycemia in Intensive Care Evaluation-Survival Using Glucose Algorithm Regulation (NICE-SUGAR) study[70] randomly assigned 6,104 patients admitted to the intensive care unit to undergo either intensive glucose control, with a target blood glucose range of 4.5–6.0 mmol/L or conventional glucose control, with a target of ≤10.0 mmol/L. The 90-day mortality was significantly higher in the intensive control group than in the conventional-control group (27.5%vs. 24.9%, P=0.02). The difference in mortality between the 2 treatment groups was still significant after adjustment for the predefined baseline risk factors (adjusted odds ratio, 1.14; 95% confidence interval 1.01–1.29; P=0.04). Severe hypoglycemia (defined as a blood glucose level ≤2.2 mmol/L) was recorded more frequently in the intensive-control group. After these studies, recent guidelines revised their recommendation from intensive glucose control to mild glucose control, avoiding hypoglycemia.

Due as an emerging risk factor for cardiovascular disease, acute hyperglycemia during cardiovascular events may be considered analogous to postprandial hyperglycemia and may carry with it similar adverse clinical implications. Accordingly, several groups, including the American Diabetes Association[71] and the American Heart Association[72], have encouraged more rigorous control of blood glucose levels during acute hospitalizations for cardiovascular diseases. The clinical trial basis for these recommendations is not yet exceedingly robust.

Although sustained chronic hyperglycemia produces excessive protein glycation, acute fluctuations of glucose may activate oxidative stress and contribute to endothelial dysfunction, which may also participate in the development of diabetes complications. Therefore, reducing postprandial hyperglycemia and glucose variability are now recognized as a priority in treatment of type 2 diabetes. Therapeutic agents acting on postprandial glucose excursions are of particular interest to diminish glucose variability. Emerging therapeutic agents such as the glucagon-like peptide 1 agonists and the dipeptidyl peptidase (DPP)-4 inhibitors are very attractive. Both increase insulin secretion and suppress glucagon release in response to meals, in a glucose-dependent manner. This review will focus on the increasing impact of postprandial hyperglycemia and glycemic variability in developing diabetes complications and the role of DPP-4 inhibitors (sitagliptin, vildagliptin, saxagliptin) in reducing both defects presenting in people with type 2 diabetes.[74]

In the more recent DIGAMI-2 study (n= 1253 patients), however, mortality did not differ significantly between diabetic patients randomized to either acute insulin infusion followed by insulin-based long-term glucose control, insulin infusion followed by standard glucose control, or standard management, probably reflecting a lack of difference in glucose control among the three groups[75]

Because hyperglycemia remained one of the most important predictors of outcome in acute coronary syndromes, however, it appears to be reasonable to keep glucose levels within normal ranges in diabetic patients. Target glucose levels between 90 and 140 mg/dL (5 and 7.8 mmol/L) have been suggested. Care needs to be taken to avoid blood glucose levels below 80–90 mg/dL (4.4–5 mmol/L), however, as hypoglycemia-induced ischemia might also affect outcome in diabetic patients with acute coronary syndromes[76]

The HI-5 study[77] attempted to rectify some of the issues that were encountered in DIGAMI-2 It was the first randomized clinical trial of intensive insulin infusion that included hyperglycemic acute myocardial infarcted patients without previously established diabetes. Patients assigned to the intensive insulin-infusion arm received standard insulin and dextrose infusion that was then adjusted to maintain glucose levels between 72 and 180 mg/dL. Patients in the conventional arm received their baseline diabetes medications (including subcutaneous insulin); additional short-acting subcutaneous insulin was permitted for those with a glucose level >288 mg/dL. There was no difference in mortality rates among the groups during hospitalization or at 3 or 6 months. There were, however, statistically and clinically significant reductions in post–myocardial infarction heart failure during hospitalization (10% absolute risk reduction) and in re infarction at 3 months (3.7% absolute risk reduction).

9. Conclusions and recommendations

Concluding, there is currently insufficient evidence to consider glucose control as a quality measure during acute myocardial infarction hospitalization, although this position may change in the future. The recommendations from a scientific statement from the American Heart Association, in hyperglycemia in acute coronary syndromes[78], are the next:

1. Glucose level should be a part of the initial laboratory evaluation in all patients with suspected or confirmed acute coronary syndrome.
2. In patients admitted to an ICU with acute myocardial infarction, glucose levels should be monitored closely. It is reasonable to consider intensive glucose control in patients with significant hyperglycemia (plasma glucose >180 mg/dL), regardless of prior diabetes history. Although efforts to optimize glucose control may also be considered in patients with milder degrees of hyperglycemia, the data regarding a benefit from this approach are not yet definitive, and regardless of diabetes status. The precise goal of treatment has not yet been defined. Until further data are available, approximation of normoglycemia appears to be a reasonable goal (suggested range for plasma glucose 90 to 140 mg/dL), as long as hypoglycemia is avoided.
3. Insulin, administered as an intravenous infusion, is currently the most effective method of controlling glucose among patients hospitalized in the ICU. Effective protocols for insulin infusion and glucose monitoring have been developed in other patient populations. Care should be taken to avoid hypoglycemia, which has been shown to have an adverse prognostic impact.
4. Treatment should be instituted as soon as feasible, without compromising the administration of life-saving and evidence-based treatments.
5. In patients hospitalized in the non-ICU setting, efforts should be directed at maintaining plasma glucose levels >180 mg/dL with subcutaneous insulin regimens.
6. Acute myocardial infarcted patients with hyperglycemia but without prior history of diabetes should have further evaluation (preferably before hospital discharge) to

determine the severity of their metabolic derangements. This evaluation may include fasting glucose and HbA1C assessment and, in some cases, a post discharge oral glucose tolerance test.

7. Before discharge, plans for optimal outpatient glucose control should be determined in those patients with established diabetes, newly diagnosed diabetes, or evidence of insulin resistance.

The chronic and acute hyperglycemia associated to acute coronary syndromes, mainly in acute myocardial infarction is an independent and determinant factor in the outcome for patients with and without diabetes mellitus. The evidence in clinical trials has showed the importance of admission glucose and glycated hemoglobin, in the evolution, risk for complications, and therapeutic response of patients with acute myocardial infarction. The control of blood glucose levels in patients with acute myocardial infarction, will lead to better outcomes regardless of diabetes status. The precise goal of treatment has not yet been defined. Until further data are available, approximation of normoglycemia appears to be a reasonable goal, as long as hypoglycemia is avoided.

Author details

Marco A. López Hernández
Internal Medicine Division, Ecatepec General Hospital, Mexico State Health Institute, Mexico

10. References

[1] Wahab NN, Cowden EA, Pearce NJ, Gardner MJ, Merry H, Cox JL. Is blood glucose an independent predictor of mortality in acute myocardial infarction in the thrombolytic era? J Am Coll Cardiol. 2002; 40:1748 –1754.

[2] Zeller M, Steg P, Ravisy J, Laurent Y, Janin- Manificat L, L'Huillier I, Beer J, Oudot A, Rioufol G, Makki H, Farnier M, Rochette L, Verges, Cottin Y. Prevalence and impact of metabolic syndrome on hospital outcomes in acute myocardial nfarction. Arch Intern Med. 2005;165:1192–1198.

[3] Raz I, Wilson PW, Strojek K. Effects of prandial versus fasting glycemia on cardiovascular outcomes in type 2 diabetes: the HEART2D trial. Diabetes Care. 2009 Mar;32(3):381-6

[4] Siegelaar SE, Kerr L, Jacober SJ. A Decrease in Glucose Variability Does Not Reduce Cardiovascular Event Rates in Type 2 Diabetic Patients After Acute Myocardial Infarction Diabetes Care 34:855–857, 2011

[5] Thom T, Haase N, Rosamond W, et al, for the American Heart Association Statistics Committee and Stroke Statistics Subcommittee. Heart disease and stroke statistics—2006 update: a report from the AHA Statistics Committee and Stroke Statistics Subcommittee. Circulation. 2006;113:e85– e151

[6] Haffner SM, Lehto S, Ronnemaa T, Pyörälä K, Laakso M. Mortality from coronary heart disease in subjects with type 2 diabetes and in nondiabetic subjects with and without prior myocardial infarction. N Engl J Med. 1998;339:229 –234
[7] Stamler J, Vaccaro O, Neaton JD, Wentworth D. Diabetes, other risk factors and 12-yr cardiovascular mortality for men screened in the Multiple Risk Factor Intervention Trial. Diabetes Care. 1993;16:434–444.
[8] Kannel WB, McGee DL. Diabetes and glucose tolerance as risk factors for cardiovascular disease: the Framingham Study. Diabetes Care. 1979;2:120 –126.
[9] Roper NA, Bilous RW, Kelly WF, Unwin NC, Connolly VM. Excess mortality in a population with diabetes and the impact of material deprivation: longitudinal, population based study. BMJ. 2001;332: 1389–1393
[10] Nicolua JC, Maia LN, vitola JV, Mahaffey KW, Machado MN, Ramires JA, Baseline glucosa and left ventricular remodeling after acute myocardial infarction. J Diabetes Complications 2007.Sep- Oct 21(5):294-9.
[11] Dandona P, Chaudhuri A, Ghanim H, Mohanty P. Effect of hyperglycemia and insulin in acute coronary syndromes. Am J Cardiol. 2007. Jun 4:99(11A);12H-18H.
[12] Gufstasson I, Kistorp CN, James NK, et al. Unrecognized glycometabolic disturbance as measured by hemoglobin A1c is associated with a poor outcome after acute myocardial infarction. Am Heart J. 2007; Sep 154(3): 470-6
[13] Ishihara M, Kagawa E, Inoue I, et al. Impact of admission hyperglycemia and diabetes mellitus in short and long term mortality after acute myocardial infarction in the coronary intervention era. Am J Cardiol. 2007; Jun 15:99 (12): 1674-9.
[14] Libby P, Plutzky J. Diabetic macrovascular disease: the glucose paradox? Circulation 2002;106:2760 –2763.
[15] Verhagen SN, Wassink AM, van der Graaf Y, et al. Insulin resistance increases the occurrence of new cardiovascular events in patients with manifest arterial disease without known diabetes. the SMART study. Cardiovasc Diabetol. 2011 Nov 21;10:100.
[16] Mathews DR, Hosker JP, Rudensky AS, et al. Homeostasis model assessment: insulin resistance and ß-cell function from fasting plasma glucose and insulin concentrations in man. Diabetologia. 1985; 28: 412–9.
[17] Haffner SM, Gonzales C, Mykkänen L, et al. Total immunoreactive proinsulin, immunoreactive insulin and specific insulin in relation to conversion to type 2 diabetes. Diabetologia. 1997;40:830–7.
[18] Young LH, Renfu Y, Russell R, Hu X, Caplan M, Ren J, Shulman GI, Sinusas AJ. Low-flow ischemia leads to translocation of canine heart GLUT-4 and GLUT-1 glucose transporters to the sarcolemma in vivo. Circulation. 1997;95:415– 422.
[19] Ceriello A, Taboga C, Tonutti L, et al. Evidence for an independent and cumulative effect of postprandial hypertriglyceridemia and hyperglycemia on endothelial dysfunction and oxidative stress generation: effects of short- and long term simvastatin treatment. Circulation. 2002;106:1211–8.
[20] Scognamiglio R, Negut C, De Kreutzenberg SV, et al. Postprandial myocardial perfusion in healthy subjects and in type 2 diabetic patients. Circulation. 2005;112:179–84.

[21] Gardner GS, Frisch DR, Murphy SA, Kirtane AJ, Giugliano RP, Antman EM, et al; TIMI Study Group. Effect of rescue or adjunctive percutaneous coronary intervention of the culprit artery after fibrinolytic administration on epicardial flow in nonculprit arteries. Am J Cardiol 2004; 94: 178– 181.

[22] Gibson CM, Ryan KA, Murphy SA, Mesley R, Marble SJ, Giugliano RP, et al. Impaired coronary blood flow in nonculprit arteries in the setting of acute myocardial infarction. J Am Coll Cardiol 1999; 34: 974–982

[23] Williams SB, Goldfine AB, Timimi FK, Roddy MA, Simonson DC, Creager MA. Acute hyperglycemia attenuates endothelium-dependent vasodilation in human in vivo. Circulation 1998; 97: 1695 – 1701.

[24] Kelley DE, Simoneau JA. Impaired free fatty acid utilization by skeletal muscle in non-insulindependent diabetes mellitus. J Clin Invest. 1994;94: 2349-2356.

[25] Cummings MH, Watts GF, Umpleby AM, et al. Increased hepatic secretion of very-low-density lipoprotein apolipoprotein B-100 in NIDDM. Diabetologia. 1995;38:959-967

[26] Esposito K, Nappo F, Marfella R, Giugliano G, Giugliano F, Ciotola M, et al. Inflammatory cytokine concentrations are acutely increased by hyperglycemia in humans: Role of oxidative stress. Circulation 2002; 106: 2067 – 2072.

[27] Cain BS, Harken AH, Meldrum DR: Therapeutic strategies to reduce TNF-alpha mediated cardiac contractile depression following ischemia and reperfusion. J Mol Cell Cardiol 1999, 31:931-947.

[28] Das UN: Possible beneficial action(s) of glucose-insulinpotassium regimen in acute myocardial infarction and inflammatory conditions: a hypothesis. Diabetologia 2000, 43: 1081-1082

[29] Ceriello A, Testa F. Antioxidant Anti-Inflammatory Treatment in Type 2 Diabetes. Diabetes care. 2009, Nov;32 Suppl 2:S232-6.

[30] Carr ME. Diabetes mellitus: a hypercoagulable state. J Diabetes Complications. 2001;15:44-54.

[31] Ceriello A, Giugliano D, Quatraro A, et al. Evidence for a hyperglycaemia-dependent decrease of antithrombin III-thrombin complex formation in humans. Diabetologia. 1990;33:163-167.

[32] Ceriello A, Giacomello R, Stel G, et al. Hyperglycemia- induced thrombin formation in diabetes. Diabetes. 1995;44:924-28.

[33] Stegenga ME, van der Crabben SN, Levi M, et al. Hyperglycemia stimulates coagulation, whereas hyperinsulinemia impairs fibrinolysis in healthy humans. Diabetes 2006;55:1807-12.

[34] Zarich SW, Nesto RW. Implications and Treatment of Acute Hyperglycemia in the Setting of Acute Myocardial Infarction. Circulation. 2007 May 8;115(18):e436-9.

[35] Dirkali A, van der Ploeg T. The impact of admission plasma glucose on long-term mortality after STEMI and NSTEMI myocardial infarction. Int J Cardiology 2007; 121(2):215–217

[36] S. Hoshida, M. Teragaki, Y. J. Lim et al. Admission with metabolic disorder is a useful predictor of the 1-year prognosis for patients with unstable angina, but not for patients

with acute myocardial infarction: East-Osaka Acute Coronary Syndrome Registry. Coronary Art Dis 2011; 22(6): 416–420

[37] Cid-Alvarez B, Gude F, Cadarso-Suarez C et al. Admission and fasting plasma glucose for estimating risk of death of diabetic and nondiabetic patients with acute coronary syndrome: nonlinearity of hazard ratios and time-dependent comparison," Am Heart J,2009;158(6) 989–997

[38] Malmberg K, Yusuf S, Gerstein HC, et al. Impact of diabetes on long-term prognosis in patients with unstable angina and non-Q-wave myocardial infarction: results of the OASIS (Organization to Assess Strategies for Ischemic Syndromes) Registry. Circulation. 2000;102:1014-1019

[39] Capes SE, Hunt D, Malmberg K, Gerstein HC.Stress hyperglycaemia and increased risk of death after myocardial infarction in patients with and without diabetes: a systematic overview. Lancet. 2000;355:773–778.

[40] Malmberg K, Norhammar A, Wedel H, Ryden L. Glycometabolic state at admission: Important risk marker of mortality in conventionally treated patients with diabetes mellitus and acute myocardial infarction: long-term results from the Diabetes and Insulin-Glucose Infusion in Acute Myocardial Infarction (DIGAMI) study. Circulation. 1999;99:2626 –2632.

[41] Stranders I, Diamant M, van Gelder R, Spruijt H, Twisk JWR, Heine RJ, Visser FC. Admission blood glucose level as risk indicator of death after myocardial infarction in patients with and without diabetes mellitus. Arch Intern Med. 2004;164:982–988.

[42] Ishihara M, Sato H, Tateishi H, Kawagoe T, Shimatani Y, Kurisu S, et al. Implications of prodromal angina pectoris in anterior wall acute myocardial infarction: Acute angiographic findings and long-term prognosis. J Am Coll Cardiol 1997; 30: 970 – 975.

[43] Maruhashi T, Ishihara M, Inoue I, Kawagoe T, Shimatani Y, Kurisu S, et al. Effect of prodromal angina pectoris on the infarct progression in patients with first ST-elevation acute myocardial infarction. Circ J 2010; 74: 1651 – 1657

[44] Oswald GA, Corcoran S, Yudkin JS. Prevalence and risk of hyperglycemia and undiagnosed diabetes in patients with acute myocardial infarction. Lancet 1984; 1: 1264 – 1267.

[45] Capes SE, Hunt D, Malmberg K, Gerstein HC. Stress hyperglycemia and increased risk after myocardial infarction in patients without diabetes: A systematic overview. Lancet 2000; 355: 773 – 778

[46] Ishihara M. Acute hyperglycemia in patients with acute myocardial infarction. Circ J. 2012 Feb 24;76(3):563-71.

[47] Sinnaeve PR, Steg PG, Fox KA, et al. Association of elevated fasting glucose with increased short term and 6 month mortaliy in ST-segment elevation and non ST-segment elevation acute coronary syndromes: the Global Registry of Acute Coronary Events. Arch Intern Med. 2009;169:402–9.

[48] Iribarren C, Karter AJ, Go AS, et al. Glycemic control and heart failure among adult patients with diabetes. Circulation. 2001;103:2668–73

[49] Sanjuan R, Nuñez J, Blasco ML.Prognostic Implications of Stress Hyperglycemia in Acute ST Elevation Myocardial Infarction. Prospective Observational Study. Rev Esp Cardiol. 2011;64(3):201–207

[50] Pinto DS, Kirtane AJ, Pride YB, Murphy SA, Sabatine MS, Cannon ChP, et al. Association of blood glucose with angiographic and clinical outcomes among patients with ST-segment elevation myocardial infarction (From the CLARITYTIMI- 28 Study). Am J Cardiol. 2008;101:303–7.

[51] Timmer J, Ottervanger J, de Boer M, Dambrink JE, Hoorntje JCA, Gosselink ATM, Suryapranata H, Zijlstra F, Van't Hof AWJ, for the Zwolle Myocardial Infarction Study Group. Hyperglycemia is an important predictor of impaired coronary flow before reperfusion therapy in ST-segment elevation myocardial infarction. J Am Coll Cardiol. 2005;45:999 –1002.

[52] Prasad A, Stone G, Stuckey T, Costantini CO, Zimetbaum PJ, McLaughlin M, Mehran R, Garcia E, Tcheng JE, Cox DA, Grines CL, Lansky AJ, Gersh BJ. Impact of diabetes mellitus on myocardial perfusion after primary angioplasty in patients with acute myocardial infarction. J Am Coll Cardiol. 45:508 –514.

[53] Iwakura K, Ito H, Ikushima M, Kawano S, Okamura A, Asano K, Kuroda T, Tanaka K, Masuyama T, Hori M, Fujii K. Association between hyperglycemia and the no-reflow phenomenon in patients with acute myocardial infarction. J Am Coll Cardiol. 2003; 41:1–7.

[54] Dziewierz A, Giszterowicz D, Siudak Z, Rakowski T, Dubiel JS, Dudek D.Admission glucose level and in-hospital outcomes in diabetic and non-diabetic patients with acute myocardial infarction. Clin Res Cardiol. 2010 Nov; 99(11):715-21

[55] Dziewierz A, Siudak Z, Rakowski T, Jakała J, Dubiel JS, Dudek D. Prognostic significance of new onset atrial fibrillation in acute coronary syndrome patients treated conservatively. Cardiol J. 2010;17(1):57-64.

[56] Sanjuan R, Blasco ML, Martinez-Maicas H, Carbonell N, Miñana G, Nuñez J, Bodí V, Sanchis J. Acute myocardial infarction: high risk ventricular tachyarrhythmias and admission glucose level in patients with and without diabetes mellitus. Curr Diabetes Rev. 2011;7 (2):126-34

[57] Bloch Thomsen PE, Jons C, Raatikainen MJ, Moerch Joergensen R, Hartikainen J, Virtanen V, Boland J, Anttonen O, Gang UJ, Hoest N, Boersma LV, Platou ES, Becker D, Messier MD, Huikuri HV; Cardiac Arrhythmias and Risk Stratification After Acute Myocardial Infarction (CARISMA) Study Group. Long-Term Recording of Cardiac Arrhythmias With an Implantable Cardiac Monitor in Patients With Reduced Ejection Fraction After Acute Myocardial Infarction. Circulation. 2010 Sep 28;122(13):1258-64.

[58] Jons C, Joergensen RM, Hassager C, Gang UJ, Dixen U, Johannesen A, Olsen NT, Hansen TF, Messier M, Huikuri HV, Thomsen PE. Diastolic dysfunction predicts new-onset atrial fibrillation and cardiovascular events in patients with acute myocardial infarction and depressed left ventricular systolic function: a CARISMA substudy. Eur J Echocardiogr. 2010 Aug;11(7):602-7

[59] Shah AM, Uno H, Køber L, Velazquez EJ, Maggioni AP, MacDonald MR, Petrie MC, McMurray JJ, Califf RM, Pfeffer MA, Solomon SD. The inter-relationship of diabetes

and left ventricular systolic function on outcome after high-risk myocardial infarction. Eur J Heart Fail. 2010 Nov;12(11):1229-37.

[60] Pfeffer MA, McMurray JJ, Velazquez EJ, Rouleau JL, Køber L, Maggioni AP, Solomon SD, Swedberg K, Van de Werf F, White H, Leimberger JD, Henis M, Edwards S, Zelenkofske S, Sellers MA, Califf RM. Valsartan in Acute Myocardial Infarction Trial Investigators. Valsartan, captopril, or both in myocardial infarction complicated by heart failure, left ventricular dysfunction, or both. N Engl J Med 2003;349:1893–906.

[61] Goyal A. Metha SR, Diaz R et al. Differential clinical outcomes associated with hypoglycemia and hyperglycemia in acute myocardial infarction. Circulation. 2009 Dec 15;120(24):2429-37.

[62] Borg R, Kuenen JC, Carstensen B, et al.; ADAG Study Group. HbA1c and mean blood glucose show stronger associations with cardiovascular disease risk factors than do postprandial glycaemia or glucose variability in persons with diabetes: the A1C-Derived Average Glucose (ADAG) study. Diabetologia 2011;54: 69–72

[63] Nalysnyk L, Hernandez-Medina M, Krishnarajah G. Glycemic variability and complications in patients with diabetes mellitus: evidence from a systematic review of the literature. Diabetes Obes Metab 2010;12:288–298

[64] Monnier L, Colette C, Mas E, et al. Regulation of oxidative stress by glycemic control: evidence for an independent inhibitory effect of insulin therapy. Diabetologia 2010;53:562–571

[65] Risso A, Mercuri F, Quagliaro L, Damante G, Ceriello A. Intermittent high glucose enhances apoptosis in human umbilical vein endothelial cells in culture. Am J Physiol Endocrinol Metab 2001; 281: E924 – E930

[66] Scognamiglio R, Negut C, Vigili S et al. Postprandial myocardial perfusión in healthy subjects and in type 2 diabetic patients. Circulation 2005;112:179-84.

[67] United Kingdom Prospective Diabetes Study Group: Intensive blood glucose control with sulphonylureas or insulin compared with conventional treatment and risk of complications in patients with type 2 diabetes (UKPDS 33). Lancet 1998;352:837-53.

[68] Ceriello A. Postprandial hyperglycemia and diabetes complications: is it time to treat? Diabetes 2005;54:1-7.

[69] Sodi-Pallares D, Testelli MR, Fishleder BL, Bisteni A, Medrano GA, Friedland C, DeMicheli A. Effects of an intravenous infusion of a potassium-insulin-glucose solution on the electrocardiographic signs of myocardial infarction: a preliminary clinical report. Am J Cardiol. 1962;9:166 –181.

[70] The NICE-SUGAR Study Investigators. Intensive versus conventional glucose control in critically ill patients. N Engl J Med 2009; 360: 1283 – 1297.

[71] American Diabetes Association. Standards of Medical Care in Diabetes—2012. Diabetes Care 2012; 35 supp 1:S11-S63.

[72] Antman EM, Hand M, Armstrong PW et al. 2007 focused update of the ACC/AHA 2004 Guidelines for the Management of Patients With ST Elevation Myocardial Infarction: a report of the American College of Cardiology/American Heart Association Task Force on Practice Guidelines. Circulation 2008;117:296-329.

[73] Mehta SR, Yusuf S, Diaz R, Zhu J, Pais P, Xavier D, Paolasso E, Ahmed R, Xie C, Kazmi K, Tai J, Orlandini A, Pogue J, Liu L, for the CEATE-ECLA Trial Group Investigators. Effect of glucose-insulin-potassium infusion on mortality in patients with acute ST-segment elevation myocardial infarction: the CREATE-ECLA Randomized Controlled Trial. JAMA. 2005;293:437– 444.

[74] Ampudia-Blasco FJ, Ceriello A. Importance of daily glycemic variability in achieving glycemic targets in type 2 diabetes: role of DPP-4 inhibitors. Med Clin (Barc). 2010 Sep;135 Suppl 2:33-9

[75] Malmberg K, Ryden L, Wedel H, Birkeland K, Bootsma A, Dickstein K, Efendic S, Fisher M, Hamsten A, Herlitz J, Hildebrandt P, MacLeod K, Laakso M, Torp-Pedersen C, Waldenstrom A. Intense metabolic control by means of insulin in patients with diabetes mellitus and acute myocardial infarction (DIGAMI 2): effects on mortality and morbidity. Eur Heart J 2005;26:650–661.

[76] Van de Werf F, Bax J, Betriu A et al. Management of acute myocardial infarction in patients presenting with persistent ST-segment elevation The Task Force on the management of ST-segment elevation acute myocardial infarction of the European Society of Cardiology. European Heart Journal (2008) 29, 2909–2945.

[77] Cheung NW, Wong VW, McLean M. The Hyperglycemia: Intensive Insulin Infusion in Infarction (HI-5) study: a randomized controlled trial of insulin infusion therapy for myocardial infarction. Diabetes Care. 2006;29:765–770..

[78] Deedwania P, Kosiborod M, Barrett E, et al. Hyperglycemia and Acute Coronary Syndrome A Scientific Statement From the American Heart Association Diabetes Committee of the Council on Nutrition, Physical Activity, and Metabolism. Circulation. 2008;117:1610-1619.

Chapter 11

Physical Activity in the Management of Diabetes Mellitus

N.A. Odunaiya and O.O. Oguntibeju

Additional information is available at the end of the chapter

http://dx.doi.org/10.5772/55522

1. Introduction

1.1. Definitions

Physical activity is any bodily movement produced by skeletal muscles that result in energy expenditure beyond resting level. This is a broad definition which involves virtually all types of activity like walking, cycling, dancing, traditional games, pastimes, gardening, housework, sports and others **(**WHO, 2012, Cavil et al, 2006**)**. Conversely, an individual is termed inactive when there is no marked increase in energy expenditure above resting level. Sedentary lifestyle include some activity, but usually not enough for gaining health effects, while active living is a way of life that integrates at least half an hour of physical activity each day into daily routines (Hagstromer, 2007).

Physical activity can be classified into two main categories. One is 'exercise' that involves structured and repetitive bodily movements. The other is 'non-exercise physical activity', such as standing, commuting to and from school or work, or participating in household chores or occupational work. Thus, sport and exercise are seen as particular types of physical activity: sport usually involve some form of competition, and exercise usually being taken to improve fitness and health. Physical activity is important for health, the levels and patterns of physical activities in a population comprise an important generic indicator in public health

The term health-enhancing physical activity is defined as any form of physical activity that benefits health and functional capacity without undue harm or risk. It emphasizes the connection between health and physical activity (Foster, 2000). Physical activity is important for health and the levels and patterns of physical activity in a population constitute an important generic indicator in public health. Physical inactivity, usually together with unhealthy food habits, is associated with the development of many of the major non-communicable diseases and conditions in the society, such as cardiovascular disease, some cancers, obesity, diabetes and osteoporosis. It has become increasingly clear that physical inactivity is a global health issue. Physical activity which is beneficial to health must be moderate or vigorous in intensity. Important favorable health effects of physical activity for adults are extensively documented and well accepted by health professionals. Reviewers have identified at least modest positive effects in the population or subsamples of youths on such health outcomes as aerobic fitness, blood lipids, blood pressure, body composition, glucose metabolism, skeletal health, and psychological health. Various levels of physical activity participation are associated with health benefits and/or health risks (Bailey et al, 1999).

2. Classification and types of physical activity

Physical activity is broadly classified using three criteria which are: intensity of activity, energy system utilized during the activity and the effect of the activity on body tissues and systems.

Classification by intensity of activity: Physical activity is classified using intensity as light or low, moderate and vigorous. It is important to provide a clear and comprehensive definition of sedentary behaviour in order to understand what a light physical activity is. Sedentary behavior refers to activities that do not increase energy expenditure substantially above the resting level and include activities such as sleeping, sitting, lying down, and watching television, and other forms of screen-based entertainment. Specifically, sedentary behavior include activities that involve energy expenditure at the level of 1.0-1.5 metabolic equivalent units (METs), where One MET is the energy cost of resting quietly, often defined in terms of oxygen uptake as 3.5mLIkg-1min-1). Light physical activity, which often is grouped with sedentary behavior but is in fact a distinct activity construct and involves energy expenditure at the level of 1.6-2.9 METs (Pate et al, 2008). It includes activities such as slow walking, sitting and writing, cooking food, and washing dishes or doing house chores. Moderate exercise generally relates to aerobic forms of exercise. These include: brisk walking, biking on flat ground, or dancing. Moderate intensity activity is exercise that requires 3 to 6 METs of effort. During moderate physical activity, breathing and heart rate become more rapid and the body burns about 3.5 to 7 calories per minute (depending on weight and fitness level). Vigorous intensity activity is intense exercise that requires more than 7 METs of effort. During vigorous physical activity, breathing and heart rate are rapid as the body exerts itself. Vigorous activity burns 8 or more calories per minute (depending on weight and fitness level). Examples of vigorous physical activity are jogging and running, in-line skating, tennis, or calisthenics such as push-ups and jumping jacks performed with intense effort (Pate et al, 2008).

Classification by energy system utilized: Three energy systems are involved in activities performed by every individual; ATP PCr system, lactic acid system and aerobic system. Activities utilizing these systems could be aerobic or anaerobic activities. There are three separate energy systems through which ATP can be produced for activity. A number of factors determine which of these energy systems is chosen, such as exercise intensity and duration.

2.1. The ATP-PCr system

ATP and creatine phosphate (also called phosphocreatine or PCr for short) make up the ATP-PCr system. PCr is broken down releasing a phosphate and energy, which is then used to rebuild ATP. ATP is rebuilt by adding a phosphate to ADP in a process called phosphorylation by an enzyme that controls the breakdown of PCr called creatine kinase (Macardle et al, 2000).

The ATP-PCr energy system can operate with or without oxygen but because it does not rely on the presence of oxygen it is said to be anaerobic. During the first 5 seconds of exercise, energy system utilized is the ATP-PCr system. ATP concentrations last only a few seconds with PCr buffering the drop in ATP for another 5-8 seconds. Combined, the ATP-PCr system can sustain all-out exercise for 3-15 seconds, so ATP- PCr system takes care of activities of short duration and high intensity (Macardle et al, 2000). If activity continues beyond this immediate period, the body must rely on another energy system to produce ATP.

2.2. The glycolytic system

Glycolysis literally means the breakdown of glucose and consists of a series of enzymatic reactions. The carbohydrates we eat supply the body with glucose, which can be stored as glycogen in the muscles or liver for later use. The end product of glycolysis is pyruvic acid. Pyruvic acid can then be either funnelled through a process called the Krebs cycle or converted into lactic acid. It is anaerobic glycolisis if the final product is lactic acid and aerobic glycolysis if the final product is pyruvic acid. Alternative terms that are often used are fast glycolysis if the final product is lactic acid and slow glycolysis for the process that leads to pyruvate being funnelled through the Krebs cycle. As its name suggest, the fast glycolitic system can produce energy at a greater rate than slow glycolysis. However, because the end product of fast glycolysis is lactic acid, it can quickly accumulate and is thought to lead to muscular fatigue. The contribution of the fast glycolytic system increases rapidly after the initial 10 seconds of exercise. This also coincides with a drop in maximal power output as the immediately available phosphogens, ATP and PCr, begin to run out. By about 30 seconds of sustained activity, the majority of energy comes from fast glycolysis. At 45 seconds of sustained activity, there is a second decline in power output (the first decline being after about 10 seconds). Activity beyond this point corresponds with a growing reliance on the oxidative system (Macardle et al, 2000).

The oxidative system consists of four processes to produce ATP: slow glycolysis (aerobic glycolysis), Krebs cycle (citric acid cycle or tricarboxylic acid cycle), electron transport chain and beta oxidation. Slow glycolysis is exactly the same series of reactions as fast glycolysis that metabolise glucose to form two ATPs. The difference, however, is that the end product pyruvic acid is converted into a substance called acetyl coenzyme A rather than lactic acid. Following glycolysis, further ATP can be produced by funnelling acetyl coenzyme A through the Krebs cycle. The Krebs cycle is a complex series of chemical reactions that continues the oxidization of glucose that was started during glycolysis. Acetyl coenzyme A enters the Krebs cycle and is broken down into carbon dioxide and hydrogen allowing more two more ATPs to be formed. However, the hydrogen produced in the Krebs cycle plus the hydrogen produced during glycolysis, left unchecked would cause cells to become too acidic, therefore hydrogen combines with two coenzymes called NAD and FAD and is transported to the electron transport chain. Hydrogen is carried to the electron transport chain, another series of chemical reactions, and here it combines with oxygen to form water thus preventing acidification. This chain, which requires the presence of oxygen, results in 34 ATPs being formed. Beta oxidation, unlike glycolysis, the Krebs cycle and electron transport chain can metabolise fat as well as carbohydrate to produce ATP. Lipolysis is the term used to describe the breakdown of fat (triglycerides) into the more basic units of glycerol and free fatty acids. Before these free fatty acids can enter the Krebs cycle they must undergo a process of beta oxidation-a series of reactions to further reduce free fatty acids to acetyl coenzyme A and hydrogen. Acetyl coenzyme A can now enter the Krebs cycle and from this point on, fat metabolism follows the same path as carbohydrate metabolism (Macardle et al, 2000).

2.3. Energy systems & training

Each of the three energy systems can generate power to different capacities and varies within individuals. Best estimates suggest that the ATP-PCR system can generate energy at a rate of roughly 36 kcal per minute. Glycolysis can generate energy only half as quickly at about 16 kcal per minute. The oxidative system has the lowest rate of power output at about 10 kcal per minute. The capacity to generate power by each of the three energy systems can vary with training. The ATP-PCr and glycolytic pathways may change by only 10-20% with training. The oxidative system seems to be far more trainable although genetics play a limiting role here too. VO2max, or aerobic power can be increased by as much as 50% but this is usually in untrained, sedentary individuals (Macardle et al, 2000).

2.3.1. Energy systems and physical activity

The three energy systems do not work independently of one another. From very short, very intense exercise, to very light, prolonged activity, all the three energy systems make a contribution however, one or two usually predominate.

3. Classification by effect on the body tissues and system

This type of physical activity includes muscle-strengthening, bone strengthening, and stretching. Exercises or activities that have a great impact on muscular strength involve weights, bands or body weight and work the muscles to maintain a specific movement. These activities are also referred to as resistance training exercises and include pushups and sit-ups, biceps curls, lifting weights, climbing stairs, and digging in the garden and calisthenics. The muscle is metabolically active tissue and this means that it utilizes calories to work, repair, and refuel itself. However, as one grows older, there is gradual loss of muscle cell as part of the natural aging process which means that the amount of calories needed each day starts to decrease, and it becomes easier to gain weight. Therefore, engaging in regular strength training exercise could decrease this loss of lean muscle tissue and even replace some that has been lost already (Macardle et al, 2000).

Strength training increases lean body mass, decrease fat mass, and increase resting metabolic rate in younger and older adults. While strength training on its own typically does not lead to weight loss, its beneficial effects on body composition may make it easier to manage one's weight and ultimately reduce the risk of disease, by slowing the gain of fat especially abdominal fat. Another beneficial effect of resistance training pertains to bone health. In addition to weight bearing, cardiovascular exercise, weight training has been shown to help fight osteoporosis. For example, a study in postmenopausal women examined whether regular strength training and high-impact aerobics sessions would help prevent osteoporosis. In some studies, researchers found that the women who participated in at least two sessions a week for three years were able to preserve bone mineral density at the spine and hip; over the same time period, a sedentary control group showed bone mineral density losses of 2 to 8 percent (Engelke et al, 2006; Katzmarzyk and Craig, 2002; Gale et al, 2007). Bone-strengthening activities strengthen the bones. This includes running, walking, jumping rope, and lifting weight. These activities make the feet, legs, or arms support the body's weight, thereby making the muscle push against the bone. Muscle-strengthening and bone-strengthening activities can also be aerobic. Whether they are depends on whether they make the heart and lungs work harder than usual. For example, running is an aerobic activity and a bone-strengthening activity. Stretching helps improve the flexibility and ability to fully move your joints. Examples of stretching is touching the toes, doing side stretches, and doing yoga exercises (NHLBI, 2011).

4. Benefits of physical activity

Regular physical activity is recognized as a key determinant of health and wellness. Strong evidence indicates that low levels of physical activity are linked with morbidity and mortality in adults, particularly the risk of chronic diseases such as type II diabetes, heart disease, osteoporosis and certain types of cancer and the risk of overweight and obesity in adults. Surveillance and monitoring are fundamental to developing evidence based programs and initiatives to combat obesity and reduce the risk for chronic disease (Chronic disease prevention Alliance of Canada,2005).

Routine physical activity has been shown to improve body composition e.g., through reduced abdominal adiposity and improved weight control; (Warburton et al, 2001, Mariona et al 2003), enhance lipid lipoprotein profiles (e.g., through reduced triglyceride levels, increased high-density lipoprotein [HDL] cholesterol levels and decreased low-density lipoprotein [LDL]-to-HDL ratios, improve glucose homeostasis and insulin sensitivity, reduce blood pressure, improve autonomic tone, reduce systemic inflammation (Adamopoulous, 2001), decrease blood coagulation, improve coronary blood flow, augment cardiac function and enhance endothelial function (Hambretch, 2000, Warburton et al, 2000).

Chronic inflammation, as indicated by elevated circulating levels of inflammatory mediators such as C-reactive protein, has been shown to be strongly associated with most of the chronic diseases whose prevention has benefited from exercise. Recent RCTs have shown that exercise training may cause marked reductions in C-reactive protein levels. Each of these factors may explain directly or indirectly the reduced incidence of chronic disease and premature death among people who engage in routine physical activity (Nicklas et al, 2005).

Routine physical activity is also associated with improved psychological well-being (e.g., through reduced stress, anxiety and depression. Psychological well-being is particularly important for the prevention and management of cardiovascular disease, but it also has important implications for the prevention and management of other chronic diseases such as diabetes, osteoporosis, hypertension, obesity, cancer and depression (Dunn et al, 2001, Warburton et al, 2011). Regular aerobic activity has been found to improve vascular function in adults independent of changes in other risk factors and has been said to result in a shear-stress–mediated improvement in endothelial function, which confers a health benefit to a number of disease states (Laughlin et al, 2004).

A study conducted by WHO European region reviewed the evidence for the health effects/benefits of physical activity and reported that it improved fitness, strength, flexibility and coordination, improved general health and assists in weight management, development of a wide range of motor skills, healthy growth and development of the cardiovascular system as well as the bones and muscles of the children. It further reported on the establishment of healthy behaviors that young people could carry throughout their lives such as better eating habits and decreased likelihood of smoking (Government of Western Australia, 2005).

Exercise has been shown to have impact on social benefits in children such as development of communication, interpersonal, leadership and co-operation skills, creation of lasting friendships, increased interest in accepting responsibility, teaches them how to deal with winning and losing, provides a vehicle for responsible risk taking, helps build social skills among children and may deter anti-social behaviours and helps young people develop self-discipline and leadership skill (Government of Western Australia, 2002).

Mental health benefits of physical activity among children includes improved self esteem and confidence, reduction in stress, anxiety and depression, improved mood and sense of wellbeing, improved concentration, enhanced memory and learning, and better performance at school, reduced feelings of fatigue and depression, and improved psychological wellbeing and mental awareness (Government Western Australia, 2005).

5. Health implications of sedentary living

Physical inactivity is a modifiable risk factor for cardiovascular disease and a widening variety of other chronic diseases, including diabetes mellitus, cancer (colon and breast), obesity, hypertension, bone and joint diseases (osteoporosis and osteoarthritis), and depression. Physical inactivity, usually together with unhealthy food habits, is associated with the development of many of the major non-communicable diseases and conditions in the society, such as cardiovascular disease, some cancers, obesity, diabetes and osteoporosis. It has become increasingly clear that physical inactivity is a global health issue among young and old(Halal et al 2012, Odunaiya et al, 2010), this is because of the technology advancement as children becomes progressively inactive as they spend more time indoor with school assignment, computer games, television and being carried to school either by bus or personal car (Sjostrom et al, 2003).

According to the World Health Organization, inactivity is responsible for a multitude of diseases, disabilities and even deaths (WHO, 2010). A dose–response relationship has been observed between time spent in sedentary behaviors (e.g., TV viewing time, sitting in a car, overall sitting time and all-cause and cardiovascular disease mortality (Katzmarzyk et al, 2009, Dunstan et al, 2010, Warren et al, 2010) This growing epidemiological evidence links sedentary behavior to health outcomes, including anxiety, diabetes mellitus, colon cancer, osteoporosis, high blood pressure, deep vein thrombosis, obesity, kidney stone, depression and cardiovascular diseases. This is shown in the epidemiological reviews of physical inactivity and it was concluded that sitting for a very long time in some particular jobs, using elevator, sitting in a car, TV viewing time and other encompassing factor is associated with some sedentary behavior).

The prevalence of childhood obesity and related health problems is increasing in many Western countries and is anticipated to continue to increase (Zaninto et al, 2010). Evidence of an association between physical activity and weight gain remains sparse (Wareham et al, 2005). However, three main benefits arising from adequate childhood physical activity have been postulated. The first is direct improvements in childhood health status and evidence is accumulating that more active children generally display healthier cardiovascular profiles, are better learner and develop higher peak bone masses than their less active counterparts. Secondly, there is a biological carryover into adulthood, whereby improved adult health status results from childhood physical activity. In particular, childhood obesity may be a precursor for a range of adverse health effects in adulthood, while higher bone masses in young people reduce the risk of osteoporosis in old age. Finally, there may be a behavioral carryover into adulthood, whereby active children are more likely to become more active (healthy) adults (Epteins, 2005) . Nevertheless, in an effort to halt or reverse trends in obesity, promotion of physical activity in children and adolescents has been identified as a key focus of efforts to promote health (Lobstein et al, 2004). Physical activity among children and adolescents is believed to be insufficient, and low levels of activity seem to persist into adulthood (WHO, 2004). This makes physical inactivity among young people a risk factor for developing cardiovascular disease, cancer, and osteoporosis in later life (Telema et al, 2005). The development and evaluation of interventions to promote physical activity in young people is therefore a priority. Physical activity which is beneficial to health must be moderate or vigorous in intensity (Hangstromer et al, 2007).

6. Measurement of physical activity

6.1. Types of measurement

Physical activity can best be measured by a combination of activity monitors, questionnaires, and analytical technique. The measures for physical activity can be organized into two categories, according to the type of information they provide: Subjective or self-report instruments and objective instruments. No one measure is capable of capturing all of the aspects related to physical activity but each has some advantages and some disadvantages (Sirard and Pate, 2001).

6.2. Objective measurement

Objective measurements are measurements that quantify levels of physical activity, producing data that are not influenced by recall ability, ethnicity, culture or socioeconomic status. Some objective instruments can also measure the duration, intensity and patterning of daily physical activity in children and youths. Objective methods for measuring physical activity make use of equipment like video, movement's counters, accelerometer, heart rate monitoring, blood pressure monitoring, electromyography, anthropometry, fitness, VO2 metabolic cart or VO2 portable equipment, respiration chamber and doubly labeled water (DLW). However, they require special equipment and are not very well adapted to a large sample study of children (Sirard and Pate, 2001).

6.3. Subjective measurement

Subjective instruments comprising self-report instruments such as questionnaires are straightforward means for population health researchers to gather information on the physical activity levels of individuals in their communities. These instruments are generally reliable, valid and are relatively simple and inexpensive to administer. These instruments should have good psychometric properties in order to be useful and such psychometric properties include validity, reliability, utility and responsiveness (Eslinger et al, 2005).

7. Effect of exercise on biochemical, metabolic and psychosocial variables in individuals with diabetes mellitus: an overview of systematic reviews, meta analysis and randomized control trial

7.1. Introduction

Physical activity (PA) is a key element in the prevention and management of type-2 diabetes mellitus. It has been observed that many persons with this chronic disease do not become or remain regularly active. High-quality studies establishing the importance of exercise and fitness in diabetes were lacking until recently, but it is now well established that participation in regular PA improves blood glucose control and can prevent or delay type-2 diabetes mellitus along with positively affecting lipids, blood pressure, cardiovascular events, mortality, and quality of life (Sigal et al, 2006). Structured interventions combining PA and modest weight loss have been shown to lower type-2 diabetes risk by up to 58% in high-risk populations. Most benefits of PA on diabetes management are realized through acute and chronic improvements in insulin action, accomplished with both aerobic and resistance training. Present recommendation includes 150 mins of aerobic exercise per week and resistance exercise 3 times a week. PA-associated blood glucose management, diabetes prevention, gestational diabetes mellitus, and safe and effective practices for PA with diabetes-related complications (Sigal et al, 2006).

In the last few years, a lot of studies have been conducted to assess the effects of exercise on several variables associated with diabetes mellitus. For effective management of individuals with diabetes mellitus using physical activity, it is critical to ensure that the type of exercise, frequency and duration most strongly associated with effectiveness are utilized. The aim of this systematic review of reviews, meta analysis, clinical trials was to identify evidence for the effectiveness/ impact of exercise/ level of evidence, exercise type, frequency and duration on biochemical, metabolic and psychosocial parameters of individuals with type 1 and type 2 diabetes mellitus.

7.2. Methods

Pedro and pubmed were searched for systematic reviews, meta-analysis, and clinical trials of interventions using physical activity in management of individuals with type 1 and type 2 diabetes mellitus from 2006 -2012. The search term used were exercise and diabetes. Literatures that addressed effectiveness to intervention components were extracted, graded for evidence and summarized. Clinical trials were assessed for methodological quality and materials that focused on effectiveness were extracted, graded and summarized. Information on effectiveness was extracted from systematic review and presented in a narrative form showing level of evidence. The RCT could not be pooled together for meta-analysis due to differences in designs and outcomes, consequently the results are presented in a narrative form.

7.3. Results

Three studies were systematic reviews, one of which included a meta analysis and 15 were randomized control trial of which one was duplicated, therefore 14 RCTs were included in the study.

Exercise has positive effect on metabolic, biochemical and psychosocial variables. Combination of aerobic and resistance exercise is more beneficial than either aerobic or resistance exercise. Daily exercise is not more beneficial than every other day exercise. Exercise of 30 mins duration every other day is as effective as 30 min exercise every day. Progressive resistance training is more effective than aerobic training and structured /supervised programme is more effective than advised exercise. Structured exercise, consisting of aerobic training, resistance training, or a combination of aerobic and resistance exercise training for at least 12 weeks, is associated with improved glycaemic control in type-2 diabetic patients. Structured weekly exercise of more than 150 minutes per week was associated with greater declines in HbA_{1c}. Structured exercise training reduced HbA_{1c} to a larger degree than physical activity advice. Physical activity advice is beneficial only if associated with dietary recommendations. Exercise improves quality of life, mental health and general health status. This is shown in Table 1

study	Author	year	population	Exec type	duration	Frequency	intensity	Impact on selected variables	Impact on psycho-social variable
SR	Umpierre et al	2011	Type 2 dia	Aerobic, resistance	30 min or more	Every day or every other day	Moderate, vigorous	Improve glycaemic control	
SR	Simpson and Singh	2008	Type 2 diab	X	X	X	X	Increase adiponectin	
SR	Thomas et al	2006	Type 2	X	X	X	X	Glucose control, increase insulin response, decrease plasma triglyceride	Reduction invisceral, sub Cute adiposity
RCT	Sigal et al	2007	Type 2	Aerobic and resistance, aerobic and resistance combined	x	Thrice weekly for 22 weeks	x	Combined aerobic and resistance has greater impact on biochemical variables	
RCT	Bacchi et al		Type 2	Aerobic, resistance compared	x	4 months intervention	x	Increase in peak vo2 max greater in aerobic, increase in strength more in resistance group. Insulin sensitivity similar in both groups and no significant difference for beta cell fuction in both groups	
RCT	Ng et al		Type 2	Aerobic, prog resistance exc compared		8 weeks 50 min aerobic at 65% of age predicted heart rate, 3 sets of 10 repetition at 65% of the assessed repetitive maximum		Both had positive effect on glycaemic control and health status but more significant changes in PRT Group in more domains of SF - 36	

study	Author	year	population	Exec type	duration	Frequency	intensity	Impact on selected variables	Impact on psycho-social variable
RCT	Gorden et al	2008	Type 2	Yoga, exercise				Decrease oxidative stress and improve anti oxidant status	
RCT	Van Dijk et al		Type 2			Daily or every other day		No difference in optimization of glycaemic control in daily or every other day hroup	
RCT	Swift et al	2012	Type 2	exer				Did not reduce C reactive protein	
RCT	Shvandi et al	2010	Type 2					Improved mental health, quality of life, and metabolic variables	
RCT	Lopez et al		Type 1	Exercise in conjunction with diet and medication				Positive influence on long term glycaemic control	
RCT	Lincoln et al		Type 2	Resistance exercise training				Improves mental health	
RCT	Adeniyi et al	2010	Type 2	Therapeutic exercise			12 week	Reduce pain, improves dermalotogical foot grade, disorders of ranges of movement but relapse when exercise was withdrawn	
RCT	Slentz et al	2009	Type 2	exercise		Moderate, vigorous		Larger significant increase with moderate exercise compared to Vigorous	
RCT	Taylor et al	2009	Type 2	Exercise and counseling directed by PT compared				No significant difference between both	

study	Author	year	population	Exec type	duration	Frequency	intensity	Impact on selected variables	Impact on psycho-social variable
				to supervised training					
RCT	Praet et al	2008	Type 2 diabetes	Brisk walking, individualized medical fitness program		3 times a week of 60 mins brisk walk, 3 sessions a week of supervised exercise using bicycle ergometer for 1 year		Improves biochemical variables and blood pressure in type 2 diabetes patients	
RCT	Winnick et al	2008	Type 2	Short term aerobic training				Improves whole body insulin sensitivity	

Table 1.

7.4. Discussion

All systematic reviews and clinical trial reviewed showed that exercise is effective in the management of both type 1 and type 2 of diabetes mellitus .Our review shows that there is limited study on the effect of exercise in the management of type 1 diabetes mellitus although exercise improves glycaemic control in conjunction with drugs and diet in type 1 diabetes mellitus. Both aerobic and resistance exercise are effective in the management of diabetes especially type-2 diabetes in improving glycaemic control However, for best management aerobic and resistance exercise should be combined as in current recommendation and moderate intensity should be preferred to vigorous intensity since vigorous exercise has no added advantage. Review shows that exercise frequency of greater than 150 mins per week is more effective than less than 150 mins per week in improving glycaemic control. However, exercise does not necessarily have to be daily as there is no significant difference in daily exercise and every other day exercise in improving glycaemic control. This is level 1 evidence.

Our review also shows that exercise improves quality of life, mental health and general health status of type-2 diabetic patients. This is level 2 evidence. Exercise also improves metabolic variables of type-2 diabetic patients with level 2 evidence. However, exercise withdrawal results in loss of all the benefits associated with exercise. It is important to note that therapeutic exercises are very effective and should be directed by experts. It is not sufficient to prescribe aerobic, resistance or both exercises for patients with type-2 diabetes but there is a need to involve exercise experts in the clinics such as physiotherapists/ exercise physiologists for therapeutic exercise especially in deconditioned and elderly patients.

7.5. Comment

For effective management of patients with diabetes mellitus, physicians should refer patients to exercise experts to enhance utilization of exercise and adherence to exercise in the management as many patients with diabetes mellitus do not participate in exercise regularly.

7.6. Limitations

Many studies were not clear on how they progress their training programmes and volumes of exercise used in many studies for comparison of aerobic and resistance exercise were not comparable. Many exercise programmes were not clear on intensity of aerobic exercise and duration per session as this could affect result by creating bias. We also recommend further studies on the effect of exercise in the management of type 1 diabetes.

Author details

N.A. Odunaiya
Department of Physiotherapy, College of Medicine, University of Ibadan, Ibadan, Nigeria
Department of Physiotherapy, Stellenbosch University, South Africa

O.O. Oguntibeju
Oxidative Stress Research Centre, Department of Biomedical Sciences, Faculty of Health & Wellness Sciences, Cape Peninsula University of Technology Bellville, South Africa

8. References

Adamopoulos, S, Piepoli, M, McCance, A (1992). Comparison of different methods for assessing sympathovagal balance in chronic congestive heart failure secondary to coronary artery disease. Am J Cardiopulmon70:1576-82.

Adamopoulos, S., Parissis, J., Kroupis, C (2001). Physical training reduces peripheral markers of inflammation in patients with chronic heart failure. Eur Heart J 22:791-7

Adeniyi, A.F., okafor, N., Adeniyi, CY (2011). Depression and physical activity in a sample of Nigerian adolescents: levels, relationships and predictors: child and adolescent psychiatry and mental health. J Mental Health 5:16-26

Bailey D. A, McKay H.A, Mirwald R.L, Crocker P.L.E & Faukner R.A (1999). A six-year longitudinal study of the relationship of physical activity to bone mineral accrual in growing children: The University of Saskatchewan bone mineral accrual study. J Bone and Mineral Res 14: 1672-1679.

Berg,A., Halle., M,Franz,I (1997). Physical activity and lipoprotein metabolism: epidemiological evidence and clinical trials. Eur J Med Res 2:259-64.

Blair, SN., Goodyear, NN., Gibbons, LW (1984). Physical fitness and incidence of hypertension in healthy normotensive men and women. JAMA 252:487-90.

Brooks, GA and Fahey T D (2000). Human energetics and its application: exercise physiology: Macmillian Publishing Company; Mayfield.

Bull, FC., Armstrong, TP, Dixon, T., Ham,S., Neiman, A., Pratt M (2004) Physical inactivity In: World Health Organization, ed. Comparative quantification of health risks Global and regional burden of disease attributable to selected major risk factors. Volume 1 Geneva, Switzerland: 729-881.

Cavill N, Kalmeirs S, Raciopp F (2006). Physical activity and health in Europe; evidence for action, Copenhagen; WHO regional office for Europe. www.who.org (Retrieved on 6th February, 2012).

The Chronic Disease Prevention Alliance of Canada (CDPAC) (2005). Newsbytes Vol: 1. Issue 3. http://www.cdpac.ca/content/pdf/CDPAC%20Newsbytes%20May_2005.pdf (Accessed on 7th October, 2012).

Dunn, AL., Trivedi, MH., O'Neal, HA (2001). Physical activity dose–response effects on outcomes of depression and anxiety. Med and Sci Sports and Exerc 33: S587-97.

Dunstan, D.W., Barr, E.L.M., Healy, G.N., Salmon, J., Shaw, J.E.,Balkau, B (2010). Television viewing time and mortality: the Australian Diabetes, Obesity and Lifestyle study (AusDiab). Circulation; 121(3): 384–391.

Engelke, K., Kemmler, W., Lauber, D., Beeskow, C., Pintag, R., Kalender, W A (2006). Exercise maintains bone density at spine and hip EFOPS: a 3-year longitudinal study in early postmenopausal women. Osteoporosis Int 17:133 42.

Eslinger D.W, Copeland JL, Barnes JD and Tremblay MS (2005). Standardizing and optimizing the use of accelerometer data for free-living physical activity monitoring. J Physical and Health 2(3): 366-383.

Foster C (2000). Guidelines for health-enhancing physical activity promotion programmes. The European Network for the Promotion of Health-Enhancing Physical Activity Tampere, the UKK Institute for Health Promotion Research.

Gale, CR., Martyn, CN, Cooper, C, Sayer, AA (2007). Grip strength, body composition and mortality. Int J Epidemiol 36:228-235.

Government of Western Australia (2OO2). http://www.dsr.wa.gov.au (Accessed 28th August, 2012).

Hallal PC, Anderson LB, Bull FC et al, 2012. Lancet Physical activity series of working group

Hagstromer M (2007). Assessment of health-enhancing physical activity at population level. Stockholm: Karolinska Institute.
http: //www.euphix.org (Retrieved 30th January, 2012).

Hambrecht, R., Wolf, A., Gielen, S (2000). Effect of exercise on coronary endothelial function in patients with coronary artery disease. N Engl J Med 342: 454-60.

Jason Karp (2009). The three metabolic energy systems; IDEA Fitness J, vol 6, no 2

Katzmarzyk, PT., Craig, CL (2002). Musculoskeletal fitness and risk of mortality. Med and Sci Sport and Exerc 34: 740-744.

Kelley, DE., Goodpaster, BH (1999). Effects of physical activity on insulin action and glucose tolerance in obesity. Med Sci Sports Exerc 31:S619-23.

Laughlin, MH, Wolfe JB (2004). Physical activity in prevention and treatment of coronary disease: the battle line is in exercise vascular cell biology. Med Sci Sports Exerc 36: 352-62.

Lobstein, T., Baur, L., Uauy, R (2004). Obesity in children and young people: a crisis in public health. Obesity Review 5 (suppl 1): 4-85.

Macardle DW, Katch FI and Katch VL (2000). Essentials of exercise physiology, 2nd edition Philadelphia, Lippincot Williams & Wilkins.

Maiorana A, O'Driscoll G, Taylor R (2003). Exercise and the nitric oxide vasodilator system. Sports Med 33: 1013-35

National heart living and blood institute (NHLBI). www.nih.gov/ health (Accessed on 6th Aug, 2012).

Nicklas, BJ., You, T., Pahor, M (2005). Behavioural treatments for chronic systemic inflammation: effects of dietary weight loss and exercise training. CMAJ 172(9):1199-209.

Odunaiya , NA., Ayodele, OA., Oguntibeju, OO,(2010). Physical activity levels of senior secondary school students in Ibadan, western Nigeria: West Ind Med J 59: 34-37.

Pate, R.R., O'Neill, J.R., and Lobelo, F (2008). The evolving definition of "sedentary. Exerc Sport Science 36 (4): 173–178.

Reilly, J.J., Dorosty, A.R. and Emmett, P.M (1999).Prevalence of overweight and obesity in British children: cohort study. Brit Med J 319: 1039.

Schmitz, KH., Hannan, PJ., Stovitz, SD., Bryan, CJ, Warren, M., Jensen, MD (2007). Strength training and adiposity in premenopausal women: Strong, Healthy, and Empowered study. Am J Clin Nutr 86: 566-572.

Sirard J.R and Pate RR (2001). Physical activity assessment in children and adolescents. Sports Med 31(6): 439-454.

SjostromM, Portvilient E, Yngve A (2003). Making way for healthier lifestyle in Europe: monitoring public health nutrition in Europe 2003. (Retrieved February 5th2012).

Sjotrom M,Oja P,Hagstromer M,Smith B.J,Bauma A (2006). Health–enhancing physical activity across European union countries the eurobarometer study. J Publ Health 14: 291-300

Warburton, DE., Gledhill, N., Quinney, A (2001). The effects of changes in musculoskeletal fitness on health. Canada J Applied Physiol 26:161-216.

Wareham, N., Van Sluijs, E., Ekelund, U (2005). Physical activity and obesity prevention: a review of the current evidence. Proc Nutr Soc 64:229-31.

Warren, T.Y., Barry, V., Hooker, S.P., Sui, X., Church, T.S., and Blair, S.N (2010). Sedentary behaviors increase risk of cardiovascular disease mortality in men. Med Sci Sports Exerc 42(5): 879–885.

World Health Organization (2012): Global strategy on diet, physical activity and health. www.who.int/di3etphysicalactivity. (Retrieved 30th February, 2012).

World Health Organization. (2004). Global strategy on diet, physical activity and health. Geneva: WHO.

Zaninotto, P., Wardle, H., Stamatakis, E., Mindell, J., Head, J (2006). Forecasting obesity to 2010. London: Depa

Chapter 12

Copper, Zinc and Magnesium in Non-Insulin-Dependent Diabetes Mellitus Treated with Metformin

Monica Daniela Dosa, Cecilia Ruxandra Adumitresi,
Laurentiu Tony Hangan and Mihai Nechifor

Additional information is available at the end of the chapter

http://dx.doi.org/10.5772/48230

1. Introduction

Non-insulin-dependent diabetes mellitus is one of the most widely spread and severe disorder currently, being the fourth mortality reason, globally. The number of patients suffering from diabetes mellitus was reported to be over 200 million people worldwide, a big part of it being NIDDM patients. Divalent cations of macro and trace elements play important roles in human body.

Magnesium (Mg) is an important divalent cation mostly localized intracellular.

Zinc (Zn) is one of the most important trace elements in the body. It is required for over 300 different cellular processes, including enzyme activity, protein synthesis and intracellular signaling [1]. It is involved in homeostasis, in immune responses, in oxidative stress, in apoptosis and in ageing [2].

Copper (Cu) is an essential trace element, capable of fluctuating between the oxidized Cu^{2+} and the reduced Cu^{+} state, being co-factor for many enzymes. This divalent cation is involved in SOD activity. Copper has the capacity to form covalent bounds and it takes part in many redox processes. Copper ions are involved in generation of reactive oxygen species through Fenton reaction, having a pro-oxidant action. Moreover, the deficiencies and the excess of Cu are associated with specific clinical manifestations [3]. Diabetes mellitus is a chronic metabolic disorder associated with the increased free radical production leading to oxidative damage, and many of the pathological effects of copper overload are consistent with an oxidative damage to membranes or macromolecules. Variation in the concentrations of those divalent cations is important to oxidative stress to which the diabetic patient's organism is submitted.

Today there is an extensive range of anti-diabetic drugs for oral intake for type 2 diabetes. The main classes are different in their mechanism of action, safety profiles and tolerability and include: agents that stimulate insulin secretion (sulphonylureas), agents that reduce hepatic glucose production (biguanides), glinides, agents that delay digestion and absorption of carbohydrate (alpha-glucosidase inhibitors) or improve insulin action (thiazolidinediones).

Metformin is one of the most used drug in the treatment of NIDDM . This drug does not promote weight gain and has beneficial effects on several cardiovascular risk factors. Metformin is widely regarded as the drug of choice for most patients with type 2 diabetes. [4] This substance is the drug of choice and should be initiated immediately after diabetes is diagnosed. If monotherapy does not provide satisfactory glucose control, other oral anti-diabetic agents or insulin are added in combination. In the metabolic syndrome, metformin is also the drug of choice. [5] The action of oral anti-diabetics at the level of vascular endothelium and the cardio-protective effect play an increasing role in the choice of anti-diabetic agents.

2. The aim of the study

This research was performed to determine the plasmatic, cellular and urinary concentration of certain divalent cations in newly diagnosed NIDDM patients that have never received any kind of oral anti-diabetic drugs or insulin and at the same time to determine the metformin effect on intracellular magnesium concentration, plasma and urinary concentrations of different divalent cations.

Our study surveyed the status of magnesium, copper, zinc, calcium in plasma and urine and erythrocyte magnesium, influenced by metformin administration, in NIDDM adult patients from the moment of diagnosis and during the therapy with oral anti-diabetic medication.

At the same time, other biochemical parameters were determined, necessary to evaluate the carbohydrate metabolism and lipidic profile and different correlations were established between carbohydrate-lipidic metabolic parameters and plasma, urinary and cellular divalent cations concentrations.

3. Material and methods

The study was performed on a group of 30 adult patients with NIDDM, 18 males and 12 females, with ages between 30 and 60 years (interval of 30-40y: 2 patients, 40-50y: 13 patients and 50-60y: 15 patients) that have never received any anti-diabetic medication, and a control group of 17 healthy subjects.

Patients with NIDDM, diagnosed in the Diabetes, Nutrition and Metabolic Diseases Clinic of Clinical County Emergency Hospital Constanta, according to the European Guide for Diabetes [6] were administered metformin (Siofor^R, Berlin Chemie) 500 mg x 2 times /day, together with a diet list comprising approximately 320 mg/day magnesium.

Subject selection criteria were: NIDDM adult subjects with absence of any previous treatment with oral anti-diabetic agents, insulin or trace elements to follow medical therapy with metformin yet without co-administration of other oral anti-diabetic agents. Non-including criteria were: pregnancy, hepatic cirrhosis, renal failure, psychosis, diuretic therapy, chronic diarrhea. An individual investigation protocol was elaborated containing the principal parameters to be investigated, and the study was performed according to the rules of clinical studies of the European Union, with the approval of the Ethical Committee of the University, and informed written consent was obtained from each subject included into the study.

The measured parameters were: glucose, HbA1c, creatinine, HDL, LDL, cholesterol, triglycerides, magnesium, copper, zinc and calcium in blood plasma; intra-erythrocyte magnesium; magnesium, copper, zinc and calcium concentration inurine/24 hours. Measurements were initially made before the administration of metformin, and after 3 months of therapy.

Material and methods: measurements were made by means of a Rx Daytona analyzer, a compact fully automated clinical analyzer, produced by Randox LTD Laboratories, UK, also used for all the other quantitative analyses, except erythrocyte magnesium.

Rx Daytona is an automated clinical chemistry analyzer with specific analyzer software, being an "in vitro diagnosis medical device" in compliance with IVD Directive and the EMC Directive of EU. The analyzer is recommended for general chemistry as photometric assay, immunology (latex reagents), with analysis methods: 1 point, 2 point end, 1 point rate, 2 point rate, and calibration options such as: factor, linear, Log Logit, exponential, spline, point to point; sample types for analysis can be: serum, plasma, urine, CSF, supernatants whole blood.

Methods of measurements for plasma divalent cations: venous blood samples from the subjects were collected in the morning after an overnight fast, into special blood collection tubes (vacutainer). There were used blood vacutainers with sodium heparin (green cup) for the measurement of zinc, copper, magnesium in plasma.

Plasma concentrations were determined through spectrophotometric method, using Randox kits, with plasma reference materials and controls, normal and abnormal level. Measurements were made by means of a Rx Daytona analyzer. Atomic absorption spectrophotometry (AAS) is the reference method for the determination of the cations in biological specimens, but it is not a usual method in clinical laboratories. The colorimetric methods used in clinical laboratories, especially for magnesium which is widely used, are fairly accurate and precise with a good correlation (r= 0.986) compared to AAS. Heparinized samples were centrifuged at 1500 g for 10 min to separate plasma from erythrocytes. Plasma was used for estimation of extracellular magnesium (without deproteinization), while trichloroacetic acid was added to precipitate proteins, the supernatant being used for analysis of zinc and copper. The measurements were initially made before the administration of metformin, and after 3 months of therapy.

Methods of measurements for urinary divalent cations: urine samples were collected in sterile, chemically clean universal containers, 30 ml, from urine / 24 h, the volume being measured. The samples were prepared in 30 minutes after collection, urine been transferred in test tubes. For estimation of calcium and magnesium the samples were used directly, for zinc and copper trichloroacetic acid was added to precipitate proteins.

The concentration of cations/24 h, was determined through spectrophotometric method, by means of Rx Daytona analyzer.

Methods of measurements for erythrocyte magnesium: blood vacutainers with sodium heparin (green cup) were used. Heparinized samples were centrifuged at 1500 g for 10 min to separate plasma from erythrocytes. The determination of erythrocyte magnesium was made using the colorimetric assay with xylidyl blue, a metallochromic dye,[3,4] after the lysis of 100 µl erythrocytes with 1500 µl double-distilled water, and deproteinization with 200 µl 0.3 mol/l Na2WO4 and 200 µl 0.35 mol/l H2SO4. The trade kit used was Human, the blue magnesium xylidyl complex, was measured at 532 nm, using a spectrophotometer (AR-Cromaline, Barcelona, Spain). Standard solutions were used along with blank solutions (1000µl working solution, 160 µl double-distilled water, 20 µl 0.3 mol/l Na2WO4 and 20 µl 0.35 mol/l H2SO4), for every analytic procedure. [7]

Methods for statistical analysis: the statistical significance and the correlations between plasmatic concentrations of the divalent cations and erythrocyte magnesium with glycemia, HbA1c, cholesterol, triglycerides, HDL were determined.

The results are expressed as means ± S.D. Differences between groups were examined using the unpaired Student's t-test, and considered statistically significant at $p<0.05$, differences in the group were examined using the paired Student's test, considered statistically significant at $p<0.05$, and to asses possible relationships between different variables, Pearson's correlation coefficient (r) was used. The statistical analyses were done using the SPSS for Windows 12.00.

4. Results

Plasma total magnesium level is reduced in NIDDM patients before treatment compared to healthy controls (1.95 ± 0.19 vs. 2.20 ±0.18 mg/dl, $p< 0.001$) and determination of plasma magnesium concentration after 3 months treatment with metformin revealed that there were not significant differences compared to the initial moment (M = 1.96, SD = 0.10 vs. M = 1.95, SD = 0.19, p= 0.735) and when compared with control group there are significant differences (M = 1.96, SD =0.105 vs M = 2.21, SD = 0.193, $p< 0.001$). Fig 1

Plasma zinc in NIDDM patients: data reveal significant differences in the NIDDM group versus the control group, for plasma zinc (67.56 ± 6.21 vs. 98.41± 20.47 µg/dl, $p<0.001$) and determination after 3 months treatment with metformin revealed that there were not significant differences compared to the initial moment (M = 64.25, SD = 5.59 vs. M = 67.56, SD = 6.21 vs. p=0.067) and when compared with control group there are still significant differences (M=64.25, SD = 5.60 vs. M = 101.65, SD = 23.14 , p< 0,001). Fig 2

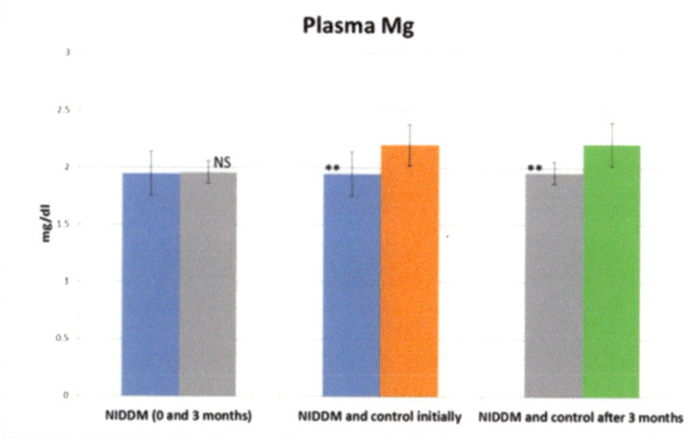

Figure 1. Plasma magnesium concentrations (NS – non-significant, * - p<0.05, ** - p<0.01)

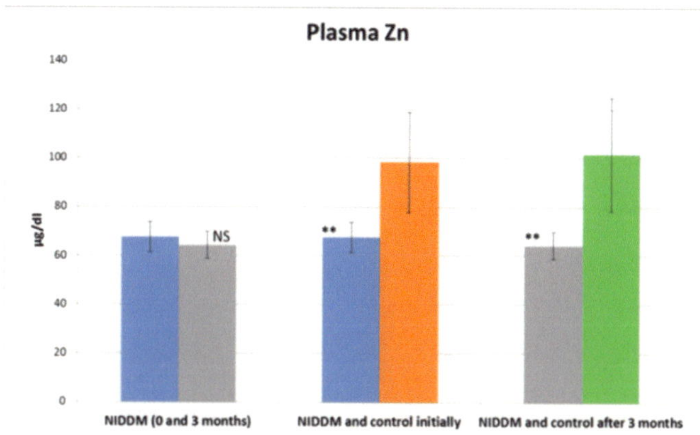

Figure 2. Plasma zinc concentrations (NS – non-significant, * - p<0.05, ** - p<0.01)

Plasma copper in NIDDM patients is increased when compared to healthy subjects (M=111.91+/-20.98 vs. M= 96.33+/- 8.56 µg/dl, p<0.001) Treatment with metformin did not modify significantly the concentration of this cation (M = 111.91, SD = 20.98 µg/dl vs. M =110.91, SD = 18.61 p= 0.413) and compared to control group there are not significant differences (M =110.08, SD = 18.61 µg/dl vs. M = 101.23, SD =21.73, p=0.147) (Fig 3) but when we compare those levels between the metabolic uncontrolled patients group (8 patients were prescribed another anti-diabetic drug after 3 months therapy with metformin) and the ones with metabolic control of metformin treatment (n=22) we see that there are significant differences (M = 127.22, SD = 22.64 µg/dl vs. M = 103.85, SD = 12.43, p= 0.023). Fig. 4

Plasma calcium in NIDDM patients before medication revealed non-significant differences when compared to healthy subjects. (M= 8.93± 0.33 mg/dl vs. 8.87 ± 0.35, p= 0.300) Treatment with metformin did not modify significantly the concentration of this cation (M = 8.987, SD = 0.44 mg/dl vs. M = 8.983, p=0.147) and compared to control group after 3 months of treatment there were not significant differences: (M = 8.98, SD = 0.44 mg/dl vs. M = 8.92, SD = 0.43, p= 0.633).

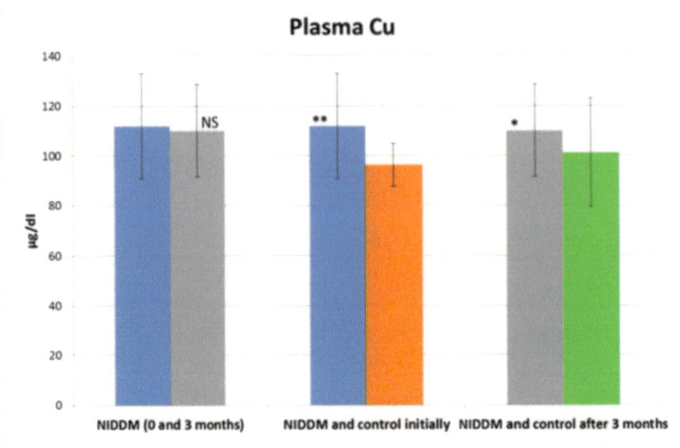

Figure 3. Plasma copper concentrations (NS – non-significant, * - p<0.05, ** - p<0.01)

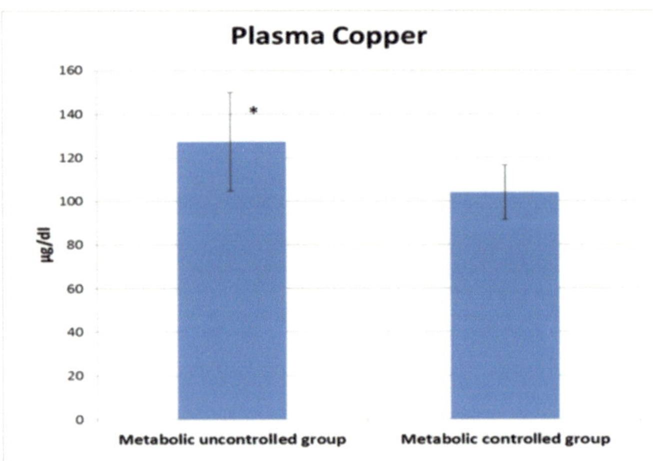

Figure 4. Plasma copper concentrations in metabolic uncontrolled patients by metformin vs metabolic controlled patients (NS – non-significant, * - p<0.05, ** - p<0.01)

Data about **intra-erythrocyte total magnesium** concentration in NIDDM patients has revealed a decreased concentration of erythrocyte magnesium in NIDDM patients before medication, when compared to healthy subjects (5.09 ± 0.63 vs. 6.38 ± 0.75 mg/dl, p< 0.001) and treatment with metformin has revealed that there were significant differences compared to the moment before medication: (M = 5.75 SD = 0.61 mg/dl vs. M = 5.09, SD =0.63, p<0.001) but compared to the control group the differences are still significant: (M = 5.75 SD =0.61 vs. M = 6.39 SD = 0.72, p=0.002) Fig 5

Urinary magnesium is increased in NIDDM patients before medication, when compared to healthy subjects (237.28±34.51 vs. 126.25±38.82 mg/24h p<0.001) and in NIDDM patients treated with metformin there were significant differences compared to the moment before medication: (M = 198.27 SD = 27.07 mg/24 h vs. M = 237.28, SD = 34.51 mg/24h p< 0.001), but compared with control group the differences are still significant M = 198.27 SD = 27.07 mg/24h vs. M = 138.39, SD = 41.37 p< 0,001). Fig 6

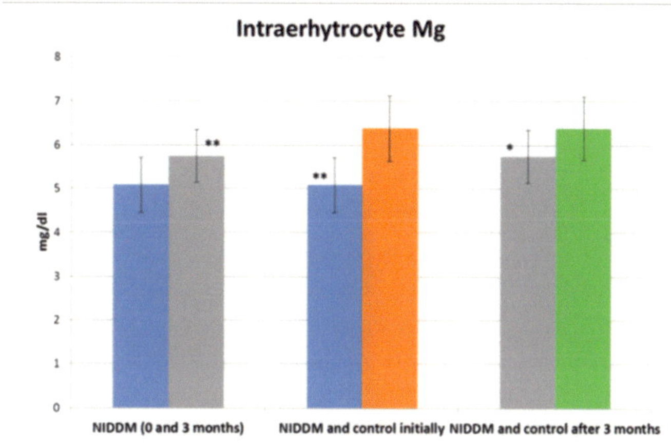

Figure 5. Intraerhytrocyte total magnesium concentrations (NS – non-significant, * - p<0.05, ** - p<0.01)

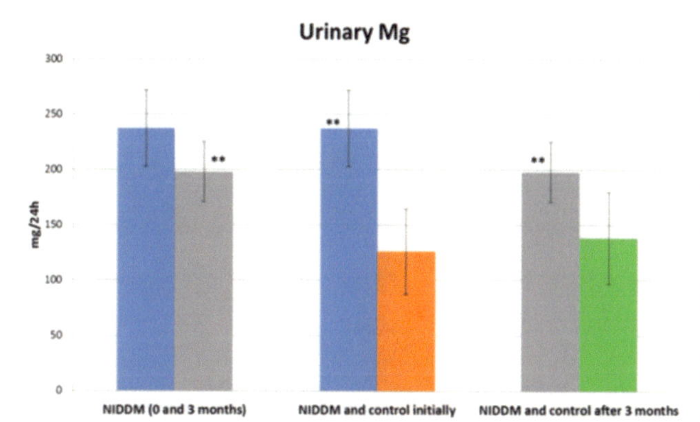

Figure 6. Urinary magnesium concentrations (NS – non-significant, * - p<0.05, ** - p<0.01)

Urinary zinc in NIDDM patients is increased before medication, when compared to healthy subjects (1347,54 ±158,24 vs. 851,65± 209,75 μg/24 h, p< 0,001) and after 3 months of medication our data has revealed that there were not significant differences compared to the moment before medication: (M = 1339,63 SD= 160,22 μg/24 h vs. M = 1347,54, SD = 158,24, p=0,530) and compared to the control group the differences are still significant (M = 1339,63, SD = 160,22 μg/24 h vs. M =880,76,SD = 186,38,p<0,001). Fig 7

Urinary copper in NIDDM patients is increased before medication, when compared to healthy subjects (51,70±23,79 vs. 36,00±11,70 μg/24h, p<0,05) and after medication data has revealed that there were not significant differences compared to the moment before medication: (M=51,705 SD = 22,13vs 53,35 μg/24 h , SD = 23,79, p= 0,301) and compared to the control group there are significant differences (M = 51,70, SD = 22,13 μg/24 h vs. M = 36,00, SD = 11,66 p= 0,009). Fig 8

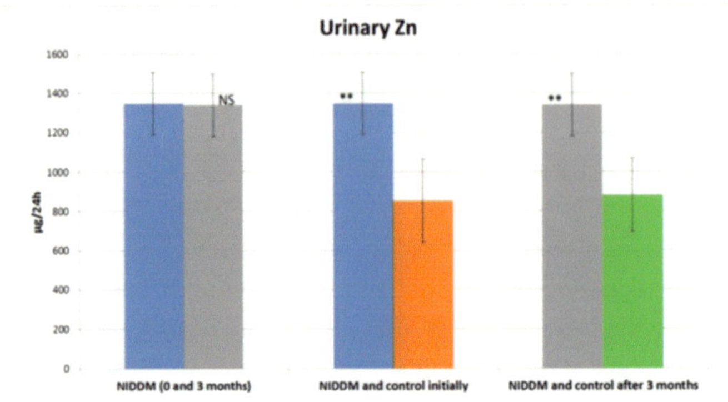

Figure 7. Urinary zinc concentrations (NS – non-significant, * - $p<0.05$, ** - $p<0.01$)

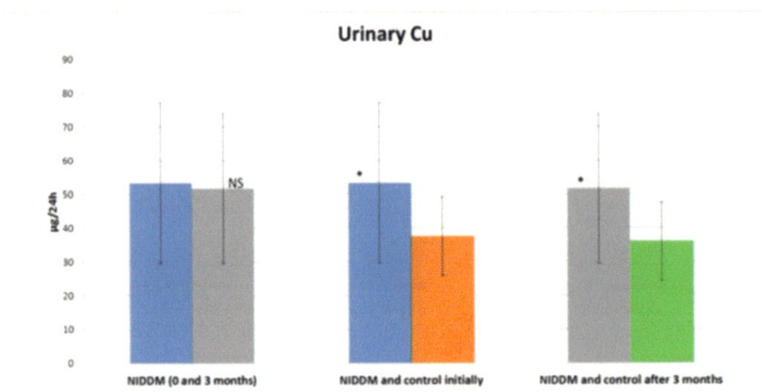

Figure 8. Urinary copper concentrations (NS – non-significant, * - $p<0.05$, ** - $p<0.01$)

Urinary calcium concentration in NIDDM patients is increased before medication, (309,23±58,41 vs. 201,51±62,13 mg/24h, p<0,001) and in NIDDM patients treated with metformin our data has revealed that there were significant differences compared to the moment before medication (M = 287,09 SD = 55,39 mg/24h vs. M = 309,23, SD = 58,41, p< 0,001) and compared to the control group: M = 287,09, SD = 55,39 mg/24h vs. M = 216,9 SD = 57,25 mg/24h, p< 0,001) Fig 9

The following correlations were obvious in metformin treated patients after 3 months: negative correlation between plasma total magnesium and glucose plasma level, positive correlation between plasma total magnesium and HbA1c, positive correlation between plasma Cu^{2+} - glucose plasma level and HbA1c, positive correlation between plasma Cu^{2+} - cholesterol plasma level and triglycerides, positive correlation between plasma Zn^{2+} and glucose plasma level, negative correlation between erythrocyte total magnesium - glucose plasma level and HbA1c, positive correlation between HbA1c and urinary Zn^{2+} concentration.

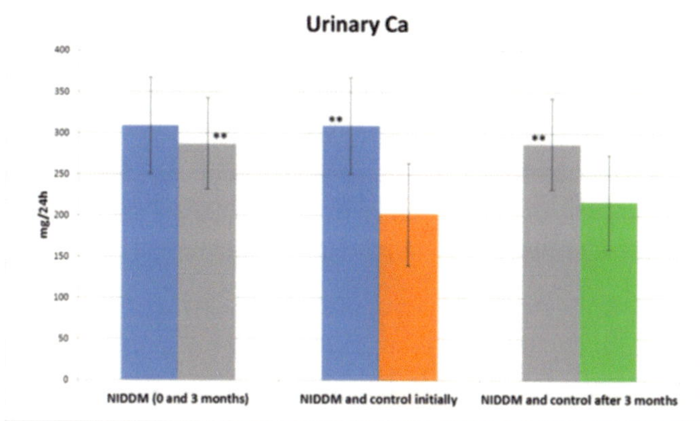

Figure 9. Urinary calcium concentrations (NS – non-significant, * - $p<0.05$, ** - $p<0.01$)

5. Discussions

The plasma magnesium level is reduced in diabetes mellitus. Our data reveals significant differences in NIDDM group versus the control group, for plasma magnesium (Fig. 1)

In accordance with other authors our data reveals the existence of plasma low total magnesium level in patients with NIDDM when compared to healthy adults. [8] Hypomagnesaemia is also involved in NIDDM pathogenesis and its complications. Both experimental and clinical studies suggest that hypermagnesemia may be the major factor involved in diabetes hypomagnesaemia. A specific renal tubular magnesium defect in diabetes together with the increased osmotic diuresis is responsible for large magnesium losses.[9] There are authors considering that serum magnesium was significantly low in diabetes with complications than in diabetes without complications ($p < 0.001$). In their study, poor glycemic control and the retinopathy were associated with hypomagnesaemia. [10]

Magnesium is cofactor in more than 300 enzymes involved in carbohydrate metabolism, required as energy bound, and it activates many enzymes involved in protein and lipids metabolism. There are data which show that hypomagnesaemia is associated to, and increase insulin resistance and we consider that magnesium can affect cellular action of insulin through: the action on the insulin receptor site, by modifying insulin-receptor binding, by affecting intracellular transduction of biologic signal; some authors [11] consider that Mg could play the role of a second messenger for insulin action by direct action on the entrance of glucose into the cell or by action on certain enzymes sites.

Magnesium deficiency may induce the increase of insulin-resistance in non-diabetic persons. [12] Deficiency of this cation can be considered a factor involved in pathogenesis and complications of type 2 diabetes mellitus.

Our data reveal significant differences for plasma zinc in NIDDM group versus the control group, for plasma zinc. (Fig. 2)

Zinc homeostasis is disturbed in patients with diabetes mellitus. Serum and intracellular zinc were significantly lower in diabetic patients compared to controls and our data are in accordance with other authors. [13] The urinary elimination of zinc is increased and intestinal absorption is decreased in patients with diabetes mellitus. Imbalances in zinc homeostasis with reduced plasmatic levels can determine deficiencies of beta pancreatic cells to produce and secrete insulin. The deficit of this cation can affect phosphorylation/ dephosphorylation of one or more steps in insulin cell signaling. [14]

Zinc ions are involved in the neutralization of free radicals and there is increasing evidence supporting the role of zinc as an antioxidant that could protect insulin and cells from being attacked by free radicals.[15] A possible mechanism of plasma zinc deficiency is due to excessive renal loss. Some authors consider that an impaired gastro-intestinal absorption in diabetics may also be involved. It is presumed that hyperglycemia may affect the tubular transport of zinc. [16] There are some clinical data that showed that zinc deficiency increased zinc occurrence of cataract among people with diabetes mellitus. [17]

Our data reveal an increased plasma level of copper in NIDDM patients when compared to healthy subjects. (Fig. 3) These data are in accordance with other studies [18] There are authors considering that excess copper is involved in type 2 diabetes mellitus pathogenesis and utilization of copper specific carriers may be a prospective therapeutic strategy in NIDDM. [19] Determination of plasma calcium in NIDDM patients, before medication, reveals non-significant differences compared to healthy subjects.

For urinary magnesium in NIDDM patients our data show an increased urinary magnesium level in NIDDM patients, before medication, when compared to healthy subjects. (Fig. 6) Our data are in accordance with other studies [20] that evidenced increased urinary levels of magnesium in newly diagnosed patients with type 2 diabetes mellitus. The possible mechanism involved in increased urinary magnesium elimination may be due to hyperglycemia that induces osmotic diuresis with decreased tubular magnesium reabsorption.

For urinary zinc in NIDDM patients our data reveal an increased urinary zinc level in NIDDM patients, before medication, when compared to healthy subjects. (Fig. 7) Hyperzincuria has been demonstrated in both type 1 and type 2 diabetes mellitus. The urinary elimination of zinc has increased and intestinal absorption has decreased in patients with diabetes mellitus. The possible mechanism involved in increased urinary zinc elimination may be due to hyperglycemia that induces osmotic diuresis. This fact is sustained by data that testified a positive correlation between HbA1c and Zn elimination being presumed that hyperglycemia interferes with the active Zn transport in tubular cells. [20, 21]

For urinary copper in NIDDM patients our data showed an increased level before medication, when compared to healthy subjects but moderate level when compared to Mg and Zn elimination, our patients having no renal disorders. (Fig. 8)

Other studies revealed urinary increased levels of copper in diabetic patients with associate disorders such as infections and neuropathy. [22]

Urinary calcium concentration in NIDDM patients has increased before medication, compared to healthy subjects, (Fig.9), our data being in accordance with other studies that evinced increased urinary levels of calcium in NIDDM patients. [23]

Determination of intra-erythrocyte total magnesium concentration has revealed a decreased concentration of this cation in NIDDM patients, before medication, when compared to healthy subjects, (fig. 5), and this is in accordance with other studies that evinced intracellular hypomagnesaemia in NIDDM patients without medication and dietary control. Insulin resistance in type 2 diabetes mellitus can negatively affect insulin capacity of stimulation for intracellular entry for both magnesium and glucose. [24] Intracellular magnesium has an important role to modulate insulin action, glucose transport and to maintain vascular tonus. Reduced intracellular concentrations of magnesium can determine deficiencies of tyrosine-kinase activity from the receptor site, also affecting intracellular transduction of biologic signal and insulin resistance in type 2 diabetic patients. [25] Magnesium may play the role of second messenger and disturbances in intracellular concentrations of this cation may contribute to insulin resistance.

In NIDDM an inverse correlation between plasma level of magnesium and insulin resistance has been determined. [26] Intracellular deficiency in Mg_{2+} and Mg ATP2 can be a genetic factor that predisposes to type 2 diabetes mellitus. It is not clear if magnesium transporters TPRMs gene expression is affected in NIDDM patients. [27] Treatment with metformin for 3 months did not modify significantly the plasma concentration of magnesium, NIDDM patients being with hypomagnesaemia. (Fig.1) The causes for the lower magnesium levels may be a deficiency in magnesium digestive absorption or an increased elimination. The patients' diet contained approximately 320 mg/day magnesium, while a daily need for adult people is about 350- 400 mg/day. Together with those factors, the increased urinary elimination of this cation, as it appears in diabetic patients, may be a cause.

It was proved that a diet with low Mg content increase the risk of NIDDM and the incidence of metabolic syndrome. [28, 29, 30]

An inefficient NIDDM metabolic control could disturb the plasma magnesium levels. Extracellular hypomagnesaemia is involved in diabetes vascular complications. [31, 32] Magnesium deficiency can increase the risk of vascular complications in diabetes. There are data from previous researches that evinced positive correlations between magnesium deficiency and oxidative stress with reduced plasmatic antioxidant profile and increased lipid oxidation. [33] GSH, a tripeptide containing thiol groups is cofactor of many enzymes as it is glutathione peroxidase , $Mg2+$ being a mandatory cofactor in GSH synthesis as it is in all processes involving ATPase, and deficiency in Mg may induce alteration in GSH synthesis.

It was proved that oral magnesium supplementation with $MgCl_2$, 2,5 g daily, increases insulin sensitivity and metabolic control in patients with type 2 diabetes mellitus [34] and patients with chronic complications such as retinopathy have decreased levels than the patients without this complication. It was proved that a low intake in magnesium increases the risk of type 2 diabetes in men and women. Treatment with metformin did not improve the plasmatic concentration of magnesium. Our data are in agreement with other authors who evinced that plasma levels of Mg have not improved at the same time with metabolic control improvement. [35]

Within experimental research, the metformin restored endothelial function and significantly improved NO bioavailability in normal and high-fat fed rats. This supports the concept of metformin as a first-line therapeutic drug to treat diabetic patients in order to protect against endothelial dysfunction associated with type 2 diabetes mellitus. [36, 37]

Metformin improved also the endothelial function in patients with metabolic syndrome. The type 2 diabetes mellitus patients who received metformin has had statistically significant improvement in endothelium-dependent vasodilatation compared to those that received placebo. [38]

Plasma zinc determination in NIDDM patients treated with metformin evinced that there were not significant differences compared to the initial moment and when compared to control group there are still significant differences.(Fig. 2)

Many studies revealed a deficiency in this divalent cation in diabetic patients.

Treatment with metformin did not improve the plasmatic concentration of zinc, patients being with hypozincemia.There are data revealing that diabetes is characterized by intracellular and extracellular imbalances of zinc. Zinc ions are involved in neutralization of ROS and nitrogen species through Cu Zn- SOD enzyme. The deficit of this cation can alter the antioxidant activity of the enzyme Cu Zn- SOD together with the expression and activity of other antioxidant biologic components, moreover, zinc deficiency can increase the fractions with oxidant activity such as ROS and RNA, and as consequence, the oxidant activity on the tissues, with oxidative capacity on the DNA, proteins and lipids. Imbalances in zinc metabolism can be involved in NIMMD pathogenesis and complications. [39]

Recent data revealed that zinc supplementation is associated with a decreased risk of diabetes appearance in women. [40] For short periods, zinc supplementation can improve the plasma glucose level in diabetic patients with increased values of HbA1c and decreased levels of zinc. [41]

A place in type 2 diabetes pathogenesis and complications is assigned to zinc transporter proteins (Zn Ts) and to metallothioneins (MTs). Many authors consider that a change in sub-cellular distribution of those may be more important than the deficiency in zinc, and those should be considered a future therapeutic target in diabetes.[42] There are some clinical data showing that zinc deficiency increased occurrence of cataract among people with diabetes mellitus. [17] Zinc and magnesium concentrations decreased in experimentally induced diabetes in rats [43].

The effect of zinc supplementation in the treatment of diabetes mellitus is controversial. [44] There is no evidence to suggest the use of zinc supplementation in the prevention of type 2 diabetes mellitus [45], but there are studies which suggest that zinc and magnesium supplementation might ameliorate diabetic neuropathy symptoms.[46] Treatment with metformin did not significantly modify the concentration of copper, but when we compare those levels between the metabolic uncontrolled patients and the ones with metabolic control of metformin treatment we see that there are significant differences. There are data revealing that increased levels of copper are not influenced by metabolic control [47]. Diabetes mellitus is a chronic metabolic disorder, which is associated with the increased free radical production leading to oxidative damage: the oxidative stress and copper both have pro-oxidant effects. This cation catalyzes the oxidative modification of LDL, in vitro and in the arterial wall and the presence of copper in high concentration can facilitate the production of free radicals through Fenton reaction [48].

The decrease of serum copper is associated to the decrease of the production of ROS on the animals with experimental diabetes. We believe that the excess of copper is involved in the pathogenesis of some complications of NIDDM. Plasma calcium determination in diabetic patients treated with metformin had showed that there were no significant differences compared to the initial moment. Intra-erythrocyte magnesium in NIDDM patients treated with metformin revealed that there were significant differences compared to the moment before medication. (Fig. 5) The results are in accordance with our previous data [49] and with few other results that revealed an increased tissue levels of magnesium associated with metformin treatment. [50] However, our study revealed there is still a decreased intra-erythrocyte magnesium level when compared to the control group. There are data revealing that hypomagnesaemia is associated to and increases insulin resistance. [26] Low levels of magnesium are associated to the increase of insulin-resistance in non-diabetic subjects as well. Treatment with metformin improved the intracellular concentration of this cation, due probably to the mechanism of action of this biguanide drug that improves the peripheral action of insulin, through an increase of GLUT 4 transporters on the plasmatic membrane, magnesium having insulin-like functions. Metformin is a drug that increases the glucose transport. Within other studies, intracellular magnesium increased after following treatment with rosiglitazone but metformin had no effect on intracellular calcium or magnesium. Ca and Mg were assessed in PBMC from healthy subjects following 72h in vitro treatment with the respective drugs and calcium content increased significantly. [51] Metformin administration improved Na(+)K(+)ATPase activity (0.28±0.08, 0.41±0.07μmol Pi/mg/h) in erythrocyte membrane, but is not clear if this action can influence bivalent cations intracellular concentrations. [52]

Metformin also improved the endothelial function in patients with metabolic syndrome. The type 2 diabetes mellitus patients who received metformin had statistically significant improvement in endothelium-dependent vasodilatation compared to those that received placebo. [53] We think that, in part, the endothelium protective effect of metformin is not produced only by NO way, but also by increasing the magnesium intracellular concentration. Good magnesium status is associated with reduced diabetes risk. The average glucose-lowering effect of the major classes of oral anti-diabetic agents is broadly similar, but the influence on the various bivalent cations concentrations and on vascular endothelium is not. Our study revealed an improvement of intra-erythrocyte magnesium by metformin medication without an improvement of plasmatic magnesium. Metformin medication improved the urinary elimination of magnesium (Fig. 6), results that are in accordance with other researchers that revealed an improvement of this cation elimination [23] but compared to the control group the diabetic patients still have hypermagnesemia. We suppose that the decreased urinary elimination of magnesium may be due to the decreased in plasma glycemia by use of metformin as well as a possible action of this drug on the renal cation transporters.

Treatment with metformin did not modify zinc elimination, patients with diabetes mellitus type 2 having hyperzincuria. (Fig. 7) The urinary elimination of zinc is increased and intestinal absorption is decreased in patients with diabetes mellitus. There are some research data confirming that patients with type 1 and type 2 diabetes mellitus have increased levels of zinc concentration in urine. [54] Increased urinary levels of this cation can be involved in the plasmatic reduced levels, and the mechanism involved may be due to hyperglycemia that can interfere with the Zn transport back in renal tubular cells, but we cannot exclude other interventions of zinc ions on the zinc transporters.

Metformin administration did not significantly modify the urinary elimination of copper when comparing the metabolic uncontrolled group of metformin administration and the group controlled by medication, there are significant differences. (Fig. 4)

Metformin administration for 3 months did not significantly modify the urinary elimination of calcium but compared to the control group there are still significant differences, diabetic patients being with hypercalciuria. (Fig. 9)

The negative correlation between plasma Mg and plasma glucose level in patients treated 3 months with metformin revealed that the treatment with metformin did not improve the plasma levels of magnesium, but increased the intracellular magnesium concentration.

The negative correlation between plasma magnesium and HbA1c evidenced the fact that the metabolic uncontrolled patients through medication have low levels of magnesium.

Our data are in accordance with other authors that revealed an inverse correlation between the metabolic control of NIDDM and plasma hypomagnesaemia. [32]

There are authors suggesting that the diabetes itself can induce hypomagnesaemia, while others revealed the fact that a supplementation of Mg can reduce the risk of development of type 2 diabetes mellitus and can improve the insulin sensitivity. [55] Our data indicated a low intracellular magnesium concentration in NIMMD patients and an increase of intra-erythrocyte magnesium after metformin treatment. This is an important point in metformin action because magnesium deficiency promotes the development of dyslipidemia and the atherogenesis. [56]

The increased oxidative stress in diabetes mellitus contribute to the development of diabetic macrovascular and microvascular complications through increased lipid oxidation, especially by increasing oxidation of LDL, which is a crucial step in the development of atherosclerosis. Magnesium can reduce the oxidative stress [57] and we consider that this is an important mechanism for antiatherogenic action of certain antidiabetes drugs.

Our results are in accordance with other authors that evinced positive correlations between plasma Cu and glycemia. [58] Once again it is proved that there is a disbalance in the copper ions in diabetes type 2 and once proved the implications of these cations in the pathogenesis and complications of diabetes.

The positive correlation between plasma copper and cholesterol, tryglicerides concentration confirms the fact that increased levels of copper are associated with lipid metabolism disturbances.The involvement of copper ions in plasma lipids metabolism are controversial. Various studies proved inverse correlations between low dietary copper and cholesterol and LDL cholesterol, in both: human and rats, and in rats with low copper diet HDL cholesterol had increased. [59]

Treatment with metformin did not modify the urinary loss nor the plasma decreased levels, all of those implying the hyperglycemia as factor involved. The issue of the correlation between copper, zinc and magnesium status and complications of diabetes mellitus is an open one. In other studies it was reported an increased plasma copper concentration in patients with specific diabetes associated complications (retinopathy, microvascular diseases or arterial hypertension) [60, 61] but no significant differences between control and diabetic patients in erythrocyte copper-zinc superoxide dismutase. The relationship between coronary risk factors in NIDDM patients is also extremely important. The plasma zinc/copper ratio is inversely associated with calculated 10 years coronary risk in non-diabetic patients. [62]

6. Conclusions

Our data are in accordance with those of other authors [32] that revealed an inverse correlation between the metabolic control of NIDDM and low plasma magnesium level.

Negative correlation between erythrocyte magnesium and HbA1c evinced that low metabolic control by medication is associated with intracellular deficit of magnesium. In our opinion, the intracellular magnesium concentration plays a more important role in prevention of the development of hypercholesterolemia and atherogenesis than plasma level of this cation.

Metformin did not modify the plasma levels of copper. About the risk for the development of vascular complication of patients with type 2 diabetes, we believe that the ratio between the concentrations of intracellular magnesium +serum zinc/serum copper is a good marker for the risk of diabetes complications development. A higher ratio indicates a more reduced risk and a low ratio an increased risk. In the evaluation of the antidiabetic effect of certain drugs must be to keep account of their influence on magnesium, zinc and copper plasma and intracellular concentrations.

We consider that magnesium and zinc administration can be of benefit in type 2 diabetes mellitus .The copper chelators could represent also a future medication in diabetes.

Author details

Monica Daniela Dosa
Pharmacology Department, Faculty of Medicine, Ovidius University of Constanta, Romania

Cecilia Ruxandra Adumitresi
Physiology Department, Faculty of Medicine, Ovidius University of Constanta, Romania

Laurentiu Tony Hangan
Medical Informatics and Biostatistics, Faculty of Medicine, Ovidius University of Constanta, Romania

Mihai Nechifor
Pharmacology Department, Gr. T. Popa University of Medicine and Pharmacy of Iasi, Romania

7. References

[1] Shannon L. Kelleher, Nicholas H. McCormick, Vanessa Velasquez, and Veronica Lopez. Zinc in Specialized Secretory Tissues: Roles in the Pancreas, Prostate, and Mammary Gland. Adv Nutr 2011; 2(2) 101–111

[2] Stefanidou M, Maravelias C, Dona A, Spiliopoulou C. Zinc: a multipurpose trace element. Arch Toxicol 2006; , Bailey CJ. Oral antidiabetic agents: current role in type 2 diabetes mellitus. Drugs 2005;65(3) 385-411

[3] Bremner I. Manifestation of copper excess. Am J Clin Nutr 1998;67:S 1069-73

[4] Krentz AJ, Bailey CJ. Oral antidiabetic agents: current role in type 2 diabetes mellitus. Drugs 2005;65(3) 385-411

[5] Pelikánova T. Treatment of diabetes in metabolic syndrome. Vnitr Lek 2009;55(7-8) 637-45.

[6] National Institute for Health and Clinical Excellence. The management of type 2 diabetes (update). (Clinical guideline 66) 2008; NICE, London Available from: URL: http://www.nice.org.uk/nicemedia/pdf/CG66NICEGuideline.pdf

[7] Zervas E, Papatheodorou G, Psathakis K, Panagou P, Georgatou N, Loukudes S. Reduced intracellular Mg concentrations in patients with acute asthma. Chest 2003;123 113-118

[8] Walti MK, Zimmermann MB, Giatgen A, Spinas A, Hurrell RF. Swiss Med Wkly 2003;133 289-292

[9] Garland HO. New experimental data on the relationship between diabetes mellitus and magnesium. Magnes Res 1992;5(3) 193-202.

[10] Sharma A, Dabla S, Agrawal RP, Barjatya H, Kochar DK, Kothari RP. Serum magnesium: an early predictor of course and complications of diabetes mellitus. J Indian Med Assoc 2007;105(1) 16-20.

[11] Takaya J, Higashino H, Kobayashi Y. Intracellular magnesium and insulin resistance. Magnes. Res 2004;171(2) 126-136

[12] Hans CP, Sialy R, Bansal DD. Magnesium deficiency and diabetes mellitus. Curr. Sci 2002;83 1456-63

[13] Kazi TG, Afridi HI, Kazi N, Jamali MK, Arain MB, Jalbani N, Kandhro GA. Copper, chromium, manganese, iron, nickel and zinc levels in biological samples of diabetes mellitus patients. Biol. Trace Elem. Res 2008;122(1) 1-18

[14] Tang XH, Shay NF. Zinc has an Insulin-Like Effect on Glucose Transport Mediated by Phosphoinositol-3-Kinase and Akt in 3T3-L1 Fibroblasts and Adipocytes. Journal of Nutrition 2001;131 1414-1420

[15] Faure P, Lafond JL, Coudray C, Rossini E, Halimi S, Favier A, Blache D. Zinc prevents the structural and functional properties of free radical treated-insulin. Biochim Biophys Acta 1994 1209(2) 260-4.

[16] Chausmer AB. Zinc, insulin and diabetes. J. Am. Coll. Nutr 1998;17 109-14.

[17] Rahim A, Iqbal K. To assess the levels of zinc in serum and changes in the lens of diabetic and senile cataract patients. J. Pak. Med. Assoc 2011; 61(9) 853-5.

[18] Kazi TG, Afridi HI, Kazi N, Jamali MK, Arain MB, Jalbani N, Kandhro GA. Copper, chromium, manganese, iron, nickel and zinc levels in biological samples of diabetes mellitus patients. Biol. Trace Elem. Res 2008;122(1) 1-18

[19] Tanaka A, Kaneto H, Miyatsura T, Yamamoto K, Yoshiuchi K, Shimomura I, Matsuoka T-A, Matsuhisa M. Role of cooper ion in the Pathogenesis of Type 2 Diabetes. Endocr. J 2009; 56(5) 699-706

[20] El-Yazigi A, Hannan N, Raines DA. Effect of diabetic state and related disorders on the urinary excretion of magnesium and zinc in patients. Diabetes Res 1993;22(2) 67-75

[21] Chausmer AB. Zinc, insulin and diabetes. J. Am. Coll. Nutr 1998;17 109-14

[22] El-Yazigi A, Hannan N, Raines DA. Urinary excretion of chromium, copper and manganese in diabetes mellitus and associated disorders. Diabets Res 1991;18(3) 129-34

[23] McBain AM, Brown IRF, Menzies DG, Campbell IW. Effects of improved glycaemic control on calcium and magnesium homeostasis intype II diabetes. J. Clin. Pathol 1988;41 933-935.

[24] Resnick L, Altura BT, Gupta RK, Laragh JH, Alderman MH, Altura BM. Intracellular and extracellular magnesium depletion in type 2 (non-insulindependent diabetes mellitus. Diabetologia 1993;36 767-770

[25] Barbagallo M, Dominquez LJ. Magnesium metabolism in type 2 diabetes mellitus, metabolic syndrome and insulin resistance. Arch. Biochem. Biophys 2007;458(1) 40-47

[26] Takaya J, Higashino H, Kobayashi Y. Intracellular magnesium and insulin resistance. Magnes Res 2004;17(2) 126-36.

[27] Wells I.C. Evidence that the etiology of the syndrome containing type 2 diabetes mellitus results from abnormal magnesium metabolism. Can. J Physiol Pharmacol 2008;86(1-2) 16-24

[28] Lopez-Ridaura R, Willett WC, Rimm EB, Liu S, Stampfer MJ, Manson JE, Hu FB. Magnesium intake and risk of type 2 diabetes in men and women. Diabetes Care 2004;27 134-140

[29] Rayssiguier Y, Gueux E, Nowacki W, Rock E, Mazur A. High fructose consumption combined with low dietary magnesium intake may increase the incidence of the metabolic syndrome by inducing inflammation. Magnesium Res 2006;19(4) 237-243

[30] Humphries S, Kushner H, Falkner B. Low dietary magnesium is associated with insulin resistance in a sample of young non diabetic black americans. Am. J. Hypertens 1999; 12 747-756

[31] Guerrero-Romero F, Rodriguez-Moran M. Hypomagnesemia, oxidative stress, inflammation, and metabolic syndrome. Diabetes Metab. Res. Rev 2006;22 471-476

[32] Sales CH, Pedrosa LdeF. Magnesium and diabetes mellitus: their relation. Clin. Nutr 2006;25(4) 554-62

[33] Hans CP, Chaudhary DP, Bansal DD. Magnesium deficiency increases oxidative stres in rats. Ind. J. Exp. Biol 2002;40 1275-9

[34] Guerrero-Romero F, Tamez-Perez HE, Gonzáles- Gonzáles G, Sarinas-Martinez AM, Montes-Villarreal J, Treviño-Ortiz JH, Rodriguez-Moran M. Oral magnesium supplementation improves insulin sensitivity in non-diabetic subjects with insulin resistance, A double-blind placebo-controlled randomized trial. Diabetes Metab 2004;30(3) 253-258

[35] Schnack C, Bauer I, Pregant P, Hopmeier P, Schernthaner G. Hypomagnesaemia in type 2 (non-insulin-dependent) diabetes mellitus is not corrected by improvement of long-term metabolic control. Diabetologia 1992;34(1) 77-9

[36] Sena CM, Matafome P, Louro T, Nunes E, FernandesSena CM, Matafome P, Louro T, Nunes E, Fernandes R, Seiça RM. Metformin restores endothelial function in aorta of diabetic rats. Br. J. Pharmacol 2011;163(2) 424-37.

[37] Mather KJ, Verma S, Anderson TJ. Improved endothelial function with metformin in type 2 diabetes mellitus. J. Am. Coll. Cardiol 2001;37(5) 1344-50.

[38] Vitale C, Mercuro G, Cornoldi A, Fini M, Volterrani M, Rosano GM. Metformin improves endothelial function in patients with metabolic syndrome. J Intern Med 2005;258(3) 250-6.

[39] Zeng Z, Li XK, Cai L. The role of zinc, copper and iron in the pathogenesis of diabetes and diabetic complications: therapeutic effects by chelators. Hemoglobin 2008;32(1-2) 135-45

[40] Sun Q, vanDam RM, Willet WC, Hu FB. Prospective study of zinc intake and risk of type 2 diabetes in women. Diabetes Care 2009;32(4) 629-34

[41] Hyun-Mee O, Jin-Sook Y. Glycemic control of type 2 diabetic patients after short-term zinc supplementation. Nutr Res Pract 2008;2(4) 283-8

[42] Mocchegiani E, Giacconi R, Malavolta M. Zinc signalling and subcellular distribution: emerging targets in type 2 diabetes.Trends Mol Med 2008;14(10) 419-28

[43] Ozcelik D, Tuncdemir M, Ozturk M, Uzun H. Evaluation of trace elements and oxidative stress levels in the liver and kidney of streptozotocin-induced experimental diabetic rat model. Gen Physiol Biophys 2011;30(4) 356-63

[44] Zampelas A. Zinc supplementation: another myth or we are heading towards a new era in the treatment of diabetes? Atherosclerosis 2011;219(1) 22-3.

[45] Beletate V, El Dib RP, Atallah AN. Zinc supplementation for the prevention of type 2 diabetes mellitus. Cochrane Database Syst Rev 2007;24(1):CD005525. Available from: URL: http://www.ncbi.nlm.nih.gov/pubmed/17253560

[46] Farvid MS, Homayouni F, Amiri Z, Adelmanesh F. Improving neuropathy scores in type 2 diabetic patients using micronutrients supplementation. Diabetes Res Clin Pract 2011;93(1) 86-94.

[47] Zargar AH, Shah NA, Masoodi SR, Laway BA, Dar FA, Khan AR, Sofi FA, Wani AI. Copper, zinc and magnesium levels in non-insulin dependent diabetes mellitus. Postgrad Med J 1998;74(877) 665-8

[48] Uriu-Adams Jy, Keen CL. Copper, oxidative stress, and human health. Mol Aspects Med 2005;26 268-298.

[49] Dosa MD, Hangan LT, Crauciuc E, Gales C, Nechifor M. Influence of therapy with Metformin on the concentration of certain divalent cations in patients with non-insulin-dependent diabetes mellitus. Biol Trace Elem Res 2011; 142 36-46

[50] Gorelik O, Efrati S, Berman S, Almozino-Sarafian D, Shteinshnaider M, Cohen N. Effect of various clinical variables on total intracellular magnesium in hospitalized normomagnesemic diabetic patients before discharge. Biol Trace Elem Res 2007;120(1-3) 102-9

[51] Alon I, Berman S, Shteinshnaider M, Efrati S, Gorelik O, Almoznino-Sarafian D, Weissgarten J, Cohen N. Total cellular calcium and magnesium content of cultured human peripheral blood mononuclear cells following exposure to antidiabetic drugs. Acta Diabetol 2006;43(2) 46-51

[52] Chakraborty A, Chowdhury S, Bhattacharyya M. Effect of metformin on oxidative stress, nitrosative stress and inflammatory biomarkers in type 2 diabetes patients. Diabetes Res Clin Pract 2011;93(1) 56-62.

[53] Vitale C, Mercuro G, Cornoldi A, Fini M, Volterrani M, Rosano GM. Metformin improves endothelial function in patients with metabolic syndrome. J Intern Med 2005; 258(3) 250-6.

[54] Nsonwu AC, Usoro CAO, Etukudo MH, Usoro IN. Glycemic control and serum and urine levels of zinc and magnesium in diabetics in Calabar, Nigeria. Pakistan J of Nutrition 2006; 5(1) 75-78

[55] van Dam RM, Hu FB, Rosenberg L, Krishan S, Palmer JR. Dietary calcium and magnesium, major food sources, and risk of type 2 diabetes in US black women. Diabetes Care 2006;29 2238-2243

[56] Shah NC, Liu JP, Iqbal J, Hussain M, Jiang XC, Li Z, Li Y, Zheng T, Li W, Sica AC, Perez-Albela JL, Altura BT, Altura BM. Mg deficiency results in modulation of serum lipids, glutathione, and NO synthase isozyme activation in cardiovascular tissues: relevance to de novo synthesis of ceramide, serum Mg and atherogenesis. Int J Clin Exp Med 2011; 4(2) 103-18.

[57] Nielsen FH. Magnesium, inflammation, and obesity in chronic disease. Nutr Rev 2010; 68(6) 333-40

[58] Zhao C, Wang H, Zhang J, Feng L. Correlations of trace elements, glucose and body composition in type 2 diabetes mellitus. Wei Sheng Yan Jiu 2008;37(5) 600-605

[59] Lefevre M, Keen CL, Lonnerdal B, Hurley LS, Schneenman BO (1986) Copper deficiency- induced hypercholesterolemia: effects on HDL subfractions and hepatic lipoprotein receptor activity in the rat. J Nutr 1986;116 1735-46

[60] Abdoljalal M. Plasma zinc and magnesium levels in type 2 diabetic patients in Gorgan City.J Med Sci 2006;6(6) 1029-32

[61] Walter RM Jr, Uriu-Hare JY, Olin KL, Oster MH, Anawalt BD, Critchfield JW, Keen CL. Copper, zinc, manganese, and magnesium status and complications of diabetes mellitus. Diabetes Care 1991;14(11) 1050-6.

[62] Ghayour-Mobarhan M, Shapouri-Moghaddam A, Azimi-Nezhad M, Esmaeili H, Parizadeh SM, Safarian M, Kazemi-Bajestani SM, Khodaei GH, Hosseini SJ, Parizadeh SM, Ferns GA (2009) The relationship between established coronary risk factors and serum copper and zinc concentrations in a large Persian cohort. J Trace Elem Med Biol 2009;23(3) 167-75.

Chapter 13

Animal Models for Study of Diabetes Mellitus

A. Lukačínová, B. Hubková, O. Rácz and F. Ništiar

Additional information is available at the end of the chapter

http://dx.doi.org/10.5772/48325

1. Introduction

Diabetes mellitus is a heterogeneous group of chronic disorders of carbohydrate, lipid and protein metabolism characterized by high blood glucose levels due to relative or absolute deficiency of insulin (Eiselein et al., 2004). Hyperglycemia, the primary clinical manifestation of diabetes, is associated with the development of diabetic complications. Several studies have suggested that hyperglycemia accelerates the development of chronic complications via several mechanisms, including increased aldose reductase related polyol pathway flux, increased formation of advanced glycation end-products (AGEs), activation of protein kinase C isoforms, increased hexosamine pathway flux, and overproduction of reactive forms of oxygen (Brownlee, 2001). AGEs are a group of complex and heterogeneous compounds, including brown and fluorescent cross-linking substances (e.g., pentosidine), non-fluorescent cross-linking products (e.g., methylglyoxal lysine dimers), or non-fluorescent, non-cross linking adducts (e.g., carboxymethyl lysine) (Dyer et al., 1991). Increasing evidence identifies AGE formation as the critical pathogenic link between hyperglycemia and long-term complications of diabetes: nephropathy, neuropathy, and retinopathy (Wada & Yagihashi, 2005). Therefore, another mode of diabetes treatment independent of blood glucose levels, inhibition of AGE formation, could be useful in the prevention or reduction of certain diabetic complications (Dong et al., 2010) in both main forms of the illness, Type 1 diabetes mellitus (T1D, insulin-dependent diabetes mellitus, IDDM) and Type 2 diabetes mellitus (T2D, noninsulin-dependent diabetes mellitus, NIDDM), and also in secondary forms related to gestation or other disorders.

In 2010, WHO estimated that 285 million people were living with diabetes (corresponding to 6.4% of the world's adult population). About 7 million people develop the disease each year and 3.9 million deaths were attributed to diabetes yearly (Shaw et al., 2010; Roglic & Unwin, 2010). Current predictions estimate that the prevalence of diabetes will reach 438 million by 2030 (corresponding to 7.8% of the adult population) and that 80% of prevalent cases will occur in the developing world (Roglic & Unwin, 2010). The increase is mainly driven by changes in dietary habits and low levels of physical activity (Wild et al., 2004). In the poorest countries, diabetes is more common among the better-off, but economic development quickly reverses this trend so that people from lower socioeconomic groups are more affected by diabetes; consequences are worse among the poor in all countries (Whiting et al., 2010, Blas & Sivasankara Kurup, 2010). Diabetes mellitus and specially diabetes with chronic complications belongs to the diseases requiring huge costs (Ettaro et al., 2004).

Diabetes mellitus is a syndrome characterized by many symptoms most typical of which is hyperglycemia. T1D is <10% of all diabetes cases, but its prevalence is constantly increasing (Green et al., 2001). This type occurs most frequently around the age of 14 years and individuals affected by this type must be treated throughout life with insulin injections (Rossini et al., 2003). Disease is the result of inflammatory islet infiltration (insulitis) and selective destruction of insulin producing β-cells (Atkinson and Eisenbarth, 2001). In general, diabetes being an autoimmune basis, T1D occurs frequently in individuals with other autoimmune diseases, especially intestinal or thyroid gland. It is strongly bound to major histocompatibility system (MHC), is dependent on T cells and can be modified by immunosuppression. When you start an autoimmune mechanism, exogenous factors play a role particularly of viral origin, but also antigens of the host cells based on molecular mimicry. These trigger tissue-specific immune response producing cross-reactive effector cells or antibodies that recognize self-proteins of β cells of the pancreas (Kukreja & Maclaren, 1999). Coxsackie B4 **virus**, for example, contains a sequence of 18 amino acids similar to enzyme glutamic acid decarboxylase (GAD) of pancreatic β-cells (Kaufman et al., 1992). At the same time viruses can cause subtle damage to the β-cells followed by autoimmune response against damaged β-damaged cells with sequestrated virus antigen. Other studies have identified endogenous retroviral genomes in diabetic islets, but whether the virus initiates or is only a marker of the disease remains unclear (Benoist & Mathis, 1997). Regardless of the type of trigger are activated specific self reactive T cell clones against pancreatic β-cells, which then infiltrate the islets of the pancreas. It is believed that these T cell clones belonging to the T helper 1 (Th1) subset. These Th1 cells produce characteristic cytokines, such as IFNγ and IL-2, which are considered as triggers of insulitis and destruction of β-cells of the pancreas (Suarez-Pinzon & Rabinovitch, 2001). Following the massive loss of pancreatic β-cells develop severe deficiency of insulin resulting in hyperglycemia. This causes glycogenolysis in the liver, activate gluconeogenetic pathways and decreases cellular uptake of glucose in peripheral tissues (muscle and adipose). Extensive degradation of fats and oxidation of fatty acids leads to hyperlipidemia and ketosis. The essential symptoms include hyperglycemia, polyuria due to osmotic diuresis, thirst due to hyperosmolar state, weight loss due to depletion of fat reserves and negative nitrogen balance, neurotoxicity due to hyperglycemia and ketoacidosis (Eiselein et al., 2004). If patients are not treated die due to circulatory collapse and coma. When initiating therapy by exogenous insulin, but are frequent hyperglycemia, develop micro- and macroangiopathies. Therefore, in diabetic patients is increased risk for coronary heart disease, stroke, gangrene of the lower limbs, chronic kidney disease, blindness and visual disturbances, and autonomic and peripheral neuropathy. These problems reduce life expectancy by up to 25% (Williams & Pickup, 2004) and the most common causes of death are diseases of heart and kidney.

In addition to people diabetes mellitus are quite often found in animals living with man (dog, cat), pets (or livestock) and laboratory animals (Malaisse & Sener, 2008).

For eliminate ethical and logistic problems in the study of T1D in connection with the heterogeneity of outbreed human populations, have been developed so many animal models of induced and spontaneous diabetes with the possibility of more frequent sampling, biopsy and autopsy samples. In these models it is possible to breeding at a controlled heredity and study of various environmental factors in relatively large and uniform populations. Animal models have a special status in the study of pathogenesis of chronic complications of diabetes, which are considered the following mechanisms: (1) non-enzymatic glycosylation, (2) intracellular hyperglycemia with associated disturbances in the polyol pathway, (3) activation of protein kinase C (PKC) and (4) increased hexosamine pathway flux (Eiselein et al., 2004). Non-enzymatic glycosylation lead to irreversible formation of advanced glycation end products (AGEs) through the Maillard reaction, and this is probably the best studied pathogenetic factor of diabetic complications. Pathological effects of AGEs are induced by impaired function of glycosylated products and by activation of AGE receptors on endothelial cells, monocytes, macrophages, lymphocytes and mesenchymal cells. Increased risk of heart diseases in diabetics is mainly attributed to the formation of AGEs (Eiselein et al., 2004). Glycosylation of collagen type IV in basement membranes of blood vessels leads to cross-links between interstitial proteins and lipoproteins, e.g., LDL. (Vlassara, 1996). LDL can be glycosylated and subsequently oxidized (Bucala et al., 1993). Modified LDL can then be bound to receptors of macrophages (CD36). The resulting foam cell formation and development of the fatty streak in the sub-endothelial space is the beginning of the atherosclerotic process (Ohgami et al., 2001). Since in diabetics the levels of AGEs of apoprotein B and phospholipids are several times higher as compared to nondiabetics, diabetics have a three- to four-fold higher risk of cardiovascular diseases (Bucala et al., 1994) and it is expected that non-enzymatic glycation is responsible also for vascular occlusions (Peppa et al., 2004). Other studies have attributed the importance of AGEs in hypertension, kidney pathology and erectile dysfunction in diabetics. These injuries are caused by AGEs present in the vascular matrix, where it inhibits the vasodilatory effect of EDRF (NO) and increased expression of endothelin-1, a potent vasoconstrictor (Quehenberger et al., 2000). Many of the effects of AGEs are dependent on the receptor. The best characterized receptor of AGEs is the receptor for advanced glycation end products (RAGE), which is a member of the immunoglobulin superfamily of cell membrane molecules (Stern et al., 2002). Studies in rodent models demonstrated that blocking RAGE can inhibit vascular hyperpermeability and reduced development of atherosclerotic lesion (Wendt et al., 2002). These results suggest that AGE-RAGE system may be a promising target for prophylaxis and treatment of late complications of diabetes mellitus. Hyperglycemia can cause various damages by changing polyol pathway, diacylglycerol-PKC pathway is important for develop of micro- and macro-angiopathy, and finally hexosamine biosynthetic pathway is also involved in the development of diabetic vascular complications (Eiselein et al., 2004).

In the study of T1D is primarily used two species of laboratory animals, rat and mouse (von Herrath and Nepom, 2009). The most commonly used model is non-obese diabetic (NOD) mouse (Serreze and Leiter, 2001). Many data in the literature explains the genetics and immunology of these animals and they were identified by at least 27 genetic loci and many immunological defects (Serreze and Leiter, 2001). Their disadvantages as a model consisted of two facts. Firstly, for this model in addition to immunosuppression also other immunomodulatory interventions showed a preventive effect on diabetes (Atkinson & Leiter, 1999), in contrast, these were ineffective in humans (Skyler et al., 2002). Second, because some of the negative factors of environment, particularly viral infections (Leiter, 1998) reduced the frequency of diabetes and often act preventively in mice (Atkinson & Leiter, 1999), while in humans viruses are known triggers. Although the original NOD mice and congenic strains derived from them provide valuable information and is necessary to keep in mind that they are not completely appropriate alternative to studying human T1D (Greiner et al., 2001). Rats provide another model. Such are BB rats (Mordes et al., 2001), a widely studied model susceptible to autoimmune destruction of pancreatic β-cells. In some experiments also nonmammal models can be exploited due they easy handling and low economic costs.

Use of animal models in diabetes research has a long tradition. Our aim was to present an overview of animal models used in research of diabetes mellitus and highlight some technological and scientific problems associated with interpretation of carrying out these experiments in accordance with current European legislation on animal protection and exploitation of animals for experimental purposes (Ništiar et al., 2006). It is based on detailed analysis of the literature, using well-known databases such as MEDLINE®, HighWire Press, PubMed and basic book, "Animal Models of Diabetes: A Primer" (Sima & Shafrir, 2000).

Already in 1890, von Mehring and Minkowski induced in dogs by removing the pancreas acute diabetes mellitus (Minkowski, 1989). In addition to partial and the total pancreatectomy, there are also non-surgical methods to induce hyperglycemia. There are five groups of diabetogenic substances: chemical and biological agents, potentiators, peptides and steroids (van der Werf et al., 2007). Among the animal models include in particular rodents, which are especially suitable for their low cost, short generation time, inherited forms of obesity and hyperglycemia. There are known animal models to study T1D also T2D (Rees & Alcolado, 2005; Yang & Santamaria, 2006). Animals with spontaneous T1D have been drawn by inbreed breeds in different laboratories. In contrast, animal models of T2D are very heterogeneous. This includes not only animals with single-gene mutation, but also other types with insulin resistant syndrome and impaired pancreatic β-cells (Matteucci & Giampietro, 2008).

More recently techniques using methods of molecular biology have produced genetically modified mouse models, including knockout and transgenic animals. Knockout animals have been defective gene in embryonic stem cells. In transgenic animals modified gene is incorporated into the pronucleus of zygote and then randomly into the genome of the animal and is transferred to the offspring.

Diabetic animal models undoubtedly have enormous benefit in clarifying the effect of insulin and insulin therapy. They also have some shortcomings, particularly when extrapolating results to humans and diabetic complications in humans (Tesch & Nikolic-Paterson, 2006) as well as some results may be misleading in the study of T1D prevention by using of model rodents (Leiter & von Herrath, 2004). It is claimed that the rodents in this area do not adequately reflect the situation in humans (Yang & Santamaria, 2006). Accordingly, these models and experiments will be necessary to standardize especially for prevention studies. Reliable results about the differences of pharmaceutical efficiency or survival of animals, delays and onset of disease, temporal relation of events require a very clear interpretation and repeatability of the experiment as well as the establishment of appropriate databases.

2. Basic considerations

Already in the Helsinki Declaration of the World Medical Association, 1964 (since been revised and amended) Rule 12 says that "to be secured by appropriate conditions, environment and care of experimental animals included in the experiment." The protection and welfare (only vertebrates) used for experimental purposes is regulated by: *Council Directive 86/609/EEC, Directive 2003/65/EC, Council Decision 1999/575/EC* and *Council Decision 2003/584/EC*. While there are considerable differences in the application of these measures in own legislation of individual countries. 23rd January 2006 the European Commission presented a modified and a new *Action Plan* for to ensure the welfare of animals in the future to a much higher level in all European Union member countries.

In 1959, zoologist William Russell and microbiologist Rex Burch presented a proposal for research on the three R: replacement, reduction and refinement (Russell & Burch, 1959). As the replacement is considered using any technique with insensitive material that replaces the use of susceptible live vertebrate animals. For the relative replacement is considered when animals are used only in certain parts of experiment thereby minimize distress during the whole experiment. Absolute replacement is if susceptible live animals are not used at any stage of the experiment. Organ and tissue cultures represent a transition between absolute and relative replacement. Reduction is one of the methods that allow researchers to reduce the number of animals used for research without reducing the statistical significance. In terms of statistical significance is extremely important to determine the number of animals needed for certain types of biomedical research (Dell et al., 2002). The significance of the test must be such as to enable to assess the clinical significance of the monitored phenomenon. Although the difference is less, we can be made certain conclusions (trends) without the need to increase the number of animals. This is necessary to meet two basic requirements, and that the differences have a normal distribution to determine the standard deviation.

Refinement is provided by better care of the animals. Fourth R, responsibility aims at increasing the accountability of scientists using animals in experiments (Bark, 1995). This area is in the forefront in recent years.

Report A2005 submitted consensus on animal experiments in the present. It also submitted a proposal for the basic procedures and compliance with conditions of four R (Perry, 2007).

Regarding diabetes mellitus is necessary to admit that the conditions regarding the extrapolation of the results of animal experiments to conditions in humans are not clearly clarified. There are neither clearly intended technical conditions for carrying animal experiments for obtaining scientific knowledge. If the technological of the performance of experiments conditions are not sufficiently clarified one cannot even assume that their moral and ethical aspects are in order. From that aspect, it is clear only that the animals were subjected to experiments at the lowest discomfort (Rees & Alcolado, 2005).

Animal models are possible principally to divide into five groups (Hau, 2008):

1. induced (experimental) models;
2. spontaneous (genetic mutant) models;
3. genetically modified models (transgenic animals);
4. negative models (strain of animals in whom the studied disease does not occur) and
5. orphan models, describing the malfunctions that occur in the model animal, but do not occur in humans (e.g., Marek's disease, bovine spongiform encephalopathy, etc.).

Induced (experimental) models are represented by animals in which a modeled phenomenon as diabetes was induced by certain agents, e.g., chemical (alloxan, streptozotocin, cow's milk), viruses (encephalomyocarditis virus) or pancreatectomy.

The use of animals for experimental purposes is always encountered negative response from the public, especially on the basis of ethical and religious reasons. These efforts led to the gradual formation of legislation towards the protection of animals used for experimental purposes. Nevertheless these experiments have contributed significantly to the current scientific knowledge of human biology, physiology, endocrinology and pharmacology (Loew, 1996). Outputs from these experiments were often not extrapolated to humans and it has also led to efforts to reduce them and to legislation guidance and control. On the other hand it should be noted that these very often contribute to a better understanding of many biological phenomena. Science on laboratory animals can be defined as a professional field focused on issues of scientific, ethical and lawful use of animals for biomedical research, i.e. interdisciplinary science involving biological and pathobiological details for optimal scientific use of animals as models for humans or other species. In general it deals with the quality of animals as susceptible objects in biomedical research. It includes comparative biology of laboratory animals, aspects of the breeding and reproduction (cross), welfare, economy of farming, anesthesia, euthanasia[1], and experimental procedures. The basic precondition for the use of animals for experimental purposes is a competence of researcher, including a solid knowledge about the biological needs, care and handling of animals.

[1] "Euthanasia" in association with the termination of life in animal experiment is a widely used term which on the other side is a mistake.

If the use of animals for experimental purposes is an essential condition a similarity of the animal with modeled objects in the light of studied phenomenon, i.e. concept the analogy of animal models. If the analogy is closer the possibility of extrapolation of results is much more reliable. Extrapolation is used to express to what extent can be used the results from animal experiments to humans (how are applicable to humans). In the analysis from big multinational pharmaceutical companies in 150 compounds were monitored compliance (concordance) between animal models and human subjects (Olson et al., 2000). Concordance determining the toxicity of the substances to humans if were tested in rodents and non-rodents was 71%, when used only non-rodents 63% and if used only rodents 43%. High concordances are detected in the cardiovascular toxicity (80%), hematological toxicity (91%) and gastrointestinal toxicity (85%). Low concordances are in the neurological manifestations. Despite the high concordances in animal experiments are often reports of damages in humans by preparations of certain pharmaceutical companies. E.g., penicillin is fatal for the guinea pig, but it is well tolerated by humans, aspirin is teratogenic for cats, dogs, guinea pigs, rats, mice and monkeys, but not teratogenic for pregnant women, despite their frequent use (Mann, 1984). Thalidomide causing malformations in 10 000 children did not cause birth defects in rats (Koppányi & Avery, 1966) nor in many other species (Miller & Strömland, 1999). The close phylogenetic or morphological similarity is not crucial for the biochemical mechanisms and physiological responses, although in many cases this is so (Beynen & Hau, 2001). A very important difference between experimental animals and human populations is their genetic variability. Experimental animals are genetically almost identical in contrast to man exhibiting great variability. It is therefore possible to lay down precise rules for extrapolation of results from one species to another species, although in the literature have been made to certain procedures (Calabrese, 1991). Under the extrapolation is necessary to bear in mind certain mathematically expressed values, although it often looks precisely from this aspect, e.g., in determining the toxicity of certain substances or to determine of pharmacologically effective doses of drugs. In our opinion, fundamental importance is the rather in detection of toxic or therapeutic efficacy of substances. For specific determination of toxic or biologically effective dose, they should be taken in extrapolating only as a possible benchmark. Therefore, for any type of research should be borne in mind that the use of animal model does not attempt to extrapolate the main objective of the immediate outcome of the man, but looking for an answer to questions of researcher. While examining the need of experiments on animals it is first necessary to determine whether the experiment gave relevant answer to the experimenter, and whether the answer to the question enriches the current knowledge about the studied phenomenon. With this reason should be hypothesis (question) subjected to analysis before the experiment (approval of animal experiments, ethics committees, input opponency), and after publishing the results (answers to questions) and by the public opinion (responses).

Selection of animal species for the experimental purpose must be based on the greatest similarity between model object and modeling object, therefore the found results showed the strong concordance and therefore extrapolation was valid. It is well known that the metabolic rate in young and small animals is much higher than in large and old animals, because body size is the one of the key indicators and benchmarks for extrapolation, and precisely on the basis that have been submitted to the methods of extrapolation for the calculation of effective or toxic doses of various compounds (Hau & Poulsen, 1988).

3. Animal models for the study of diabetes mellitus

Recently almost 140 years passed from the excellent experiments of Mehring and Minkowski with pancreatectomized dogs. There have been many experiments with this model on rabbits and dogs when Banting and Best came to experiment, which led to the beginning of the isolation and purification of insulin (Bliss, 1982). Dog Marjorie, who was first treated with exogenous insulin, is probably one of the most famous experimental animal in the history, comparable only with Dolly the sheep from genetic studies at the end of the last century. The early experimental models of diabetes were focused on pancreatectomized (partial or total) animals. Selection of species was more or less spontaneous. Usually used by small animals (mostly rats and mice), both because of handling or space needs and the affordable price. These experiments have often been questioned that the extrapolation to humans is appropriate from experiments on larger animals such as cats, dogs, pigs and primates (McNamara et al., 2009).

Among the non-surgical method inducing hyperglycemia after pancreatic damage with toxic substances, the most famous are streptozotocin (Junod et al., 1969) and alloxan (Lenzen & Panten, 1988; Lenzen, 2008). Surgical and non-surgical methods are a good model for studying the consequences of chronic hyperglycemia and the development of diabetic complications (Salgado et al., 2001). Using female animals it is also possible to study the effects of hyperglycemia to the offspring (Caluwaerts et al., 2003). Problems related to control of hyperglycemia, application of insulin or oral antidiabetic drugs require further improvements of experiments (Herrera et al., 1985). It should be noted that euglycemia cannot be reached in pancreatectomized animals (Harder et al., 2003). In pancreatectomized animals also transplantation of Langerhans' islet cells was studied. Islets cells can be transplanted without capsules or in capsules that protect them from rejection (Lanza et al., 1999), either subcutaneously (Wang et al., 2011), or under the kidney capsule (Korec, 1991, Carlsson et al., 2000) or via the portal vein to the liver (Trimble et al., 1980). Transplanted animals must receive antirejection therapy (Kobayashi et al., 2008). Like in humans is a key event in many successful interventions should be carried out (how many animals to be used) so that we can draw on the basis of their results, conclusions appropriate for transplantation programs.

Rodents are commonly used models for testing the new pharmacologically active substances not only in the context of transplantation (immunosuppressives), but also with regard to therapy or prevention of human diseases. Rats and mice are commonly used in safety and effectiveness testing of new orally active compounds. These experiments also led to unexpected findings about how the PPAR γ agonists may have a protective effect on the β-cells (Bonora et al., 2008). Similarly, in such experiments were also identified the effects of insulin analogues for the development of tumors (Sandow, 2009).

Experimental animals used to study of diabetes mellitus can be essentially classified into several groups (Shafrir, 2003):

1. Animals with chemically induced destruction of pancreatic β-cells:
    a. Alloxan model
    b. Streptozotocin (single dose)
    c. Streptozotocín (more subdiabetogenic doses).
2. Animals with spontaneous autoimmune diabetes:
    a. BB rats
    b. NOD mice
    c. Akita mice
    d. LETL rats
    e. Torii rats
    f. LEW.1AR1/ZTM.
3. Genetically altered animals (transgenic models) with various form of diabetes
4. Insulin resistant mutants of rodents with potent diabetogenity:
    a. C57BKs *db* mice ($lepr^{db}$)
    b. C57BL6J *ob* mice (lep^{ob})
    c. Yellow A^{v} a A^{vy} mice
    d. KK mice
    e. NZO mice
    f. Zucker *fa* rats ($lepr^{fa}$) and BB/Wor rats
    g. Zdf/Drt-*fa* rats
    h. Wistar-Kyoto diabetic/fatty rats
    i. Obese (corpulent, *cp*) rats of strains SHR/N-*cp*, LA/N-*cp*, SHHF/Mcc-*cp* and JCR.LA-*cp*.
5. Rodents with spontaneous diabetes of various etiology:
    a. NON mice
    b. WBN/Kob rats
    c. ESS rats
    d. BHE/Cdb rats
    e. OLETF rats
    f. NSY mice
    g. Koletzky (SHROB) rats (fa^{K})
    h. Hypertriglyceridemic (HTG) rats
6. Rodents by overfeed induced diabetogenity:
    a. *Psammomys obesus* (sand rats, gerbil)
    b. Acromys cahirinus (spiny mice)
    c. C57BL/6J mice

Diabetic rodents obtained by selective crossbreeding from normal strains:

   d. GK (Goto-Kakizaki) rats
   e. Cohen diabetic rats (induced by diabetogenic diet rich in sucrose and poor in copper).
7. Diabetic non-rodents:
   a. Primates
   b. Pigs
   c. Dogs
   d. Cats.

3.1. Models of spontaneous type 1 diabetes mellitus (T1D)

The most known models of spontaneous T1D include NOD (non-obese diabetic) mice and BB (BioBreeding) rats, having a many common features with human T1D (von Herrath & Nepom, 2009). In addition to these we include here LETL (Long Evans Tokushima Leans) and KDP (Komeda diabetes prone) rats, LEW congenic rats, New Zealand white rabbits, Keeshond dogs (long haired dog of Dutch race), Chinese hamster and Celebes black apes. It should be noted that these animals are kept as inbred in laboratory conditions for many generations and gradually selected to hyperglycemia.

An excellent overview and classification of animal models of T1D is in von Herrath & Nepom (2009):

- Spontaneous or genetically modified diabetic animals:
  - Non-obese:
    - *NOD* mice
    - Akita mice
    - *BB* rats
    - *LETL* (Long-Evans Tokushima Lean) rats
    - *KDP* (Komeda diabetes prone) rats
    - LEW.1AR1/Ztm-*iddm* rats
    - Monkeys
    - Keeshond dogs
    - Some races of cats (feline models).
- Chemically induced diabetic animals:
  - Non-obese:
    - Single dose of ALX, respectively, more low doses of STZ
    - Vacor (rodenticide, which acts as an antagonist of B vitamins, particularly nicotinamide), dithizone, dehydroascorbic acid, pentamidine and 8-hydroxyquinoline.
- Surgically prepared diabetic animals:
  - Non-obese:
    - Totally pancreatectomized animals, e.g., dogs, primates, pigs and rats.
- Virus-induced models.

3.2. Models of spontaneous type 2 diabetes mellitus (T2D) and monogenic forms of diabetes

T2D is a heterogeneous group of disorders characterized by insulin resistance and impaired insulin secretion, defined by elevated fasting glycemia and hyperglycemia after load of glucose. Some newer subtypes of diabetes are based on single-gene defect, called MODY (Maturity Onset Diabetes of the Young) syndromes (Vaxillaire & Froguel, 2008), syndromes with severe insulin resistance (Semple et al., 2011) and a mitochondrial diabetes (Berdanier, 2007). In most patients, diabetes is caused by several genetic and environmental factors and disease development in all leads to chronic complications.

Animal models of T2D are complex and heterogeneous as in humans (Kaplan & Wagner, 2006). Advances in the interpretation of the problem coming from various sources and models (*ob/ob* mice – monogenic model of obesity with leptin deficiency, db/db mice – monogenic model of obesity with leptin resistance, Zucker [*fa/fa* rats] – monogenic model of obesity with resistance to leptin; Goto Kakizaki rats, KK mice, NSY mice, OLETF rats, Israeli sand [desert] rats, streptozotocin-treated rats receiving fat diet, CBA/Ca mice, New Zealand obese mouse). In some animals, is dominated insulin resistance, compared to other it is damage of pancreatic β-cells (Cefalu, 2006). Animals with glucose intolerance and phenotypically more obese with dyslipidemia and hypertension are a good model of human T2DM. Similar to NOD mice and BB rats for T1D, selective inbreeding increases the spontaneous incidence of T2D. Most of the studies come from monogenic models of *ob/ob*, *db/db*, *fa/fa* and agouti strains (Franconi et al., 2008).

Obesity and subsequent insulin resistance are the main triggers of T2D in humans. Due to strong similarities with humans animal models must be obese. Some strains maintain euglycemic status with a strong and sustained compensatory response to β-cells, leading to insulin resistance and hyperinsulinemia. Similarly, *ob/ob* mice and *fa/fa* rats are a good example of this phenomenon. For others, such as *db/db* mice and *Psammomys obesus* which were rapidly develops hyperglycemia and therefore β-cells are not able to maintain high levels of insulin. The study of these different animal models may be helpful in explaining why some people with morbid obesity never develop T2D while in others hyperglycemia is already at relatively mild insulin resistance and obesity (Tirabassi et al., 2004).

These models have also contributed significantly to the study of obesity (Srinivasan & Ramarao, 2007). In 1994, Friedman with coworkers cloned ob/ob mice with a mutant gene for severe obesity (Zhang et al., 1994). Normal ob gene encodes a protein secreted by adipocytes and called leptin. In *db/db* mice and *fa/fa* rats was found mutations in the gene for the hypothalamic leptin receptor (Lee et al., 1996).

Recent classification of animals for modeling of T2D:

- Spontaneous or genetically modified diabetic animals:
    - Obese:

    - *ob/ob* mice
    - *db/db* mice
    - KK (Kuo Kondo) mice
    - KK/A^y (yellow obese) mice
    - NZO mice
    - NONcNZO10 mice
    - TSOD (Tsumura Suzuki obese diabetic) mice
    - M16 mice
    - Nagoya-Shibata-Yasuda (NSY) mice
    - Zucker fatty rats
    - ZDF (Zucker diabetic fatty) rats
    - Obese-hyperglycemic Wistar Kyoto rats
    - SHR/N-cp rats
    - SHHF/Mcc-*cp* rats
    - JCR/LA-*cp* rats
    - OLETF rats
    - eSS rats
    - BHE/C*db* rats
    - Koletzky (SHROB) rats
    - Yucatan miniature pigs
    - Sinclair miniature pigs
    - Göttingen miniature pigs
    - Ossabaw pigs
    - Familial hypercholesterolinemic pigs (FHP)
    - Obese rhesus monkeys
    - Macaca fascicularis
    - Macaca radiata
    - Papo anobis.
  - Non-obese:
    - WBN/Kob rats
    - Goto Kakizaki (GK) rats
    - Hypertriglyceridemic (HTG) rats
    - Torii rats (SDT, spontaneously diabetic Torii)
    - Torii non-obese mice C57BL/6
    - ALS/Lt mice
    - Non-obese mutant C57BL/6 (Akita) mice.
- With diet/nutrition induced diabetic animals:
  - Cohen diabetic rats
  - Psammomys obesus
  - Acomys cahirinus
  - Ctenomys talarum (tuco tuco)
  - Guinea pigs (Cricetulus griseus)
  - C57/BL 6J mice

        - *Macaca* mullata
        - Dogs
        - Cats
        - Chinese Guizhou mini-pigs.
- Chemically induced diabetic animals:
    - Obese:
        - GTG (gold thioglucose)–treated obese mice
        - Yorkshire and with Yorkshire crossbred strains of pigs (STZ-induced diabetes).
    - Non-obese:
        - Single low dose of ALX or single dose of STZ to adult rats, mice and etc.
        - Neonatal STZ-treated rats.
- Surgically prepared diabetic animals:
    - Obese:
        - VMH (ventromedial hypothalamus)–damaged dietetically obese diabetic rats.
    - Non-obese:
        - partially pancreatectomized animals, e.g., dogs, primates, pigs and rats.
- Transgenic/knockout diabetic animals:
    - Obese:
        - β_3 receptor knockout mice
        - UCP1 knockout mice.
    - Non-obese:
        - transgenic or knockout mice in genes for insulin, insulin receptor and their components in the direction of insulin signaling, i.e., IRS-1, IRS-2, GLUT-4, PTP-1B and other
        - PPAR-γ tissue specific knockout mice
        - Glukokinase or GLUT-2 gene knockout mice
        - HIP rats (rats with overexpession of human islet amyloid polypeptide).

3.3. Models of spontaneous type 2 diabetes mellitus – Advantages and disadvatages

In view of advantages and disadvantages of different models of T2D animal models, we can say that:

- Spontaneous or genetically modified diabetic animals have:
    - Advantages:
        - Development of T2D is a spontaneous and provides genetic factors. In animals developed the similar features as in human T2D.
        - Animal models are mostly inbred in which is homogeneous genetic background and environmental factors are well controllable.
        - Variability of the results is minimal and requires a small number of animals.

- Disadvantages:
  - They are highly inbred, homogeneous, and often with monogenic inheritance therefore development of diabetes is strongly genetically determined versus heterogeneity in humans.
  - Limited life span and the time dimension of diabetes study.
  - In animals with brittle pancreas (db/db, ZDF rats, *P. obesus*, and other) is high mortality caused by ketosis and therefore need insulin treatment to prolong their life.
  - Require more sophisticated forms of breeding purposes and care.
- With diet/nutrition induced diabetic animals:
  - Advantages:
    - The development of diabetes associated with obesity is the result of overfeed, as it is also in diabetes in human populations.
    - Toxicity of chemical (diabetogenic) compounds to other vital organs and tissues can be eliminated.
  - Disadvantages:
    - Animal models often require long periods of dietary treatment.
    - Not too significant hyperglycemia are after a simple dietary treatment in genetically normal animals and are therefore unsuitable for studying antidiabetogenic substances by determining of blood glucose.
- Chemically induced diabetic animals:
  - Advantages:
    - Selective loss of β-cells of the pancreas (alloxan/STZ), while maintaining of intact α - and δ-cells.
    - Residual insulin secretion allows animals to live without insulin therapy a relative long time.
    - Ketosis and subsequent mortality is relatively low.
    - They are cheaper and easier to maintain.
  - Disadvantages:
    - Hyperglycemia develops primarily as a result of direct cytotoxic effects on β-cells and subsequent insulin deficiency and not as a result of insulin resistance.
    - Chemically induced diabetes is less stable and often occurs spontaneously regeneration of pancreatic β-cell, which is a disadvantage of long-term studies.
    - In chemically induced diabetes can be toxic substance damaged other molecular structures, and may result to the general toxic effects.
    - Variability of results with regard of hyperglycemia is very high.
- Surgically prepared diabetic animals:
  - Advantages:
    - Eliminates the cytotoxic effect of chemical diabetogenic substances to other organs and tissues.
    - Strongly resembles regarding reduction of β-cell mass to human T2D.

    - Disadvantages:
        - Technical complexity and cumbersome, postoperative procedures.
        - The occurrence of certain digestive problems (as result of excision of the exocrine pancreas, amylase deficiency, etc.).
        - Removal of α-cells (glucagon producing) together with β-cells leads to problems in regulation of hypoglycemic events.
        - Mortality is relatively high.
- Transgenic/knockout diabetic animals:
    - Advantages:
        - The effect of a single gene or their mutations on diabetes can be studied *in vivo.*
        - Greatly facilitate the resolution of the genetic complexity of T2D.
    - Disadvantages:
        - Highly sophisticated and expensive procedures for production and breeding.
        - Very expensive for routine screening tests.

Spontaneous T2D diabetic animals are normally obtained from animals with mutations in one or more genes that are transmitted from generation to generation (e.g., *ob*/*ob*, *db*/*db* mice) or the selection from non-diabetic outbred animals selectively crosses over several generations (e.g., GK rats, TSOD mice). These animals have congenital diabetes with the monogenic or polygenic defects. Metabolic peculiarities may be due to a single gene defect (monogenic) with a dominant phenotype (e.g., yellow obese KK/Ay mice) and the recessive phenotype (diabetic *db*/*db* mice, Zucker fatty rats) or may have polygenic origin (i.e. KK mice, NZO mouse) (**Aerts & Van Assche**, 2006). T2D in humans is the result of interaction of different environmental factors and many genes which under certain conditions may manifest as diabetes with very contrasting symptomatology (e.g., MODY), single-gene defects with clinically overt diabetes are rare. Therefore, animals with polygenic defects are more objective for a modeling study of T2D in humans (Lofty et al., 2011).

4. Problems of evaluation and interpretation of the results from animal experiments

Long-term fluctuations in blood glucose levels can lead to loss of consciousness in animals. Both hyperglycemia and hypoglycemia can lead to diabetic coma, which is characterized by disorientation and convulsions. Diabetic coma is a life-threatening event. Without therapy of diabetic rats, blood glucose levels rising significantly, there is dehydration and electrolyte losses by urine, is not stores the fat and protein, even significantly break down protein and fat reserves. This dysregulation leads to ketosis and the release of ketone bodies in blood. It is unethical not treated animals with glycemia above 25 mM/L. Therefore, certain authors rejected animals from experiment with glycemia above 25 mM/L (Matteucci & Giampietro, 2008).

Similarly, non-treatment of significant hypoglycemia in the initial phase of alloxan diabetes is unethical. Some authors reported that animals are treated by glucose solution to alleviate complications and death due to hypoglycemia during the first 6 hours after administration of alloxan (de Carvalho et al., 2008).

Induction of diabetes after administration of diabetogenic substances is confirmed by the determination of glucose in blood. After blood collection are blood cells separated within one hour with the addition of glycolytic inhibitors. Glucose is then determined in plasma by using of standard enzymatic methods (Sacks et al., 2002). The concentration of glucose in plasma is 11% higher than in whole blood and glucose concentration in heparinized plasma may be 5% lower than in serum. Glucose concentrations during the oral glucose tolerance test in capillary blood are higher (about 20–25%) than in venous blood. Variation coefficient for glucose in plasma is ≤2.2%. Transmissible glucometers have a much lower sensitivity than the above coefficient of variation. There are similar differences between values measured by different glucometers. American Diabetes Association has built a development goal for blood glucose monitors with analytical deviations <5%. The diagnosis of diabetes in humans is based on the following criteria (ECDCDM, 2003):

- symptoms of diabetes and casual glycemia above 11.1 mM/L;
- fasting glycemia (FPG, *Fasting Plasma Glucose*) ≥7.0 mM/L;
- glycemia after glucose load increases over 2 h ≥11.1 mM/L.

These values can be confirmed the next day by re-examination. It must be noted that these criteria are applicable if the rules for determining the glucose levels are sufficiently accurate and sensitive beyond the range of between 7 and 11.1 mM/L.

When using the blood glucose monitors is needed just a drop of blood (less traumatized animals), although reproducibility and statistical accuracy is lower (needs more tests). As is to harmonize with the principle of the four R?

Oral glucose tolerance test (oGTT) provides information on ability to cope with the load by glucose. In adults, it is used in 3 hours arrangement and applied to 100 g of glucose in the diagnosis of gestational diabetes mellitus, compared with 2 hours arrangement and the application of 75 g glucose was used to confirm a diagnosis of diabetes (prediabetes) in the previous dubious blood glucose levels. In children used 1.75 g glucose/kg of b.w. maximum of 75 g glucose. It is a sensitive test for detection of disorders of glucose metabolism, especially if fasting blood glucose are in the dubious areas. For its correct implementation is necessary to respect a several principles:

- does not reduce the glucose uptake three days before the test;
- test should be performed after fasting overnight (10–14 h);
- 25–30% glucose solution is administered orally;
- glucose levels are measured before and 30, 60 and 120 minutes after administration of glucose;
- during the test do not receive food and water.

In rats given 25–30% aqueous solution of anhydrous glucose at a dose of 1-10 g/kg of b.w. Sampling are quite different before glucose administration and every 30 minutes up to 300 minutes after glucose administration (Matteucci & Giampietro, 2008).

In rats, it would be appropriate to use a similar arrangement of the test than in children with a completed at 120 min, in the case of dubious glucose levels at 8–12 mM/L.

If in rats are found blood glucose levels (between 12–16 mM/L), they can be considered as mild diabetic (or as prediabetic condition). Usually they have after a short period increased blood glucose above 16 mM/L, rats with glycemia above this level are considered as clearly diabetic (Lukačínová et al., 2008).

In the oGTT in rats and humans is difference in glucose load in terms of 1 kg of body weight. These differences are not indicated anything substantial cause.

Intravenous glucose tolerance test (ivGTT) used to determine of insulin secretion and determination of the first phase of insulin response (FPIR, *First Phase Insulin Response*), which is considered a risk factor for T1D in humans (Culina et al., 2011). When studying the prevention of T1D showed that 2 h oGTT was sensitive about 6 months before diagnosis of diabetes compared with FPIR, which was lower and declined with age. Higher sensitivity was achieved using both tests (Barker et al., 2007). Dextrose was administered at a dose of 0.5 g/kg (maximum 35 g) intravenously over 3 minutes. Blood was taken with the -10, -4, 1, 3, 5, 7 and 10 minutes before and after load with dextrose and analyzed for glucose and insulin. FPIR is expressed on the basis of the sum of values - 1 and 3-minute insulin levels.

In rats, using anhydrous glucose at a dose of 0.001 to 1.0 g/kg of b.w. and blood glucose and insulin are evaluated at different time periods typically from -15 min within 30-120 minutes from the load with glucose. It should be noted that these tests in animals do not have such importance and predictive value as in humans (mainly the system of food intake and fasting before the test). Deprivation of food in animals from the evening before the examination is a powerful stress stimulus (due to their nocturnal activity), which has a significant influence on interindividual differences. Of course it is difficult to determine what dose of load in humans corresponds to a similar stress in rats, what is the possibility of extrapolation of results between these species. Probably there should be a 35 g aliquot of the maximum load in humans (but how and when to realize?). We believe that this model could be accepted to study of impact assessment of preventive or therapeutically active substances.

Intraperitoneal glucose tolerance test (ipGTT) is not used in humans. In rats, the dose of glucose ranging from 0.2 to 2.0 g/kg of b.w. and monitored for three to seven time periods from 0 to 60–120 minutes after load of glucose (Matteucci & Giampietro, 2008). It should therefore be considered only as an experimental model without real impact for extrapolation. This model may be interesting for studies comparing of load by different agents as a possible methodological model.

When studying the problem of diabetes plays an experimental protocol and the possibility of extrapolating a very important role. The experimental protocol must include a detailed description of the methods of research, in an experiment to be included animals suitable for this study and must be chosen a good system of controls, used substances must be best defined and used appropriate methods of statistical analysis of results. E.g., in the case of research in herbal medicine has been submitted WHO guidelines specifying the some principles of experiment (WHO, 1993). The primary aims of non-clinical studies are: (1) determine whether the substance has a beneficial effect in terms of herbal medicine (2) characterize the range of pharmacological effects, (3) define the chemical characteristics of the pharmacologically active natural products and their mechanisms of action.

Pharmacodynamic and current pharmacological investigations used animal models or bioassays which are good models for modeling of human disease. As an experimental object (test system) can be used live animals, isolated organs or tissues, blood and its components, tissue and cell cultures, and various subcellular structures. A very important point is determining the appropriate doses for a given system from viewpoints of study of dose-effect relationship and their extrapolation to human (Resjö et al., 2008). In all studies must be a negative control (vehicle without active substance) and positive control (known drug/substance). The series of examinations should be tests to clarify the biological activity of the herbal preparation. For example, plasma insulin concentrations in relation to blood glucose, liver glycogen and triglyceride levels may help in understanding the absorption and utilization of glucose and the like. Toxicological methods include tests of toxicity (topical, systemic and special). Acute toxicity tests require a sufficient number of dose levels to determine the lethal dose and monitoring should take at least 7–14 days. In chronic tests of toxicity is application period lasts from the 2 weeks to 12 months. Particularly difficult are lifelong toxicity tests (Lukačínová et al., 2011). When rodents are used it is recommended that each group has at least 5–10 animals for both sexes.

In most animal studies, the experimenters assessed the effect of intervention on the basis of the null hypothesis, i.e. assume that the experimental intervention had no effect. Guidelines for construction of animal experiments is why strictly rules necessary for adequate control by using the smallest number of animals (Festing & Altman, 2002). Randomization and the use of blanks are rarer and therefore animal experiments indicate much more positive effects of treatment (Perel et al., 2007). Random choice of animals is essential for selection of animals to experimental (treated) and control groups (usually all individuals are healthy!) and despite does not reflect adequately to human population. Groups are designated by researcher and he knew what was that group treated and has been these groups intervened. In this area, animal experiments will be necessary to objectify (one divided and treated groups, and other these groups evaluated).

Since safety and efficacy of drugs before clinical examination are tested on animals, there are important all efforts to eliminate bias and random errors. Moreover, animal models should be as much as possible related clinical conditions. This is particularly important in extrapolation of dose (g/kg, g/m^2 of body surface, resp.). Similarly, when comparing in drug already in use, in animal experiments should be used of dosage as in humans.

5. Conclusion

The dawn and the subsequent development of experimental medicine in the second half of the XIXth century was unimaginable without the use of animals. Nobody cared about their fate and suffering – they were sacrificed in the war against diseases and for the development of science. The rules of experiment were simple and represented only the needs of the experimentator. The discovery of pancreatic diabetes and the subsequent isolation of insulin are the best examples of this era.

The situation changed dramatically in the second half of the XXth century in the development of new methods on laboratory analysis, in the development of new preventive and therapeutic procedures but especially in the new non-animal and animal models for the study in this area. For this analysis shows that are not yet standardized animal experiments even in the study of diabetes. These differences can lead to different conclusions regarding the pharmacologically active substances used in particular in the prevention but also in treatment of diabetes mellitus, e.g., hypoglycemic effect and dose relations in the application of vanadium or bioflavonoids (Lukačínová et al., 2008). It will be important to present a unified experimental approaches for testing of different substances on animals, both from the aspect of arrangement the experiment (control groups, conditions of experiment, statistical evaluation) as well as the selection of the studied parameters (markers) for individual type of test (acute, chronic, etc.) or the test substance. In this consideration is necessary increased attention to the requirements for the application of 4R. In this case, it can be expected the significant reduction in the need for experimental animals, does not need to repeat certain experiments only because they were not considered some of the basic conditions (often simple parameters such as the weight of the animals, water intake, food intake, urine output, etc.). Therefore, further work is needed to improve and refine existing guidelines for their specific needs for testing of biologically active substances for medical use. Especially at present when more and more come to the forefront of evidence-based medicine (Borgerson, 2005) should become a standard working method in animal experiments.

In any case, in the future is expected many new findings from animal models, particularly in the pathogenesis of human diseases. The immediate benefit of such experiments was the introduction to testing of insulin therapy, as well as testing of other drugs. It is necessary to calculate that there can also lead to no thoroughfares of research, and it should be remembered the reproducibility and extrapolation of results for the human population. We expect the most benefit but in the verification of preventive strategies with various drugs.

Author details

A. Lukačínová
Department of Physiology, Faculty of Medicine, Šafárik University, Košice, Slovak Republic

B. Hubková
Department of Medical and Clinical Biochemistry,
Faculty of Medicine, Šafárik University, Košice, Slovak Republic

O. Rácz
Department of Pathological Physiology,
Faculty of Medicine, Šafárik University, Košice, Slovak Republic
Department of Nanobiotechnology and Regenerative Medicine,
Faculty of Healthcare, Miskolc University, Hungary

F. Ništiar
Department of Pathological Physiology,
Faculty of Medicine, Šafárik University, Košice, Slovak Republic

Acknowledgement

This work was supported by Grant Agency VEGA No. 1/3494/06.

6. References

Aerts, L., Van Assche, F.A. (2006): Animal evidence for the transgenerational development of diabetes mellitus. *Intern. J. Biochem. Cell Biol.*, vol. 38, No. 3-4 (May-June 2006), pp. 894–903. ISSN 1357-2725.

Atkinson, M.A., Eisenbarth, G.S. (2001): Type 1 diabetes: New perspectives on disease pathogenesis and treatment. *Lancet*, vol. 358, No. 9277 (21 July 2001), pp. 221–229. ISSN 0140-6736.

Atkinson, M.A., Leiter, E.H. (1999): The NOD mouse model of insulin dependent diabetes: As good as it gets? *Nature Med.*, vol. 5, No. 6 (June 1999), pp. 601–604. ISSN 1078-8956.

Bark, R.E. (1995): The fourth R of research. *Am. Assoc. Lab. Anim. Sci.*, Vol. 54, No. 2 (March 1995), p. 50. ISSN 1559-6109

Barker, J.M., McFann, K., Harrison, L.C., Fourlanos, S., Krischer, J., Cuthbertson, D., Chase, H.P., Eisenbarth, G.S. (2007): Pre-type 1 diabetes dysmetabolism: maximal sensitivity achieved with both oral and intravenous glucose tolerance testing. *J. Pediatrics*, Vol. 150, No. 1 (January 2007), pp. 31–36. ISSN 0340-6199

Benoist, C., Mathis, D. (1997): Autoimmune diabetes: Retrovirus as trigger, precipitator or marker? *Nature*, Vol. 388, No. 6645 (28 August 1997), pp. 833–834. ISSN 0028-0836

Berdanier, C.D. (2007): Linking mitochondrial function to diabetes mellitus: an animal's tale. *Am. J. Physiol. Cell Physiol.*, Vol. 293, No. 3 (September 2007), pp. C830–C836. ISSN 0363-6143

Beynen, A.C., Hau, J. (2001): Animal models. In: *Principles of Laboratory Animal Science*. van Zutphen, L.F.M., Baumans, V., Beynen, A.C. (Eds): *Principles of Laboratory Animal Science*. Elsevier, ISBN 0444506128, Amsterdam, pp. 197–205.

Blas, E., Sivasankara Kurup, A. (Eds.) (2010): *Priority Public Health Conditions: From Learning to Action on Social Determinants of Health*. World Health Organization, ISBN 9789241563970, Geneva, pp. 77–94.

Bliss, M. (1982): *The discovery of insulin*. Chicago Univ. Press, ISBN 0-226-05897-2, Chicago, pp. 1–304.

Bonora, E. (2008): Protection of pancreatic beta-cells: is it feasible? *Nutr. Metab. Cardiovasc. Dis.*, Vol. 18, No. 1 (January 2008), pp. 74–83. ISSN 0939-4753

Borgerson, K. (2005): Evidence-Based Alternative Medicine? *Perspect. Biol. Med.*, Vol. 48, No. 4 (Autumn 2005), pp. 502–515. ISSN 0031-5982

Brownlee, M. (2001): Biochemistry and molecular cell biology of diabetic complications. *Nature*, Vol. 414, No. 6865 (13 December 2001), pp. 813–820. ISSN 0028-0836

Bucala, R., Makita, Z., Koschinsky, T., Cerami, A., Vlassara, H. (1993): Lipid advanced glycosylation: pathway for lipid oxidation in vivo. *Proc. Natl. Acad. Sci. USA*, Vol. 90, No. 14 (15 July 1993), pp. 6434–6438. ISSN 0027-8424

Bucala, R., Vlassara, H., Cerami, A. (1994): Advanced glycosylation end products: role in diabetic and non-diabetic vascular disease. *Drug Develop. Res.*, Vol. 32, No. 2 (June 1994), pp. 77–89. ISSN 1098-2299

Carlsson, P.-O., Palm, F., Andersson, A., Liss, P. (2000): Chronically decreased oxygen tension in rat pancreatic islets transplanted under the kidney capsule. *Transplantation*, Vol. 69, No. 5 (15 March 2000), pp. 761–766. ISSN 0041-1337

Calabrese, E.J. (1991): *Principles of Animal Extrapolation: Predicting Human Responses from Animal Studies*. Lewis Publishers, Inc., ISBN 0-87371-410-5, Chelsea, MI., pp. 1–616.

Caluwaerts, S., Holenmans, K., Van Bree, R., Verhaeghe, J., Van Assche, F.A. (2003): Is low-dose streptozotocin in rats an adequate model for gestational diabetes mellitus? *J. Soc. Gynecol. Investig.*, Vol. 10, No. 4 (May 2003), pp. 216–221. ISSN 1071-5576

Carvalho, V.F., Campos, L.V., Farias-Filho, F.A., Florim, L.T., Barreto, E.O., Pirmez, C., Savino, W., Martins, M.A., Silva, P.M.R. (2008): Suppression of allergic inflammatory response in the skin of alloxan-diabetic rats: relationship with reduced local mast cell numbers. *Int. Arch. Allergy Immunol.*, Vol. 147, No. 3 (October 2008), pp. 246–254. ISSN 1018-2438

Cefalu, W.T. (2006): Animal models of type 2 diabetes: clinical presentation and pathophysiological relevance to the human condition. *ILAR J.*, Vol. 47, No. 3, pp. 186–198. ISSN 1084-2020

Culina, S., Boitard, C., Mallone, R. (2011): Antigen-based immune therapeutics for type 1 diabetes: magic bullets or ordinary blanks? *Clin. Develop. Immunol.*, doi:10.1155/2011/286248. ISSN 1740-2522

Dell, R.B., Hollevan, S., Ramakrishnan, R. (2002): Sample size determination. *ILAR J.*, Vol. 43, No. 4, pp. 207–213. ISSN 1084-2020

Dong, W., Shil, H.B., Ma, H., Miao, Y.B., Liu, T.J., Wang, W. (2010): Homoisoflavanones from *Polygonatum odoratum* rhizomes inhibit advanced glycation end product formation. *Arch. Pharm. Res.*, Vol. 33, No. 5 (May 2010), pp. 669–674. ISSN 0253-6269

Dyer, D.G., Blackledge, J.A., Thorpe, S.R., Baynes, J.W. (1991): Formation of pentosidine during nonenzymatic browning of proteins by glucose. *J. Biol. Chem.*, Vol. 266, No. 18 (25 June 1991), pp. 11654–11660. ISSN 0021-9258

Eiselein, L., Schwartz, H.J., Rutledge, J.C. (2004): The challenge of type 1 diabetes mellitus. *ILAR J.*, Vol. 45, No. 3, pp. 231–236. ISSN 1084-2020

Ettaro, L., Songer, T.J., Zhang, P., Engelgau, M.M. (2004): Cost-of-illness studies in diabetes mellitus. *Pharmacoeconomics*, Vol. 22, No. 3, pp. 149–164. ISSN 1170-7690

ECDCDM (Expert Committee on the Diagnosis and Classification of Diabetes Mellitus) (2003): Report of the expert committee on the diagnosis and classification of diabetes mellitus. *Diabetes Care,* Vol. 26, Suppl. 1 (January 2003), pp. S5–S20. ISSN 0149-5992

Festing, M.F.W., Altman, D.G. (2002): Guidelines for the design and statistical analysis of experiments using laboratory animals. *ILAR J.*, Vol. 43, No. 4, pp. 244–258. ISSN 1084-2020

Franconi, F., Seghieri, G., Canu, S., Straface, E., Campesi, I., Malorni, W. (2008): Are the available experimental models of type 2 diabetes appropriate for a gender perspective? *Pharmacol. Res.*, Vol. 57, No. 1 (January 2008). pp. 6–18. ISSN 1043-6618

Green, A., Patterson, C.C., EURODIAB TIGER SG (2001): Trends in the incidence of childhood-onset diabetes in Europe 1989-1998. *Diabetologia*, Vol. 44, Suppl. 3 (October 2001), pp. B3–B8. ISSN 0012-186X

Greiner, D.L., Rossini, A.A., Mordes, J.P. (2001): Translating data from animal models into methods for preventing human autoimmune diabetes mellitus: *caveat emptor* and *primum non nocere. Clin. Immunol.*, Vol. 100, No. 2 (August 2001), pp. 134–143. ISSN 1521-6616

Harder, T., Franke, K., Fahrenkrog, S., Aerts, L., Van Bree, R., Van Assche, F.A., Plagemann, A. (2003): Prevention by maternal pancreatic islet transplantation of hypothalamic malformation in offspring of diabetic mother rats is already detectable at weaning. Neurosci. Lett., *Vol.* 352, No. 3 (11 December 2003), pp. 163–166. *ISSN 0304-3940*

Hau, J. (2008): Animal models for human disease: an overview. In: *Sourcebook of Models for Biomedical Research*. Conn, M.P. (Ed.): Humana Press, ISBN 978-1-58829-933-8, Totowa, New Jersey, pp. 3–8.

Hau, J., Poulsen, O.M. (1988): Doses for laboratory animals based on metabolic rates. *Scand. J. Lab. Anim. Sci.*, Vol. 15, No. 2, pp. 81–84. ISSN 0901-3393

Herrera, E., Palacin, M., Martin, A., Lasuncion, M.A. (1985): Relationship between maternal and fetal fuels and placental glucose transfer in rats with maternal diabetes of varying severity. *Diabetes,* Vol. 34, Suppl. 2, pp. 42–46. ISSN 0012-1797

Junod, A., Lambert, A. E., Stauffacher, W. and Renold, A. E. (1969): Diabetogenic action of streptozotocin: Relationship of dose to metabolic response. *J. Clin. Invest.*, Vol. 48, No. 11 (1 November 1969), pp. 2129–2139. ISSN 0021.9738

Kaplan, J.R., Wagner, J.D. (2006): Type 2 diabetes – an introduction to the development and use of animal models. *ILAR J.*, Vol. 47, No. 3, pp. 181–185. ISSN 1084-2020

Kaufman, D.L., Erlander, M.G., Clare-Salzler, M., Atkinson, M.A., Maclaren, N.K., Tobin, A.J. (1992): Autoimmunity to two forms of glutamate decarboxylase in insulin-dependent diabetes mellitus. *J. Clin. Invest.,* Vol. 89, No. 1 (1 January 1992) pp. 283–292. ISSN 0021.9738

Kobayashi, T., Arefanian, H., Harb, G., Tredget, E.B., Rajotte, R.V., Korbutt, G.S., Rayat, G.R. (2008): Prolonged survival of microencapsulated neonatal porcine islet xenografts in immune-competent mice without antirejection therapy. *Cell Transplant.*, Vol. 17, No. 11/12, pp. 1243–1256. ISSN 0963-6897

Koppányi, T., Avery, M.A. (1966): Species differences and the clinical trial of new drugs: a review. *Clin. Pharmacol. Ther.*, Vol. 7, No. 2 (February 1966), pp. 250–270. ISSN 0009-9236

Korec, R. (1991): *Experimental and Spontaneous Diabetes Mellitus in the Rat and Mouse.* Edition Center of Šafarik University, ISBN 80-7097-123-1, Košice, pp. 1–248.

Kukreja, A., Maclaren, N.K. (1999): Autoimmunity and diabetes. *J. Clin. Endocrinol. Metab.,* Vol. 84, No. 12 (1 December 1999), pp. 4371–4378. ISSN 0021-972X

Lanza, R.P., Ecker, D.M., Kühtreiber, W.M., Marsh, J.P., Ringeling, J., Chick, W.L. (1999): Transplantation of islets using microencapsulation: studies in diabetic rodents and dogs. *J. Molecular Medicine,* Vol. 77, No. 1 (January 1999), pp. 206–210. ISSN 0946-2716

Lee, G.H., Proenca, R., Montez, J.M., Carroll, K.M., Darvishzadeh, J.G., Lee, J.I., Friedman, J.M. (1996): Abnormal splicing of the leptin receptor in diabetic mice. *Nature,* Vol. 379, No. 6566 (15 February 1996), pp. 632–635. ISSN 0028-0836

Leiter, E.H. (1998): NOD mice and related strains: Origins, husbandry, and biology. In: *NOD Mice and Related Strains: Research Applications in Diabetes, AIDS, Cancer and Other Diseases.* Leiter, E.H., Atkinson, M.A. (Eds.): Internet: R.G. Landes Co., ISBN 157059466X, pp. 1–36.

Leiter, E. H., von Herrath, M. (2004): Animal models have little to teach us about type 1 diabetes: 2. In opposition to this proposal. *Diabetologia,* Vol. 47, No. 10 (October 2004), pp. 1657–1660. ISSN 0012-186X

Lenzen, S. (2008): The mechanisms of alloxan- and streptozotocin-induced diabetes. *Diabetologia,* Vol. 51, No. 2 (February 2008), pp. 216–226. ISSN 0012-186X

Lenzen, S., Panten, U. (1988): Alloxan: history and mechanism of action. *Diabetologia,* Vol. 31, No. 6 (June 1988), pp. 337–342. ISSN 0012-186X

Loew, F.M. (1996): Using animals in research. In: *Birth to Death: Science and Bioethics.* Thomasma, D.C., Kushner, T. (Eds): Cambridge University Press, ISBN 0521555566, Cambridge, pp. 301–312.

Lotfy, M., Singh, J., Kalász, H., Tekes, K., Adeghate, E. (2011): Medicinal chemistry and applications of incretins and DPP-4 inhibitors in the treatment of type 2 diabetes mellitus. *Open Med. Chem. J.,* Vol. 5, Supple 2-M4 (9 September 2011), pp. 82–92. ISSN 1874-1045

Lukačínová, A., Mojžiš, J., Beňačka, R., Keller, J., Maguth, T., Kurila, P., Vaško, L., Rácz, O., Ništiar, F. (2008): Preventive effects of flavonoids on alloxan-induced diabetes mellitus in rats. *Acta Vet. Brno,* Vol. 77, No. 2 (June 2008), pp. 175–182. ISSN 0001-7213

Lukačínová, A., Rácz, O., Lovásová, E., Ništiar, F. (2011): Effect of lifetime low dose exposure to heavy metals on selected serum proteins of Wistar rats during three subsequent generations. *Ecotoxicol. Environ. Saf.,* Vol. 74, No. 6 (September 2011), pp. 1747–1755. ISSN 0147-6513

Mann, R. D. (1984): *Modern Drug Use; An Enquiry on Historical Principles.* MTP Press Ltd., ISBN 0852007175, Lancaster and London, pp. 1–769.

Matteucci, E., Giampietro, O. (2008): Proposal open for discussion: defining agreed diagnostic procedures in experimental diabetes research. *J. Ethnopharm.,* Vol. 115, No. 2 (17 January 2008), pp. 163–172. ISSN 0378-8741

McNamara, J.M., Stephens, P.A., Dall, S.R.X., Houston, A. I. (2009): Evolution of trust and trustworthiness: social awareness favours personality differences. *Proc. R. Soc. B,* Vol. 276, No. 1657 (22 February 2009), pp. 605–613. ISSN 1471-2954

Miller, M.T., Strömland, K. (1999): Teratogen update: Thalidomide: a review, with a focus on ocular findings and now potentional uses. *Teratology*, Vol. 60, No. 5 (November 1999), pp. 306–321. ISSN 1542-0760

Minkowski, O. (1989): Historical development of the theory of pancreatic diabetes. *Diabetes*, Vol. 38, No. 1 (January 1989), pp. 1–6. ISSN 0012-1797

Mordes, J.P., Bortell, R., Groen, H., Guberski, D.L., Rossini, A.A., Greiner, D.L. (2001): Autoimmune diabetes mellitus in the BB rat. In: *Animal Models of Diabetes: A Primer.* Sima, A.A.F., Shafrir, E. (Eds.). Harwood Academic Publishers, ISBN 9058230961, Warsaw, pp. 1–41.

Ništiar, F., Ništiarová, A., Beňačka, R., Rácz, O., Lukačínová, A. (2006): *Quo vadis* experiments on animals in the university education and tesearch? *Slovak Veter. J.*, Vol. 31, No. 5, pp. 289–291. ISSN 1335-0099

Ohgami, N., Nagai, R., Ikemoto, M., Arai, H., Kuniyasu, A., Horiuchi, S., Nakayama, H. (2001): Cd36, a member of the class b scavenger receptor family, as a receptor for advanced glycation end products. *J. Biol. Chem.*, Vol. 276, No. 2 (2 February 2001), pp. 3195–3202. ISSN 0021-9258

Olson, H., Betton, G., Robinson, D., Thomas, K., Monro, A., Kolaja, G., Lilly, P., Sanders, J., Sipes, G., Bracken, W., Dorato, M., Van Deun, K., Smith, P., Berger, B., Heller. A. (2000): Concordance of the toxicity of pharmaceuticals in humans and in animals. *Regul. Toxicol. Pharmacol.*, Vol. 32, No. 1 (August 2000), pp. 56–67. ISSN 0273-2300

Peppa, M., Uribarri, J., Vlassara, H. (2004): The role of advanced glycation end products in the development of atherosclerosis. *Curr. Diabetes Rep.*, Vol. 4, No. 1 (February 2004), pp. 31–36. ISSN 1534-4827

Perel, P., Roberts, I., Sena, E., Wheble, P., Briscoe, C., Sandercock, P., Macleod, M., Mignini, L.E., Jayaram, P., Khan, K.S. (2007): Comparison of treatment effects between animal experiments and clinical trials: systematic review. *BMJ*, Vol. 334, No. 7586 (27. January 2007), pp. 197–202. ISSN 0959-8138

Perry, P. (2007): The ethics of animal research: a UK perspective. *ILAR J.*, Vol. 48, No. 1, pp. 42–46. ISSN 1084-2020

Quehenberger, P., Bierhaus, A., Fasching, P., Muellner, C., Klevesath, M., Hong, M., Stier, G., Sattler, M., Schleicher, E., Speiser, W., Nawroth, P.P. (2000): Endothelin-1 transcription is controlled by nuclear factor-kappa B in AGE-stimulated cultured endothelial cells. *Diabetes*, Vol. 49, No. 9 (September 2000), pp. 1561–1570. ISSN 0012-1797

Rees, D.A., Alcolado, J.C. (2005): Animal models of diabetes mellitus. *Diabetic Medicine,* Vol. 22, No. 4 (April 2005), pp. 359–370. ISSN 1464-5491

Resjö, R., Berger, K., Fex, M., Hansson, O. (2008): Proteomic studies in animal models of diabetes. *Proteomics Clin. Appl.*, Vol. 2, No. 5 (5 May 2008), pp. 654–669. ISSN 1862-8354

Roglic, G., Unwin, N. (2010): Mortality attributable to diabetes: estimates for the year 2010. *Diabetes Res. Clin. Pract.*, Vol. 87, No. 1 (January 2010), pp. 15–19. ISSN 0168-8227

Rossini, A.A., Thompson, M.J., Mordes, J.P. (2003): Diabetes mellitus. In: *Office Practice of Medicine.* 4th ed., Branch, W.T. Jr. (Ed.): Saunders, ISBN 0721676723, Philadelphia, pp. 695–740.

Russell, W.M.S., Burch, R.L. (1959): *The Principles of Humane Experimental Technique*. Methuen & Co. Ltd., ISBN 0900767782, London, pp. 1–238.

Sacks, D.B., Bruns, D.E., Goldstein, D.E., Maclaren, N.K., McDonald, J.M., Parrott, M. (2002): Guidelines and recommendations for laboratory analysis in the diagnosis and management of diabetes mellitus. *Clin. Chem.*, Vol. 48, No. 3 (March 2002), pp. 436–472. ISSN 1434-6621

Salgado, H.C., Fazan, R., Fazan, V.P.S., Dias da Silva, V.J., Barreira, A.A. (2001): Arterial baroreceptors and experimental diabetes. *Ann. N. Y. Acad. Sci.*, Vol. 940, No. 1 (September 2001), pp. 20–27. ISSN 1749-6632

Sandow, J. (2009): Growth effects of insulin and insulin analogues. *Arch. Physiol. Biochem.*, Vol. 115, No. 2 (May 2009), pp. 72–85. ISSN 1744-4160

Semple, R.K., Savage, D.B., Cochran, E.K., Gorden, P., O'Rahilly, S. (2011): Genetic syndromes of severe insulin resistance. *Endocr. Rev.*, Vol. 32, No. 4 (1 August 2011), pp. 498–514. ISSN 0163-769X

Serreze, D.V., Leiter, E.H. (2001): Genes and pathways underlying autoimmune diabetes in NOD mice. In: *Molecular Pathology of Insulin Dependent Diabetes Mellitus*. Von Herrath M.G. (Ed.): Karger Press, ISBN 3805572409, Basel, pp. 31–67.

Shafrir, E. (2003): Diabetes in animals: contribution to the understanding of diabetes by study of its etiopathology in animal models. *In: Diabetes Mellitus*, Porte, D., Sherwin, R.S., Baron, A. *(Eds.)*, McGraw-Hill, ISBN 0838520413, New York, *pp.* 231–255.

Shaw, J., Sicree, R., Zimmet, P. (2010): Global estimates of the prevalence of diabetes for 2010 and 2030. *Diabetes Res. Clin. Pract.*, 87, pp. 4–14.

Sima, A.A.F., Shafrir, E. (Eds.) (2000): *Animal Models of Diabetes: A Primer*. Harwood Academic Publishers, ISBN 9058230961, Amsterdam, pp. 1-364.

Skyler, J.S., Brown, D., Chase, H.P., Collier, E., Cowie, C., Eisenbarth, G.S., Fradkin, J., Grave, G., Greenbaum, C., Jackson, R.A., Kaufman, F.R., Krischer, J.P., Marks, J.B., Palmer, J.P., Ricker, A., Schatz, D.A., Wilson, D., Winter, W.E., Wolfsdorf, J., Zeidler, A., Dickler, H., Eastman, R.C., Maclaren, N.K., Malone, J.I. (2002): Effects of insulin in relatives of patients with type 1 diabetes mellitus. *N. Engl. J. Med.*, Vol. 346, No. 22 (30 May 2002). pp. 1685B–1691B. ISSN 0028-4793

Srinivasan, K., Ramarao, P. (2007): Animal models in type 2 diabetes research: an overview. *Indian J. Med. Res.*, Vol. 125, No. 3 (March 2007), pp. 451–472. ISSN 0971-5916

Stern, D.M., Yan, S.D., Yan, S.F., Schmidt, A.M. (2002): Receptor for advanced glycation end products (RAGE) and the complications for diabetes. *Ageing Res. Rev.*, Vol. 1, No. 1 (February 2002), pp. 1–15. ISSN 1568-1637

Suarez-Pinzon, W.L., Rabinovitch, A. (2001): Approaches to type 1 diabetes prevention by intervention in cytokine immunoregulatory circuits. *Int. J. Exp. Diabetes Res.*, Vol. 2, No. 1, pp. 3–17. ISSN 1560-4284

Tesch, G. H., Nikolic-Paterson, D. J. (2006): Recent Insights into experimental mouse models of diabetic nephropathy, *The Nephron Journals*, Vol. 104, No. 2 (September 2006), pp. 57–62. ISSN 1660-8151

Tirabassi, R.S., Flanagan, J.F., Wu, T., Kislauskis, E.H., Birckbichler, P.J., Guberski, D.L. (2004): The BBZDR/Wor rat model for investigating the complications of type 2 diabetes mellitus. *ILAR J.*, Vol. 45, No. 3, pp. 292–302. ISSN 1084-2020

Trimble, E.R., Siegel, E.G., Berthoud, H.-R., Renold, A.E. (1980): Intraportal islet transplantation: functional assessment in conscious unrestrained rats. *Endocrinology*, Vol. 106, No. 3 (1 March 1980), pp. 791–797. ISSN 0013-7227

Van der Werf, N., Kroese, F.G., Rozing, J., Hillebrands, J.L. (2007): Viral infections as potential triggers of type 1 diabetes. *Diabetes Metab. Res. Rev.*, Vol. 23, No. 3 (March/April 2007), pp. 169–183. ISSN 1520-7552

Vaxillaire, M., Froguel, P. (2008): Monogenic diabetes in the young, pharmacogenetics and relevance to multifactorial forms of Type 2 diabetes. *Endocr. Rev.*, Vol. 29, No. 3 (1 May 2008), pp. 254–264. ISSN 0163-769X

Vlassara, H. (1997): Recent progress in advanced glycation end products and diabetic complications. *Diabetes*, Vol. 46, Suppl. 2, pp. S19–S25. ISSN 0012-1797

Von Herrath, M., Nepom, G.T. (2009): Animal models of human type 1 diabetes. *Nature Immunol.*, Vol. 10, No. 2 (February 2009), pp. 129–132. ISSN 1529-2908

Wada, R., Yagihashi, S. (2005): Role of advanced glycation end products and their receptors in development of diabetic neuropathy. *Ann. N. Y. Acad. Sci.*, Vol. 1043, No. 1 (June 2005), pp. 598–604. ISSN 1749-6632

Wang, P., Yigit, M.V., Medarova, Z., Wei, L., Dai, G., Schuetz, C., Moore, A. (2011): Combined small interfering RNA therapy and in vivo magnetic resonance imaging in islet transplantation. *Diabetes*, Vol. 60, No. 2 (February 2011), pp. 565–571. ISSN 0012-1797

Wendt, T., Bucciarelli, L., Qu, W., Lu, Y., Yan, S.F., Stern, D.M., Schmidt, A.M. (2002): Receptor for advanced glycation endproducts (RAGE) and vascular inflammation: Insights into the pathogenesis of macrovascular complications in diabetes. *Curr. Atheroscler. Rep.*, Vol. 4, No. 3 (May 2002), pp. 228–237. ISSN 1523-3804

Whiting, D., Unwin, N., Roglic, G. (2010): Diabetes: equity and social determinants. In: *Priority Public Health Conditions: From Learning to Action on Social Determinants of Health.* Blas, E., Sivasankara Kurup A. (Eds.). World Health Organization, ISBN 9789241563970, Geneva, pp. 77–94.

WHO (World Health Organization) (1993): *Research Guidelines for Evaluating the Safety and Efficacy of Herbal Medicines.* Regional Office for the Western Pacific, ISBN 9290611103, Manila, pp. 1–94.

Wild, S. Roglic, G., Green, A., Sicree, R., King, H. (2004): Global prevalence of diabetes: estimates for the year 2000 and projections for 2030. *Diabetes Care*, Vol. 27, No. 5 (May 2994), pp. 1047–1053. ISSN 0149-5992

Williams, G., Pickup, J.C. (2004): *Handbook of Diabetes.* 3rd ed., Blackwell Publishing Ltd., ISBN 1405120525, Malden MA, pp. 1-288.

Yang, Y., Santamaria, P. (2006): Lessons of autoimmune diabetes from animal models. *Clinic. Sci.*, Vol. 110, No. 6 (June 2006), pp. 627–639. ISSN 0143-5221

Zhang, Y., Proenca, R., Maffei, M., Barone, M., Leopold, L., Friedman, J.M. (1994): Positional cloning of the mouse obese gene and its human homologue. *Nature (Lond.)*, Vol. 372, No. 6505 (1 December 1994), pp. 425–432. ISSN 0028-0836

Chapter 14

Essentials of Diabetes Care in Family Practice

Hakan Demirci, Ilhan Satman, Yıldırım Çınar and Nazan Bilgel

Additional information is available at the end of the chapter

http://dx.doi.org/10.5772/48616

1. Introduction

Worldwide there are a large number of patients with diabetes mellitus (DM) and the prevalence is increasing rapidly. About 20-30% of patients visiting family practice units suffer from DM or its complications. Family physicians require in-depth knowledge of DM. A family physician is expected to know about the disease as well as the drugs prescribed to treat the disease. They should provide practical and comprehensive care to DM patients. The diagnosis of a disease must be easy and less costly and should provide an estimation of the risks facing a patient in the future if precautions and recommendations are not adhered to. Family physicians need standard algorithms to follow their patients with DM. This chapter summarizes simple definitions, routine assessments, standard treatment and preventive options that should be known, easily recognized and applied by family physicians providing daily care to patients with DM.

2. History

Symptoms of DM have been reported since very old times. Diabetes is a word of Greek origin and means a "siphon". Aretus the Cappadocian, a Greek physician who lived in the 2nd century, named the condition such because his patients had polyuria and passed water like a siphon. Mellitus is a Latin word and means "honey". The combination of these two words describes an illness that is associated with frequent and sweet urination. Current medical knowledge supports the ancient definition because it is now known that plasma glucose levels over 180-200 mg/dL impair glomerular filtration and pollakiuria and glycosuria are the result.

In 2009, the American Diabetes Association (ADA) and European Association for the Study of Diabetes (EASD) published a consensus report stating that the A1C can be used as a criterion for the diagnosis of DM [ADA, 2012]. Table 1 summarizes the current diagnosis approach. The A1C measure defines DM clearly for family physicians and prevents confusion in the diagnosis of patients with DM. There are some other well established tests, including the oral glucose tolerance test. However, it takes time to obtain a definitive result from this test as repeated blood samples (3-4 over 2-3 hours) are required to measure plasma glucose. In addition to diagnosis of DM, the A1C provides clues about the possible complications that the diabetic patients may be faced with. The A1C is also used to direct treatment options. If the A1C values are within normal limits then a decision whether to continue with the ongoing treatment is made. This criterion has been the topic of much debate in Medical arena as many authorities do not agree with the use of A1C as a diagnostic criterion. It has been argued that the A1C may not able to detect DM characterized by postprandial hyperglycemia. Another argument relates to the standardization of the A1C measurement techniques used by laboratories. Therefore, a standardized method needs to be used, and it is recommended that the A1C should be confirmed with fasting plasma glucose (FPG ≥126 mg/dL). However, laboratories that serve family physicians are not always set up to measure the A1C. In addition, the A1C values may vary depending on race and ethnicity [Ziemer et al. 2010 & Kumar et al. 2010].

	FPG	OGTT 2-h PG	Random PG	A1C
Diabetes Mellitus	≥126 mg/dL (7.0 mmol/L)	≥200 mg/dl (11.1 mmol/L)	≥200 mg/dl (11.1 mmol/L) and classic symptoms of hyperglycemia	≥6.5% (≥48 mmol/mol)
Increased risk for DM (prediabetes)	100-125 mg/dL (5.6-6.9 mmol/L)	140-199 mg/dL (7.8-11 mmol/L)		5.7-6.4% (39-46 mmol/mol)

*[ADA, 2012]

Table 1. Current criteria for diabetes mellitus diagnosis and increased risk for diabetes mellitus*

Over the last decade we have observed some major modifications in the treatment options related to DM. In 2006, the ADA reported that life-style changes alone are not sufficient to overcome DM in individuals recently diagnosed with the disease. Based on meta-analyses studies, Metformin has been included as a first line treatment option, if no contraindications are present [Nathan et al., 2006]. Metformin has many beneficial effects in the treatment of DM and it is very cost effective. Metformin decrease plasma glucose (PG) and has been shown to slightly alleviate obesity and reduce elevated blood lipids. However, it is well known that metformin is not always well tolerated and therefore half the target dose is recommended during the initial stages of metformin therapy. Metformin therapy is not recommended for patients with creatinine levels exceeding the upper limit of normal range (>1.4 mg/dL) or if eGFR less than 60 mL/minute.

The ADA, supported by the EASD, indicated that a global target for reasonable glycemic control should be A1C <7%. However, International Diabetes Federation (IDF), the local societies, like Society of Endocrinology and Metabolism of Turkey (SEMT) and others suggested a slightly lower target (A1CA1C ≤6.5%) [ADA, 2012; IDF, 2005; SEMT, 2011]. However, from 2010, individual specifications such as diabetes duration, life expectancy, and previous glycemic control status, associated co-morbidities, and complications are advised to be taken into account before setting the target of glycemic control.

3. Pathogenesis

Diabetes Mellitus is characterized by hyperglycemia that results from defects in the secretion and/or action of insulin. DM is primarily classified into two groups, type 1 DM and type 2 DM. Generally, type 1 DM is accepted as an autoimmune disease with some triggering factors usually responsible for the development of autoimmunity. Destruction of pancreatic β-cells by several autoantibodies (i.e. islet cell cytoplasmic antibodies; ICA, antibodies against glutamic acid decarboxylase; Anti-GAD, islet associated or anti-tyrosine phosphatase antibodies; IA2, anti-fogrin antibodies; IA2-β, insulin autoantibodies; IAA, and antibodies against zinc transporter-8; Anti-ZnT8) is the typical explanation regarding the mechanism for the development of type 1 DM. On the other hand, peripheral insulin resistance, loss of β-cell reserve or β-cell exhaustion, problems in hepatic glucose production, abnormalities in glucose absorption and obesity are the main pathological characteristics of type 2 DM [Barnet & Braunstein, 2007].

4. Epidemiology

DM is a major epidemic of the 21st century. However, reports published in 2010 demonstrated that the estimated targets for 2025 have already been reached, 15-20 years earlier than expected. According to the recent estimates by IDF (IDF Fifth Atlas, 2011), there are 366 million people with DM worldwide, and the population with DM is expected to increase to 552 million by the year 2030.

It has been shown that the risk for DM is higher in individuals who have not completed formal education as compared with those who received a high school or university education. In cross-sectional studies current smoking has been suggested to have a protective effect that may be explained by lower caloric intake or weight loss associated with smoking. However, ex-smokers are more prone to developing DM compared with non-smokers due rapid weight gain [Amorosa et al., 2011]. Recent guidelines decreased the diagnostic level for FPG and this increased the number of people diagnosed with DM. In addition, a sedentary life-style, poor diet, obesity and the lack of regular physical activity contributed to reaching the 2030 DM estimates early [Satman et al., 2010]. The increased prevalence of childhood obesity has been associated with insulin resistance. For children born after the year 2000 there is a 32.8% risk of developing DM in males and 38.5% risk in females [Amorosa et al., 2011].

5. Routine assessments

Routine assessments are very important in DM because these allow physicians to monitor the development of the disease and associated complications. These assessments provide early identification of co-morbidity, risk factors as well as complications of DM that include coronary artery disease (CAD), impotence, neuropathy, nephropathy, retinopathy and blindness. The combination of neuropathy, retinopathy and nephropathy in DM is termed the "triopathy". Awareness of retinopathy is typically found in individuals who have had a family member who experienced the same complication or those actively seeking information relating to the complications of DM. Family doctors should inform their patients about the danger of complications. They should ensure that the appropriate laboratory examinations are performed in time and refer patients to specialists or colleagues if required. A plan for the management of DM should be developed and maintained between the physician and the patient. Compliance of the patient to the plan should be monitored by the physician.

5.1. Glycosylated hemoglobin A1C

The A1C percentage may reflect average glycemic control over several months [Sacks et al., 2002]. The A1C test helps in the diagnosis of DM and is also valuable for the determining the efficacy of treatment. In addition, the test is useful for determining DM complications (Table2).

As we mentioned previously, A1C target levels differ from patient to patient. For the elderly and children the aim is not to have a tight control of the A1C level. Tight control may disturb quality of life of the patient and it may increase health risks. Immaturity in children <6 or 7 years and their inability to recognize hypoglycemia leads to modifications in glycemic goals. There is small data available to show benefits of intensive glycemic, blood pressure, and lipid control in the elderly [ADA, 2012].

Type 1 DM (DCCT study)	Retinopathy 35% ↓ Neuropathy 30% ↓ Nephropathy 24-44% ↓
Type 2 DM (UKPDS study)	Micro vascular complications 35% ↓ Death rate in DM 25% ↓ MI 18% ↓ Mortality of all causes 7% ↓
DM, diabetes mellitus; DCCT, Diabetes Control and Complication Trial; UKPDS, United Kingdom prospective Diabetes Study; MI, myocardial infarction.	

Table 2. Relationship between complications and 1% decrease in A1C

5.2. Microalbuminuria and estimated glomerular filtration rate (eGFR)

Microalbuminuria measurements can be performed using different methods. Albumin and creatinine determination in spot (preferably first morning) urine sample is preferred to 24 hour urine analyses [Eknoyan et al., 2003, Levey et al., 2003]. Determination of early morning microalbuminuria in spot urine is an easy method that can be obtained in a family practice setting but a limitation is that this method is associated with false positives. In addition, hydration status affects the test results. However, albumin to creatinine ratio (ACR) is less affected by dehydration. Classification of microalbuminuria state is shown in table 3.

Diagnosis of persistent microalbuminuria should occur if positive in two out of three urine samples over six months. It should be remembered that exercise in the previous 24 hours, infections, congestive heart failure and uncontrolled hypertension may interfere with the results. The ADA and EASD recommend microalbuminuria testing at least once a year.

Normal	<30
Microalbuminuria	30-299
Macroalbuminuria	≥300

Table 3. Microalbuminuria (ACR; early morning spot urine albumin [μg]/creatinine [g])

Estimated glomerular filtration rate (eGFR) is another method for evaluating renal function. The Modification of Diet in Renal Disease (MDRD) formula can be used to estimate GFR. There are websites for calculating eGFR on the internet. Some laboratories note the results of eGFR together with creatinine measurements [Levey et al., 1999]. eGFR <90 mL/minute indicates renal failure.

5.3. Serum cholesterol

"Diabetic dyslipidemia" is considered in individuals with low HDL-cholesterol and high TG. The targets for HDL-cholesterol should be ≥50 for females and ≥40 mg/dL for females, and <150 mg/dL for TG. Hyperlipidemia is a common co-morbidity seen in DM. The Framingham Heart Study found that DM and hyperlipidemia are major risk factors for the development of coronary artery disease. Lipid profiles should be checked every year in patients with DM. Precautions should be taken if there is an elevated lipid profile. Low density lipoprotein cholesterol (LDL-cholesterol) levels <100 mg/dL must be achieved as soon as possible. If there is already a history of coronary artery event then the target for LDL-cholesterol should be revised to <70 mg/dL [Grundy et al., 2004].

5.4. Fundus examination

Screening for diabetic retinopathy gained importance after reports that laser photocoagulation was very effective in preventing visual loss (DRS Group, 1976). Fundus examination by an ophthalmologist at least once in a year is recommended. Some family physicians may have experience examining the retina; however it would be better to do so in a hospital setting. Examination can be performed using an ophthalmoscope or a slit lamp. Fluorescein angiography (FFA) can be used to determine the location of the leakage in suspected cases.

Diabetic retinopathy is classified as non-proliferative or proliferative in nature. Once a retinal hemorrhage has been identified it is recommended, especially for individuals with proliferative retinopathy, the assessment should be performed more frequently.

5.5. Foot examination

Physicians should examine the feet of DM patients preferably in every visit to help prevent the development of the "diabetic foot ulcers". A careful inspection and palpation of lower extremity pulses is required. Skin temperature must be checked and increases or decreases in the regular temperature, suggests the existence of an underlying problem. Skin hair loss, atrophy, cracked skin, or poor circulation suggests neurotropic or autonomic changes. Cracked skin is a haven for infections and a loss of circulation delays wound healing. Patients should be educated about these changes. If they notice something abnormal they should inform their family physicians about the problem.

6. Microvascular complications

Microvascular complications of DM worsen the quality of life and cause increased morbidity in patients. These complications include diabetic foot ulcers that family physicians should be aware of as well as prevent their progression. In the case of DM related end stage renal disease (ESRD), hemodialysis is usually considered. This situation also worsens the quality of life for patients with DM. Diabetic retinopathy is the most common cause of blindness. However, before reaching the stage of blindness it causes occupational and some other serious problems. This in turn affects other members of the family if the patient was the only one who works outside. Considering complications in DM it should be kept in mind that the first thing to do is to control PG levels and regulate hypertension if it is present. This approach will not only prevent most of the complications but also stops the progression of the pre-existing complications.

6.1. Retinopathy

Excluding traumatic cases, DM is the most common cause of blindness. During the first two decades of DM, nearly all the patients with type 1 DM and more than half of the patients with type 2 DM experience retinopathy to some degree [Budak et al., 2004].

It is possible to diagnose retinopathy while performing routine ophthalmologic examination but family doctors should suspect diabetic retinopathy when microalbuminuria is detected in the urine. In addition, patients with known CAD have a greater risk of retinopathy.

Early detection of retinopathy should be one of the priorities when assessing DM patients. Early detection ensures a beneficial response to treatment. A FFA verifies the suspected retinopathy and photocoagulation is the preferred treatment if the diagnosis is evident. Ophthalmologists attempt to coagulate leaking retinal vessels to prevent the progression of retinal edema. Improvement in DM retinopathy is associated with reduced PG regulation [Klein (1995)] and blood pressure [Leske et al., 2005].

6.2. Neuropathy

Neuropathy is one of the most common chronic complications of DM (the prevalence over 20 years duration of DM is approximately 70%) but is usually under diagnosed [Barnett & Braunstein 2007]. Duration of DM and poor PG control correlates with the occurrence of diabetic neuropathy. Peripheral neuropathy is seen in 30% of cases. Neuropathy of nerves in the feet provides the earliest symptoms. Neuropathy has been sub-divided into three groups (autonomic, focal, and diffuse). Autonomic neuropathy has three components, cardiovascular, gastrointestinal and genitourinary. Examples of focal neuropathies are mononeuritis and carpal tunnel syndrome. Proximal motor neuropathy and distal symmetric polyneuropathies are diffuse neuropathies. Paresthesia can be described as numbness, burning or pins and needles in extremities. A characteristic of paresthesia is that the pain increases at night [Amorosa et al., 2011].

Analgesics, antiepileptic drugs and antidepressants can be used in the treatment of painful neuropathies. Amitriptilin, an antidepressant drug, has been used widely for pain relief in painful neuropathic cases. Anticonvulsants such as gabapentin, and pregabalin or SSRIs such as duloxetine, are modern pain relief drugs commonly used in painful neuropathies. B complex vitamins have also been used to treat neuropathy; however recent studies do not support their use. It has been suggested that long term metformin use may cause iatrogenic neuropathy due to malabsorption of vitamin B12 [Attarian 2011].

6.3. Diabetic foot ulcers

Diabetic foot ulcers are due to impaired nerve innervations in the lower extremities. This in turn causes decreased circulation that result in deficient migration of leukocytes to infected areas. Dryness of the extremity causes cracked skin that increases the risk of microorganisms settling there. Insufficient immune responses prevent local inflammation and subsequent healing.

Management of mild to moderate cases of diabetic foot should be provided by a foot care team including a physician, vascular surgeon, orthopedist, plastic surgeon, podiatrist, nutritionist, and physiotherapist. Treatment of advanced diabetic foot ulcers requires long hospitalization periods, and is costly. Treatment often requires surgery and in some cases the amputation of the affected finger or foot. In certain situations, an amputation or revised amputation at a higher level is indicated. Hyperbaric oxygen therapy is considered an adjuvant therapy and may be effective in some cases [Cimşit et al., 2009]. This therapy enables accelerated circulation to hypoxic, infected or ulcerated parts of the foot. Anemia should also be corrected as soon as possible to enhance wound healing. A neglected, small injury may cause the loss of a finger, foot or a leg.

The basic approach in DM patients suffering from any complication is prevention. Family physicians stand at the center of treatment. They should educate their patients about foot care and inform them about importance of PG regulation and advise the cessation of smoking. Patient education also includes information and training about topics such as foot inspection, appropriate shoes and socks, nail cutting and the importance of consulting a podiatrist [Barnett & Braunstein 2007].

6.4. Nephropathy

The incidence of DM related nephropathy is 20-30% [Barnett & Braunstein 2007]. Microalbuminuria and eGFR should be measured every year in patients with DM. When macroalbuminuria is diagnosed then a protein restriction diet is recommended. Blocking the renin–angiotensin system (RAS) by drugs such as ACE inhibitor or ARB is advised to reduce BP, established microalbuminuria and CAD outcomes [HOPE study group 2000]. ESRD is the undesired complication if the recommended treatment does not work. ESRD is usually treated by hemodialysis. Nephropathy of different stages is not rare in a population, but it is often undiagnosed. It is possible to evaluate eGFR if serum creatinine is measured. The eGFR results can be used effectively by family physicians for preventing the progression to renal failure. Hemodialysis on top of DM can make the life more difficult for diabetic patients.

6.5. Erectile dysfunction

Erectile dysfunction affects over 50% of men with diabetes >60 years old. Its etiology is multifactorial. It was shown that erectile dysfunction may be a signal for silent CAD [Phe & Rhoupret 2012]. Sildenafil may be effective in its treatment. However, risk of accompanying cardiovascular problems limits sildenafil use. Cessation of smoking should be strongly recommended.

7. Macrovascular complications

Accelerated atherosclerosis causes macrovascular complications that include CAD, cerebral and peripheral vascular diseases. It is not unusual for DM patients to experience a stroke more than once. Macrovascular complications are the primary cause of death in patients with DM.

7.1. Hypertension

When considering macrovascular complications, controlling hypertension is even more important than the regulation of hyperglycemia. ACE inhibitors are the first line of therapy, despite the finding that ARB and calcium channel blocker drugs may be as effective. The target for the reduction of blood pressure is slightly lower than normal (systolic <130 and diastolic <80 mmHg). Studies have shown that blood pressure over 115/75 mmHg carries a high risk for CAD [Chobanian et al., 2003].

On average about three different types of drugs are needed to decrease blood pressure in patients with DM.

7.2. Coronary artery disease

The most important complication related to mortality and morbidity in DM is CAD. DM is considered a cardiovascular disease equivalent. Major CAD risk factors should be evaluated once a year and identified risks (e.g. hyperlipidemia, hypertension, smoking and microalbuminuria) should be treated. In general, asymptomatic patients and/or patients with a "normal" resting electrocardiogram (ECG) are not recommended for further screening for CAD. However, DM patients who have not been diagnosed with CAD are considered to have the same risk as non-diabetic CAD patients [Barnett & Braunstein 2007]. DM patients diagnosed with CAD risk are recommended to use aspirin. However, based on recent meta-analyses aspirin is not routinely recommended for primary prevention of CAD. ACE inhibitors and statins should be added to therapy for DM patients with CAD. Post Myocardial Infarction (MI) patients are advised to use a β-blocker for at least two years if tolerable.

7.3. Stroke

About 80% of patients with DM die from stroke or CAD. During a stroke blood supply to the brain is reduced resulting in brain tissue damage. Sudden onset paralysis, cognitive and speech impairments are observed. Clot dissolving treatment must be started as soon as possible. Stroke prevention and treatment requires the reduction of lipids and hypertension. Cessation of smoking is mandatory.

Usually it is not advised to decrease PG levels too quickly especially if long-term poor glycemic control exists.

8. Treatment

Treatment of DM is multidisciplinary and unique for every patient. The first step of treatment in DM is acceptance of the disease. Every patient should receive comprehensive information about the seriousness of the disease. Importance of self-care in DM must be stressed. Establishment of confidence between the physician and patient should be established before treatment algorithms are implemented. The patient should accept that with the help of the family physician the disease can be controlled. During face to face interviews patients must be made aware that the disease is chronic and that treatment will be life-long. It should be emphasized that if precautions are not taken this will increase the risk of complications that may increase morbidity and mortality. The patient should be informed that DM may affect their quality of life as well as that of their family. On the other hand, the patient should also be made aware that DM is a common condition. Its prevalence is assumed to be more than 10% worldwide and this means that the patient is not alone. The above general considerations regarding acceptance of the disease takes time, patience and experience.

The conventional treatment guidelines recommend metformin administration as soon as the diagnosis has been established. Metformin therapy is cost effective. However, for cases where the A1C values >10% and/or FPG >300 mg/dL and/or complaining about severe hyperglycemic symptoms then insulin therapy must be commenced immediately. Recently, a common approach has been to use a long acting insulin analog injection once daily with or without an oral antidiabetic drug.

Persuading a patient to transfer to the use of insulin is difficult and sometimes impossible. The public perception of insulin therapy is poor. Insulin is considered the end of the road and some individuals see it as a "poison".

In medicine the existence of treatment "fads" or "myths" is ever present. Over-time the truth we believe in may turn out to be a false. Physicians should work with evidence-based science. Family physicians must be up to date with current DM treatment practices. Insulin is the accepted drug used in the treatment of DM. It is claimed that high dose insulins such as glargine or NPH, and pioglitazone may be associated with slightly increased risk of some kinds of malignancies. Researchers have not been able to link between the development of breast cancer and glargine insulin or between bladder cancer cases and pioglitazone. Both of these medications are very successful treatment options.

In daily practice it is not surprising to observe patients that are using two or more different kinds of oral antidiabetic drugs despite this not being recommended in the treatment guidelines. Unfortunately, patients sometimes use drugs that have the same mechanism of action. This may result in hypoglycemia. It is not possible for family physicians to know every disease and every drug. However, DM is a common chronic disease and therefore family physicians should have comprehensive knowledge of the medication used for all stage of the disease. This will increase the physician's confidence and increase the level of confidence between the patient and the physician.

Resistance to insulin can be classified into three types: Clinical insulin resistance, patient's resistance to insulin injection and physician's resistance to prescribe insulin. Of these the first type is the true biological resistance that plays a role in the development of DM. Physicians who are not confident in prescribing insulin therapy should refer their patients to an experienced specialist. Any delay in referral may result in harm to the patient and an increased risk of developing complications. Research has shown that a 1% drops in the A1C will result in a 21% decrease in complications and decrease mortality and morbidity rates in DM patients. Keeping patients unaware of suitable therapy such as insulin is not ethical and may be considered as malpractice. Hospitalization is not a rule when transferring to insulin. If the patient is not critically ill then education about insulin injections can be given at the family practice. A physician and/or a nurse trained that has received training in DM care can educate the patient.

It is a common approach to start injecting basal insulin using a dose of 0.2 Units/day. If the insulin is a premixed human short acting and long acting then 2/3 of the total dose is injected in the morning and 1/3 in the evening. Human insulin mixtures are preferably injected 15-30 minutes before the main meal but insulin analogs are injected just 5-15 minutes before the meal. If a mixture of analog insulins is prescribed, then about 50-60% can be given in the morning, and the rest before dinner. Patients should self-monitor their glucose levels and share the results with their physician. Postprandial measures are obtained at the end of the second hour following the meal. At the start of treatment, if there are no extraordinary problems, the physician evaluates the self monitored results every three days and based on these results decides on how to manage the optimal dose of insulin.

Insulin injections are administered using a special pen that can be adjusted to comfortably inject the desired doses. Education on the use of the pen should be provided to the DM patients. Family physicians should instruct patients to keep insulin in refrigerator at an optimal temperature and not to allow it to freeze. Injection methods should be explained and demonstrated in person. A description regarding the use of the insulin pen is provided in the pen boxes. However, this may confuse beginners as well as individuals who are scared of injections. During the insulin education interview patients may be asked to write down the steps one by one in their own words so that at the time of application there is no confusion. It is known that insulin absorption is faster around the umbilicus where there is a large amount of vessels.

Patients must be informed about hypoglycemia. Hypoglycemia usually occurs in response to fasting for a long time and/or when individuals perform with extra effort compared with normal. Signs of hypoglycemia are cold sweating, tachycardia, blurred vision and changes in consciousness. If the physician informs patients about the risk of hypoglycemia before they experience it, this may help in the management of hypoglycemia treatment, improving trust between the patient and physician. In addition, a better compliance to the treatment will be achieved.

Attempting to determine the optimal insulin dose as soon as possible is not recommended. In cases of stroke and retinopathy, smooth increases in insulin doses are advised. Target A1C levels may differ in different groups. For example, for the children and the elderly, targets are not as low as in adults. Diabetes treatment should not be based on a single individual. It must be acknowledged that the diagnosis of DM in a small baby will obviously affect the whole family. Sometimes a diabetic woman may be forced to give up insulin injections by her husband. If this is the case, family physicians must provide extra attention to these patients. Care in DM needs to be directed not only to the patient but also to the family and at times, the public.

9. Noninsulin therapy (drugs)

9.1. Insulin sensitizers: Biguanids (metformin)

This medication is recommended as first line therapy in addition to life style modifications. It is important to check creatinine levels when using the drug. A creatinine level that is >1.4 mg/dL, or an eGFR >60 mL/minute is critical when making a decision to discontinue the drug. When the drug is used for the first time by a patient a stepwise manner is recommended. Half or sometimes one quarter of the dose is started for 3-7 days and then increased gradually until the total dose is administered. Gastrointestinal symptoms are common if the drug has not been taken 1-2 hours after a meal. Metformin may have a mild positive effect on weight loss and is therefore its use is preferred in obese individuals.

9.2. Insulin secretagogues: Sulfonylureas (gliclazide)

Gliclazide is an alternative group of oral antidiabetic drugs. The risk of hypoglycemia is the major adverse effect and it may last more than 24 hours. It is usually preferred in patients older than 30 years old, who are relatively thin and have had DM for no longer than 5 years.

Others:

α-Glucosidase inhibitors (acarbose)

It has mechanism of action on glucose absorption from gastrointestinal tract. Gastrointestinal side effects like flatulence, abdominal discomfort and diarrhea have been observed. In elderly it is preferred because there are no serious side effects like hypoglycemia when the drug is used alone.

DPP-4 inhibitors (Sitagliptin)

These are known as insulin like oral glucose-lowering drugs. They selectively and reversibly block degradation of GLP-1 and other incretins. They promote insulin sensitivity and improve β-cell function.

10. Insulin therapy

10.1. Long acting insulin

NPH insulin, Glargine insulin and detemir insulin are classified as long acting insulin. The first two are recommended once a day but detemir insulin can be used twice a day. If the patient is recommended to use insulin once a day, depending on the patient's reaction, it can be injected in the morning or in the evening. To avoid hypoglycemia while sleeping the insulin can be injected in the evening but sometimes it works better when injected in the morning.

10.2. Short acting insulin

Short acting insulin is primarily used as a part of intensive insulin therapy. Usually it is administered three times a day before the meals. Insulin analogues can be injected just before the meal.

10.3. Mixed insulin

There are different formulations for insulin mixtures. Probably the most commonly used formulation is the 30/70 insulin mix that is composed of 30% short acting and 70% long acting insulin. It is advised that the insulin is mixed well before use. In general, 2/3 of the total daily dose is injected before breakfast and the remaining 1/3 before dinner. The reason why it is important to follow this protocol is because during the daytime the patient continues to eat but after dinner there may only be a small snack eaten just prior to sleeping.

Therefore, to prevent hypoglycemia during the sleep a smaller dose is injected at dinner. There are also 50/50, 25/75 and 20/80 combinations. Preferably, the 20/80insulin mix is administered in the elderly while the 50/50 combination may be beneficial in diabetic patients who perform heavy work as well as individuals who have poor dietary habits. In these individuals the mix is injected three times a day.

10.4. Intensive insulin therapy

Intensive insulin therapy is indicated on some occasions. Probably the most effective method for injecting insulin injection is dividing the total dose into 4-5 administrations. In practice this is not comfortable. Physicians usually prefer to divide the total dose of insulin into 4 or more administrations when it exceeds 100 Units per day. It is recommended that family physicians consult with endocrinologists when intensive insulin therapy is considered.

11. Gestational diabetes mellitus

Gestational diabetes mellitus (GDM) is diagnosed during the pregnancy and may sometimes persist after the baby is born. Family physicians should screen for GDM as soon as possible. Screening for GMD is recommended in the general population if risks for diabetes are present. If there is no DM risk in the pregnant women a75 g oral glucose tolerance test is recommended at 24-28 weeks of gestation. Following labor checking for the persistence of DM is recommended.

GDM carries risks for the mother and baby. Treatment options during the pregnancy are limited.

If GDM cannot be controlled by diet then insulin administration must be considered. Oral antidiabetic drugs may be teratogenic. Conventional insulin should be selected for treatment because there are not enough clinical data regarding the use of modern insulin analogs.

12. Immunization

The Centers of Disease Control and Prevention (CDC) recommend both influenza and pneumococcal vaccines for all patients with DM. The ADA also recommends that DM patients should be vaccinated against influenza and pneumonia because they are more susceptible to these diseases and are typically hospitalized for a longer time than non-diabetics and have an increased risk of dying. Therefore, the World Health Organization has a target to increase the number of DM patients that receive vaccinations to75% against influenza and 50% against pneumonia.

12.1. Influenza vaccine

Hospitalization due to influenza is three times more common among diabetics who have not been vaccinated [Colquhoun et al., 1997]. Hospitalization in intensive care units is four times more likely in unvaccinated cases. Trivalent influenza vaccine is available and contains the expected subgroups of influenza in the region for a particular year. A history of anaphylactic egg allergy is a contraindication for influenza vaccines. Children under 36 months are vaccinated with an infant dose that is half the normal dose. If a child is less than nine years old and is being is vaccinated for the first time a vaccination is repeated one month after the initial vaccination. It is recommended that family members of diabetics are also vaccinated.

12.2. Pneumococcal pneumonia vaccine

Pneumococcal pneumonia is an important cause of morbidity and mortality in patients with DM. Patients over 65 years and who had an additional pulmonary or cardiovascular problem are at an increased risk. This vaccine is recommended every five years. Half of the patients may suffer from local irritation at injection sites. The vaccine can be injected at the same time as other vaccines (e.g. influenza vaccine) but preferably in the other deltoid muscle.

12.3. Hepatitis B vaccine

Currently, there are studies examining recommendations for Hepatitis B vaccinations in DM. The Advisory Committee on Immunization Practices (ACIP) recommended that all of the unvaccinated adults aged 19 through 59 years with DM be vaccinated against hepatitis B [CDC 2011].

13. Conflicts of interest

The authors state that there are no conflicts of interest.

Author details

Hakan Demirci
Department of Family Medicine, Sevket Yilmaz Training & Research Hospital, Bursa, Turkey

Ilhan Satman
Division of Endocrinology and Metabolism, Department of Internal Medicine, Istanbul Faculty of Medicine, Istanbul University, Istanbul, Turkey

Yıldırım Çınar
Department of Internal Medicine, Trakya University, Edirne, Turkey

Nazan Bilgel
Department of Family Medicine, Uludag University, Bursa, Turkey

Acknowledgement

The authors express their thanks to Mrs Nazlı Demirci (philologist) for her support in editing the English language of this chapter.

14. References

American Diabetes Association. (2012). Diagnosis and classification of diabetes mellitus. Diabetes Care. Vol. 35, No. 1, pp. 64-71.

Amorosa LF, Lee EJ, Swee DE (2011). Diabetes Mellitus. Rakel & Rakel Textbook of Family Medicine 8th Edition. Chapter 34, pp. 731-755.

Attarian S. (2011). Original articles on axonal neuropathy. Rev Neurol (Paris). Vol. 167, pp. 951-954.

Barnett PS, Braunstein GD. (2007). Diabetes Mellitus. Andreoli and Carpenter's Cecil Essentials of medicine 7th Edition. Chapter 68, pp. 676-707.

Budak Y, Demirci H, Akdogan M, Yavuz D. (2004). Erythrocyte membrane anionic charge in type 2 diabetic patients with retinopathy. BMC Ophthalmology http://www.biomedcentral.com/1471-2415/4/14. Accessed 2004 Oct.

Centers of Disease Control and Prevention (CDC). (2011). Use of hepatitis B vaccination for adults with diabetes mellitus: recommendations of the Advisory Committee on Immunization Practices (ACIP). MMWR Morb Mortal Wkly Rep. Vol. 60 No.50, pp. 1709-11.

Cimşit M, Uzun G, Yildiz S. (2009) Hyperbaric oxygen therapy as an anti-infective agent. Expert Rev Anti Infect Ther. Vol. 7, No. 8, pp. 1015-1028.

Chobanian AV, Bakris GL, Black HR, et al. (2003). National Heart, Lung, and Blood Institute Joint National Committee on Prevention, Detection, Evaluation, and Treatment of High Blood Pressure; National High Blood Pressure Education Program Coordinating Committee. The Seventh Report of the Joint National Committee on Prevention, Detection, Evaluation, and Treatment of High Blood Pressure: the JNC 7 report. JAMA. Vol. 289, pp.2560–2572.

Colquhoun AJ, Nicholson KG, Botha JL, Raymond NT. (1997). Effectiveness of influenza vaccine in reducing hospital admissions in people with diabetes. Epidemiol Infect. Vol. 119, pp.335–341.

Eknoyan G, Hostetter T, Bakris GL, et al. (2003). Proteinuria and other markers of chronic kidney disease: a position statement of the national kidney foundation (NKF) and the national institute of diabetes and digestive and kidney diseases (NIDDK). Am J Kidney Dis. Vol. 42, pp. 617–622.

Grundy SM, Cleeman JI, Merz CN et al. (2004). National Heart, Lung, and Blood Institute; American College of Cardiology Foundation; American Heart Association. Implications of recent clinical trials for the National Cholesterol Education Program Adult Treatment Panel III guidelines. Circulation. Vol. 110, pp. 227–239.

Heart Outcomes Prevention Evaluation Study Investigators. (2000). Effects of ramipril on cardiovascular and microvascular outcomes in people with diabetes mellitus: results of the HOPE study and MICRO-HOPE sub study. Lancet. Vol. 355, pp. 253–259.

Klein R. (1995). Hyperglycemia and microvascular and macrovascular disease in diabetes. Diabetes Care. Vol. 18, pp. 258–268

Kumar PR, Bhansali A, Ravikiran M. et al. (2010) Utility of glycated hemoglobin in diagnosing type 2 diabetes mellitus: a community-based study. J Clin Endocrinol Metab. Vol. 95, pp. 2832-2835.

Leske MC, Wu SY, Hennis A, et al. Barbados Eye Study Group. (2005) Hyperglycemia, blood pressure, and the 9-year incidence of diabetic retinopathy: the Barbados Eye Studies. Ophthalmology. Vol. 112, pp.799-805.

Nathan DM, Buse JB, Davidson MB et al. (2006) Management of hyperglycemia in type 2 diabetes: A consensus algorithm for the initiation and adjustment of therapy: a consensus statement from ADA and EASD. Diabetes Care. Vol. 29, pp.1963-1972.

Levey AS, Coresh J, Balk E, et al. (2003). National Kidney Foundation. National Kidney Foundation practice guidelines for chronic kidney disease: evaluation, classification, and stratification. Ann Intern Med. Vol. 139, pp. 137–147

Levey AS, Bosch JP, Lewis JB, Greene T, Rogers N, Roth D. (1999). Modification of Diet in Renal Disease Study Group. A more accurate method to estimate glomerular filtration rate from serum creatinine: a new prediction equation. Ann Intern Med. Vol. 130, pp.461–470.

Satman I and TURDEP II study group report (2011). 48. Ulusal Diyabet Kongresi, Antalya.

Sacks DB, Bruns DE, Goldstein DE, Maclaren NK, McDonald JM, Parrott M. (2002). Guidelines and recommendations for laboratory analysis in the diagnosis and management of diabetes mellitus. Clin Chem. Vol. 48, pp. 436-472.

The Diabetic Retinopathy Study Research Group. (1976). Preliminary report on effects of photocoagulation therapy. Am J Ophthalmol. Vol. 81, pp. 383–396.

Ziemer DC, Kolm p, Weintraub WS. et al. (2010) Glucose independent, black-white differences in hemoglobin A1c levels: a cross sectional analysis of 2 studies. Ann Intern Med. Vol. 153, pp. 770-777.

Chapter 15

Spontaneous Diabetes Mellitus in Animals

Emilia Ciobotaru

Additional information is available at the end of the chapter

http://dx.doi.org/10.5772/48170

1. Introduction

Diabetes mellitus is considered as a common metabolic disease diagnosed frequently in canine and feline pathology. On the other hand, clinical syndrome of diabetes is described rarely in other domestic species (cattle, small ruminants, swine and horses) [1-3]. Many similarities with human counterpart are clearly emphasized in the literature, considering the mechanism of this disease. This is the reason why the animals are frequently used in many research studies with respect to etiopathogenesis and treatment [4]. The most of the cases present as main clinical sign the failure of β-cells to produce insulin to support the metabolic needs of the organism. The insidious onset of diabetes may be induced by various causes: diminished synthesis of insulin, decreased sensitivity of target cells and organs to insulin, excess of other hormones and drugs or multiple combinations of these causes [1].

Polyphagia, polyuria and polydipsia are mentioned as the most common clinical signs of uncomplicated *diabetes mellitus* (non-ketoacidotic). The animal presents persistent hyperglycemia generated by a low cellular uptake of glucose, increased glycogenolisis and gluconeogenesis from amino acid source. All these metabolic disorders are linked with a diminished glucose oxidation. Abnormal gluconeogenesis from amino acids will be clinically expressed as atrophy of the muscles and weight loss. High level of serum lipids is generated by increased lipolysis and decrease entry of fatty acid into adipocytes. Subsequently, the liver exhibits large quantities of mobilized lipids that cannot be used or transformed in lipoproteins. Grossly, the liver appears enlarged, even with hepatomegaly. Prolonged hyperglycemia will generate persistent high level of glucose in primary urine; these levels exceed the threshold of glucose resorption in renal tubes, thus leading to subsequent glucosuria, osmotic diuresis, polyuria and compensatory polydipsia. Despite of persistent hyperglycemia, the animal presents an increased appetite generated by the failure of neurons from hypothalamic satiety center to uptake the glucose [1].

The classification of diabetes in animals is the one used for the humans, although it is not entirely applicable to domestic animals.

Type 1 (insulin dependent diabetes mellitus - IDDM) and 2 diabetes mellitus (non-insulin dependent diabetes mellitus - NIDDM) are generally accepted as the main form of this disease in animals. Specific types of diabetes (previously framed as type 3 or secondary diabetes mellitus) include the cases which are the consequence of insulin antagonism or other situation when destruction of pancreatic islets was generated by pancreatitis, pancreatic necrosis and tumoral processes. Gestational diabetes is a particular clinical expression of this condition, the occurrence being reported in dogs [5].

2. Diabetes mellitus in horses

Despite all the controversies reported in the literature, it is generally accepted that horses develop all three forms of diabetes: insulin dependent diabetes mellitus, non-insulin dependent diabetes mellitus and secondary diabetes. Recent observation and studies recommend paying further attention and investigation to the resemblance between human and equine insulin resistance, which particularly develops in horses with clinical signs of equine metabolic syndrome (EMS). This may be expressed as obesity, associated with prior or concurrent rhabdomiolysis, ostechondrosis and laminitis (inflammation of the hoof wall), the onset of diabetes being exceptional [6-10].

Diabetes mellitus was diagnosed in horse and pony, all cases being described in individuals with pancreatitis or pars intermedia pituitary tumors [11-13]. IDDM was reported mainly in young horses, but elderly horses are also affected (the age ranges between 5 and 18 years). Gender is not considered as a predisposing factor, but many of the cases were diagnosed in mare. Affected individuals with IDDM develop rapid weight loss despite polyphagia, as well as hyperglycemia, glucosuria, low insulin levels, high glycosylated hemoglobin and fructosamine, polydipsia and compensatory polyuria. Hepatomegaly due to hepatic lipidosis may occur. The pancreas exhibits segmental shrinkage, effacement of lobule demarcation by lymphocytic infiltrates and same inflammatory population into the pancreatic islets which causes severe decrease of β-cells [14]. Sometimes inflammation is not observed, especially in old individuals, the number of β-cells being reduced and confined to the periphery of the islets [15]. A case was featured by concurrent lymphocytic thyroiditis and adrenalitis. Thus, considering polyendocrine involvement it is postulated that autoimmune cause of IDDM may be suspected [14].

Non-insulin dependent diabetes mellitus in horse have less resemblance to human counterpart, comparing to cats. Particularly, insulin resistance as one of the major features of the type 2 diabetes in human and cats is less important for the onset of diabetes in a horse and more attributable to obesity, inflammation and vascular diseases. The factors which interfere with the effectiveness of insulin in horse are the excess of glucocorticoides, free fatty acids and adipokynes. Hyperinsulinemia as the result of insulin resistance may be maintained for years, without exhaustion of β-cell [7]. This is the reason why non-insulin dependent diabetes mellitus is rarely diagnosed in horses. A minimal model of analysis of type 2 diabetes in horse has been presented. Insulin versus glucose dynamics has been monitored, insulin resistance and impaired β-cell functioning being obtained [16].

Transient IDDM may occur in neonates. Concomitant hyperglycemia, hypoinsulinemia and intestinal infection with Coronavirus was reported, the foal becoming euglycemic in less than a year [17].

3. Type 1 diabetes mellitus in cattle

Diabetes mellitus has been reported in various breeds of cattle: Holstein Fresian and Hereford [18, 19], Aberdeen Angus and Jersey [20], Brangus cattle [21], Charolais [22], Japanese brown and Japanese black [23-26]. Young individuals are constantly affected, the age ranging between 6 months and 5 years of age. Although there is no evidence of sex predilection, most of the data report cases of diabetes in females. Mild weight loss to severe emaciation, polyuria, polydipsia, dehydration, hyperglycemia, glucosuria and kenonuria are the most important clinical signs described. Previous studies mention diagnostic tests used in cattle: glucose tolerance test and measurements of serum fructosamine to prove that the most important signs of diabetes (hyperglycemia, glucosuria and kenonuria) have been induced by insulin deficiency. The results of these tests proved that the glucose disappearance rate and half time were longer than in normal control cows. Elevated values of serum fructosamine were also observed [22, 25].

At necropsy, the pancreas presents normal volume or various degree of atrophy, granular surface due to interstitial fibrosis and yellowish-brown color of the parenchyma. The liver is friable and pale. The kidneys present the same discoloration, observed mainly in the cortex. Histologically, lymphocytic insulitis is the most important feature diagnosed. Pancreatic islets are reduced in size and number. The inflammatory infiltrate is represented dominantly by lymphocytes, few plasma cells and neutrophils being occasionally observed. The atrophied islets are composed by small cells, without aldehyde-fucsin and Masson-Goldner positive granules, proving that insulin secretion is ceased. This was supplementary proved by immunohistochemical investigation, almost all cells of atrophied islets being rarely reactive to anti-insulin antibody and poorly reactive to anti-glucagon and anti-somatostatin. Residual pancreatic islets present vacuolization of cytoplasm and a decreased synthesis of insulin. Unaffected islets may contain mitotic figures of cell nuclei. The lesions of exocrine components are interlobular and interacinar fibrosis, lymphocytic infiltrates around small pancreatic ducts and glycogen accumulation into the cytoplasm of ductal epithelial cells [23, 25].

Several possible mechanisms of insulin-dependent diabetes mellitus onset in cattle are described, such as viral infection, metabolic disorders (fatty liver, fat cow syndrome), parturition and chronic insulitis [2].

Considering viral infection, many studies were focused on foreign antigens exposure of genetically susceptible individuals. These molecules have similar biochemical structure with some of the components of β-cells. This way, a cell-immune mediated response is triggered also against islet cells. The viruses are the most suitable source of antigenic protein, bovine viral diarrhea virus (BVDV) and foot and mouth disease virus (FMDV) being subjected for extensive studies [2].

It is suspected that human IDDM is strongly related with viral infection as in bovine counterpart and include group B Coxsackie, Epstein-Bar, cytomegalovirus, herpesvirus, enteric rotavirus, influenza virus, rubella viruses, and mumps. This concept is highly supported by the results which prove epitope homology between Coxsackie B viral protein and glutamic acid decarboxylase – GAD (this enzyme mediates decarboxylation of glutamate and forms γ-aminobutiric acid - GABA). Furthermore, the cattle with IDDM do not express GAD in the cytoplasm of cells of atrophied islets [27-29].

Destruction of β-cells via apoptosis seems to be controversial, generated by many pathways (perforin/granzyme, FasL, and other members of the necrosis factor superfamily), each of those mentioned being dominant or redundant in initial or late stage of cell death. Thus, perforin/granzyme pathway mediated by CD8+ T-lymphocytes is preferentially active during onset of autoimmunity. FasL is dominant in CD4+ T-cell mediated insulitis [30-32]. In addition, ongoing lymphocytic insulitis is preceded by releasing of many cytokines (IL-1β, INF-γ, TNF-α) and free radicals [18, 27, 33]. Damaged proteic structures of β-cells result in molecules with enhanced antigenic properties, being initiated a self-perpetuating destruction of the cells. INF-γ and TNF-α are both responsible for increased expression of class I MHC molecules on β-cells [34, 35]. Combined effects of those molecules results in expression of class II MHC molecules on β-cells surface. Elevated expression of MHC molecules induces homing of lymphocytes into the islets. Activation of lymphocytes is initiated by INF- γ, engaging this way the responsiveness of these cells to local antigens. Differentiation of T-lymphocytes in IDDM shifts towards T helper lymphocytes type 1 (Th1) pathway. Although, Th2 pathway cytokine (IL-10) may be also involved by the effect on local vessels and promoting local release of other cytokines [33].

4. Type 1 diabetes mellitus in dog

Spontaneous cases of insulin-dependent diabetes mellitus in dog were mentioned for the first time in 1861 by Leblanc and Thiernesse [36]. Later, in depth studies subjected on dog considered a large numbers of individuals and concluded that this condition is specific for older dogs and also for females [36]. Sex predilection in diabetes was further associated with increased incidence shortly after estrus period and in pregnant females [36-38]. A major breakthrough in canine diabetes mellitus was the identification of the diabetogenic effect of progesterone induced mammary growth hormone (GH) [39]. During the last ten years a big number of studies have focused on etiology of dog diabetes, especially on dog leukocyte antigen (DLA) and their association, candidate genes and autoantibodies [40-43].

Epidemiological studies on canine diabetes conducted in different part of the world concluded that the disease is diagnosed mainly in Samoyed, Cairn Terrier, Tibetan Terrier, Australian Terrier, Miniature Poodle and Schnauzer, Bichon Frise, Border Collie and some of the Scandinavian breeds (table 1) [37, 44, 45]. In addition, other papers complete the list with Labrador retriever, Yorkshire terrier, Spitz, Lhasa Apso, Beagle and Dachshund. Keeshonds and probably Golden retriever are potential candidate breeds due to islet hypoplasia, the onset of diabetes being recorded in the first months of life. Popular breeds as

Boxer and German shepherd seem to be resistant. Generally, canine diabetes mellitus is clinically diagnosed in dogs with 4-18 years of age, the median age at diagnosis being 7-9 years [37, 44-46].

Swedish study [37]	**UK study [44]**	**North America study[45]**
Australian Terrier	Samoyed,	Miniature Schnauzer
Samoyed	Tibetan Terrier	Bichon Frise
Swedish Lapphund	Cairn Terrier	Miniature Poodle
Swedish Elkhound		Samoyed
Border Collie		Cairn Terrier

Table 1. The breeds commonly affected by diabetes mellitus

Juvenile onset of the disease is an uncommon event and it has been recorded in dogs with less than 12 months of age [47-49]. Several studies concluded that females are prone to diabetes (more than 70% of diagnosed cases) [37]. These results are controversial with other studies which conclude that the number of females and male with diabetes is almost equal [44]. The aforementioned studies highlight that ovariohisterectomy in the first year of life seems to eradicate diabetes, the particular hormonal status of the dam being the cause of diabetes onset. These can also explain the high incidence of this condition in diestrous and pregnant bitches.

The etiopathogenesis of diabetes mellitus in dog remains unclear for the majority of diagnosed cases. The difficulties in framing the type of diabetes come from the possible multifactorial etiology of the condition. Unfortunately, the human system of classification of diabetes is not entirely applicable to dog. The existence of NIDDM in dog is questionable, being known that insulin must be provided sooner or later for almost all diabetic dogs. In this context, it was suggested that classification of diabetes in dog would consider the underlying pathogenesis rather than response to insulin treatment [50]. Current diagnosis and therapy consider a classification system based on underlying cause of hyperglycemia: insulin deficiency diabetes and insulin resistance diabetes (Table 2). It is noteworthy that insulin resistance diabetes will be replaced progressively by insulin deficiency diabetes due to glucotoxicity and β-cell exhaustion [50].

Insulin deficiency diabetes (progressive destruction of β-cells, absolute insulin deficiency)	β-cell hypoplasia Immune mediated β-cell destruction β-cell cell loss associated with exocrine pancreatic lesions (pancreatic necrosis, pancreatitis) Idiopathic processes
Insulin resistance diabetes (relative insulin deficiency produced by insulin antagonists or concurrent disorders)	Diestrus/gestational diabetes Secondary to other endocrinopathies (acromegaly, hyperadrenocorticism) Obesity Iatrogenic (synthetic progestagens and glucocorticoids)

Table 2. Classification system of diabetes mellitus in dog [50]

Most of the diabetic dogs present unspecific destruction of Langerhans islets. Destruction of β-cells via autoantibodies may be considered, this being characteristic for 50% of newly diagnosed dogs [51]. Comparing with IDDM in human and cattle some diabetic dog express serological reactivity to 65kDa isoform of GAD and/or insulinoma antigen 2 (IA-2) [44, 52].

Furthermore, there have been described some gene associations with increase susceptibility to diabetes in dog similar with human counterpart such as INF-γ, IL-10, IL-12β, IL-6, insulin, protein tyrosine phosphatase non-receptor type 22 (PTPN22), IL-4 and TNF-α, comparing with protective association between IL-4, PTPN22, IL-6, insulin, IGF2, TNFα [43]. Canine major histocompatibility complex gene known as dog leukocyte antigen (DLA) is also linked with the onset and progression of diabetes. Samoyed, Cairn Terrier and Tibetan Terrier known as prone to diabetes express DLA-DRB1*009/DQA1*001/DQB1*008 haplotype of MHC, comparing with resistant breeds [50].

Inheritance of IDDM was studied and previously mentioned in Keeshonds, the genotype being described as autosomal recessive [41, 53].

Statistical analysis on a large canine population established a significant correlation between obesity and diabetes mellitus in Shetland Sheepdog, Dachshund, and Golden Retriever [54]. Hyperinsulinemia and glucose intolerance reaches the highest values in dogs with the highest degree of obesity [55]. The same authors concluded later that obese diabetic dogs can be subdivided in two groups according to the response to glucose administration: first group with fasting hypeinsulinemia which have a good response to glucose by increasing the level of insulin secretion and a second one with decompensate status featured by fasting hyperinsulinemia and lack of response to glucose administration. The results of the same study highlight that the obese dogs from this study present lower levels of insulin comparing with obese non-diabetic dogs [56]. It was also concluded that a high-fat diet generates subsequent insulin resistance which is not followed by compensatory hyperinsulinemia and create the premises for the onset of glucose intolerance and diabetes [57]. Despite to these reports, diabetes induced by insulin resistance and hyperinsulinemia in dog seems to be a rare condition.

Gestational diabetes mellitus (GDM) and diestrus diabetes are rare conditions in dog, thus being reported only in few cases [38, 58, 59]. Pregnancy is essentially dominated be tremendous metabolic changes which are set for supporting fetal development. Thus, caloric intake, insulin secretion, peripheral insulin resistance and lipid metabolism record higher levels and values in pregnant dam. These metabolic changes are focused to direct glucose and amino acids towards fetal development, lipids being used as alternative energetic supply for the female. Considering this new metabolic status, β-cells from the existing Langerhans islets undergo hypertrophy and hyperplasia [60]. These morphological and functional adaptations permit high level of insulin which maintains normal glycemia. GDM results from the failure of this adaptive process. It is described that peripheral insulin resistance is upregulated by hormones such as progesterone, prolactine, cortisol and placental lactogens. Progesterone induced mammary growth factor hormone (GH) generates anti-insulin activity, being one of the most important diabetogenic hormones involved in the pathogenesis of GDM [61]. Destruction of β-cells and termination of insulin secretion is engaged by glucotoxicity. Both pregnant and diestrous nonpregnant dams have higher levels of GH and lack of GAD-65 autoantibodies [38]. These findings prove that the onset of the diabetes is induced via ovarian hormones. Furthermore, ovariohisterectomy and/or termination of gestation provide a substantial improvement of the prognosis, almost a half of affected animals returning to normal after these surgical procedures. It is possible for diabetes to become a permanent status in aging animals, because of senile diminishing of β-cells secretion and a shortened period of tolerance to hyperglycemia [38].

Similar pathogenic pathways to gestational diabetes mellitus are described in females with persistent corpora luteal and associated pseudopregnancy. Long term administration of synthetic progestagenes (medroxyprogesterone and megestrol acetate) initiates diabetes by vacuolization of β-cells [62].

5. Type 2 diabetes mellitus in cat

Non insulin dependent diabetes mellitus (NIDDM) is one of the most frequently encountered endocrinopathy in cats. Many research studies concluded that diabetic cat mimic some of the clinical and pathological features of human diabetes type 2: occurrence in obese, indoor confined, middle-aged and old individuals (highest incidence in cats with 8 years of age), with residual and subsequent decline of insulin secretion, deposits of amyloid in Langerhans islets associated with loss of β-cells and onset of complications such as peripheral neuropathy and retinopathy. Diseases or drugs which increase the risk of insulin resistance such as hyperadrenocorticism, acromegaly, hyperthyroidism, renal and cardiac disease, administration of corticosteroids and progestagenes were also considered. Cats express supplementary ketoacidosis and insulin-dependence [63-67]. It is quite difficult to estimate the incidence of IDDM in cat: β-cell antibody did not prove any involvement in pathogenesis of diabetes in cat [68] and require further investigation and lymphocytic insulitis is rare [69].

The synergy between hyperinsulinemia and exaggerated response to glucose feature the early stages of the disease and countervail basal insulin resistance. When diabetes becomes overt, the compensatory insulin synthesis and secretion decline, this being usually accompanied by exhaustion of β-cells and amyloid deposition into the islets. Cats may express clinically insulin independence at the beginning of the condition, but insulin requirement is very probable later [67].

The frequency of diabetes mellitus in cats records different values in a given population, ranging to 0.43 to 2.24%, with significant prevalence in Burmese cats. The mean age was significantly higher for the same breed (more than 13 years of age) comparing with short and longhaired domestic breeds. Males seem to be prone to diabetes, comparing with the incidence of the disease in females [70-72]. Juvenile diabetes is rarely described. The condition is clinically featured by classical symptoms, islet hypoplasia and diabetic bilateral cataract with both cortex and nucleus involvement [73].

As in humans, diabetic cats present islet amyloidosis, progressive loss of number of β and α-cells and normal number of δ-cells. Nevertheless, these lesions are not capital for inducing impaired glucose tolerance in cat and also for the onset of diabetes, but it have an important contribution to the progression of the disease [74].

Early stages of the disease are particularly featured by a first-phase attenuated secretion of insulin as response to glucose administration, followed by an exaggerated second-phase response. Deleterious effects as glucose toxicity, lipotoxicity and islet amyloidosis are the mechanism incriminated in gradual onset of diabetes.

The onset of type 2 diabetes in cats is strongly related with glucose toxicity. Intraperitoneal administration of the glucose for a long time produce vacuolation of islet cells and even diabetes mellitus, this being one of the first experimental model in cats which prove toxic effect of glucose on Langerhans islets [75]. Glucotoxicity may be used as a major target of handling the therapy protocol of hyperglycemia, allows obtaining further preservation of β-cells and even succeed remission of the condition. In normal individuals, glucose stimulates synthesis of insulin via initiating transcription of insulin gene by phosphorylation of PDX1. Downregulation of glucose transporters on the membrane of β-cells and decreased expression of insulin and PDX1 genes usually mediate hyperglycemia and subsequent glucose toxicity. Persistence of hyperglycemia (for at least 10 days) leads to overloading of β-cells with glycogen and cell death. Toxic effect of glucose is enhanced by overburden secretion of insulin and initiation of β-cells destruction [76, 77].

Lipotoxicity concerns disturbances provoked by the excessive quantities of triacylglycerol and subsequent deposition in other non-adipose tissues (myocardium, liver, pancreas, skeletal muscle). Furthermore, the excess of triacylglycerol in β-cells will be expressed as loss of these cells and impaired synthesis of insulin; accumulation of triacylglycerol in muscles and liver leads to insulin resistance. The presence of triacylglycerol in the cytoplasm may be not sufficient to induce low levels of insulin and insulin resistance. It is presumed that lipolysis and synthesis of triacylglycerol are prone to produce fatty acids generating peroxidation compounds or other toxic lipid intermediates. Finally, these will initiate the expression of death receptor gene and alter insulin signaling in liver and β-cells. Long-chain acyl coenzyme A has been suggested as a major mediator of lipotoxicity and insulin resistance in non-adipose tissues [78]. The most reliable proof of this mechanism is offered by the skeletal muscles. High level of long-chain acyl coenzyme A into the sarcoplasm was correlated with decreased glucose entry. In addition, intramuscular content is higher in insulin-resistant animals and human [78].

Islet amyloidosis is the dominant feature in non-insulin dependent diabetes mellitus, being diagnosed in more than 80% of affected domestic and wild cats [79, 80]. Amyloid deposition is usually detected in healthy cats, the amount increasing with the age. The prevalace of amyloidosis is higher in diabetic animals than in non-diabetics. The presence of amyloid is a hallmark for impaired β-cells function and proves previous overstimulation and exhausting of β-cells. The deposits are mainly extracellular, although intracellular amyloid is possible in non-endocrine cells of the islets, generating further disruption of the cellular membrane and cell death [81]. The major component of islet amyloid is islet amyloid polypeptide or amylin (IAPP), based on identification of a residual fragment of this hormone [82-84]. High levels of IAPP are identified in obese cat and also in euglicemic cats with impaired glucose tolerance. Although, increased concentration of IAPP is mandatory but not exclusive in insular amyloid formation, other accompanying mechanisms such as defective synthesis of β-cells and failure of secretion, transport and degradation of IAPP are probably implicated [85]. There is a strong correlation between IAPP levels and pathogenesis of type 2 diabetes in human and cats. As a premise of the onset of diabetes in cat, increased body condition score in correlated with increased levels of circulating IAPP and insulin in non-diabetic cats [86].

Increased levels of IAPP will generate impaired glucose tolerance. Inhibitory effect of IAPP on glucose-stimulating insulin synthesis and increased gluconeogenesis will contribute to hyperglycemia. Insulin resistance of the muscle is also induced by IAPP and it results in inhibition of glucose uptake and further glycogenolysis. Fat tissue seems to be insensitive to IAPP. It is suspected that glucose resulted from muscle glicogenolysis is used in lipogenesis causing secondary obesity [87].

Obesity is rightly considered as an important predisposing factor to NIDDM, being equally involved in the individual genetic predisposition to insulin resistance and impaired glucose tolerance [88]. The risk of disease results from obesity induced low sensitivity of tissues to insulin and compensatory hyperinsulinemia. The onset of obesity is multifactorial, with genetic and environmental origin. One of the cause is the presence of active "thrifty genotype" which allows lipogenesis when the food is plentiful and lipid mobilization when the food supply is diminished or absent [89]. Still, intake of large amount of highly palatable food with high concentration of carbohydrates, aging, neutering, and low physical exercises are considered important [90]. The onset of obesity is responsible of high levels of leptin and resistin, inflammatory cytokines such as tumor necrosis factor alpha (TNFα), interleukins 1β and 6, and C-reactive protein. Particularly, TNFα interfere insulin sensitivity by blocking activation of insulin receptors [88]. It is documented that weight gain in lean cats is followed by insulin sensitivity comparable with the range recorded in cats with overt diabetes. Furthermore, fasting-induced hyperinsulinemia in lean cats is considered to be the greatest risk for the onset of impaired glucose tolerance with obesity.

Male cats have a propensity to become obese comparing female, adipose tissue mass being larger than obese female [70, 91]. The lack of effectiveness of insulin to reduce basal glucose level is proportional with mass of adipose tissue. Lean male are less insulin sensitive than lean female, these sensitivity recording decline when the male have weight gain. Fasting hyperinsulinemia is more likely to develop in obese male than obese female cats.

Abdominal fat deposition is correlated with a more severe insulin resistance. This is also observed in diabetic Burmese cats which particularly have large amount of abdominal fat tissue and less subcutaneously [71].

Although obesity alone cannot induce diabetes, it is known that small increases of body weight and size of adipocytes result in higher risk of overt diabetes. Thus, 25% of cats which have weight gain have values of insulin sensitivity comparable with diabetic cats [92].

Insulin resistance is the expression of internalization of insulin receptors, low affinity of these receptors to insulin and disturbances of intracellular oxidative glucose metabolism. Skeletal muscle and liver present the highest expression of insulin resistance, which finally results into a low glycogen synthesis within the sarcoplasm and hepatocyte cytoplasm. As it was previously mentioned, IAPP prevents glucose uptake, inhibits glycogen synthetase and induce glycogenolysis followed by lactate production. The liver take lactate and initiates gluconeogenesis. In addition, three important insulin signaling genes are downregulated in liver and muscle of the moderate obese cats: insulin receptor substrate (IRS)-1, IRS-2, and phosphatidylinositol 3'-kinase (PI3-K) p85alpha. These data add a new resemblance between human and feline insulin resistance specific for NIDDM [93].

6. Pancreatic disease and diabetes mellitus

The destruction of Langerhans islets via pancreatic necrosis, acute or chronic inflammation and tumors are presented in dogs, cats, cattle and horses.

Particularly, canine acute pancreatitis and acute pancreatic necrosis are differentially framed as long as inflammation or necrosis is dominant. Thus, necrosis may be consistently represented comparing with inflammation and supports using the term of acute pancreatic necrosis (APN). This lesion is considered the common cause of diabetes mellitus in dog, knowing that APN is occasionally encountered in cats and sporadic in pigs and horses. Interestingly, the most of predisposing factors of APN are generally considered in the pathogenesis of diabetes mellitus. Obesity, hyperadrenocorticism, prolonged therapy with glucocorticoids are linked with APN and also with impaired glucose tolerance, insulin resistance and insulin antagonism. Most of the dogs with fatal APN express ketonuria while diabetic ketoacidosis can coexist with acute inflammatory lesions of the pancreas. Usually, all ketonuric dogs with APN or acute pancreatitis are diabetic. It is important to bear in mind that diabetes mellitus may create conditions for an increased risk for developing pancreatitis. Diabetic dogs express hypertriglyceridemia, which is a risk factor for acute pancreatitis [94, 95].

Chronic pancreatitis is featured by fibrosis, atrophy of parenchyma, lymphocytic infiltrate and cyst of pancreatic ducts [96, 97]. The onset of chronic inflammation is a common consequence of the repeated mild episodes of APN or acute pancreatitis. Chronic pancreatitis in dogs, cats, cattle and horses is not always sufficient to induce massive destruction of the islets with subsequent onset of diabetes. If the magnitude of the fibrosis, atrophy and lymphoplasmacytic infiltrate is sufficient enough to involve large areas of the pancreas, than exocrine and endocrine insufficiency may develop. Nevertheless, it is considered that chronic pancreatitis claims an important percentage from the canine patients with diabetes mellitus, almost 30% of diagnosed cases were linked with histological features attributable to chronic inflammation of the pancreas [98]. The incidence can be higher when is correlated with breed predisposition [99].

Various morphological types of pancreatic adenocarcinoma may determine extensive destruction of the parenchyma and secondary diabetes in old cats and dogs [3]. The tumors of islet cells are rarely described, most being diagnosed in dog. Adenomas and carcinomas of pancreatic islets induce hormonal hypersecretion. The dogs and also cattle, and ferrets can present more than one hormone in histological sections in the majority of diagnosed cases. Pancreatic or extrapancreatic glucagonoma is linked with diabetes mellitus and is featured by antagonism of glucagon with insulin. Although not pathognomonic, the condition is also clinically recognized by the superficial necrolytic dermatitis which affect muzzle, mucocutaneous junctions, ears and frictional and pressure points of the body. The excessive secretion of glucagon determines hyperglycemia due to the high level of hepatic gluconeogenesis and glycogenolysis [3, 95, 100].

7. Diabetogenic hormones and drugs

Antagonists of insulin such as hormones and drugs represent an important mechanism of diabetes in animals. Thus, glucocorticoids, growth factor, thyroxine, glucagon, epinephrine, progesterone and synthetic progestagens are frequently involved. Antagonic effect is triggered on peripheral tissues, followed by sustained hyperglycemia and further exhaustion of islets. Early clinical management to monitor diabetes may be followed by resolution of secondary diabetes if remaining β-cells are sufficient. Finally, when antagonism can no longer be controlled the animals present a permanent insulin-dependent status.

Hyperadrenocorticism (tumorally induced or by administration of corticosteroids as dexamethasone and prednisolone) [101] is one of the antagonist in dog and rarely encountered in cats [102-104], the new abnormal hormonal status being concurrent with insulin resistance. Functional adenomas or adenocarcinomas of either pituitary gland or adrenal cortex are responsible for hyperadrenocorticism, more than a half of affected animals being diabetic at the time of diagnosis. Systemic control of glycemia is poorly developed and expressed by classical signs. Supplementary, the animals present bad condition of hair coat (bilateral alopecia) and skeletal muscles, excessive fragility of the skin, enlarged abdomen (pot belly), bacterial infection of skin, urinary and respiratory tract [64]. ACTH secreting adenoma of pars intermedia associated with hyperplasia of adrenal cortex and reduced β-cell population was diagnosed in horse, although reference to hormonal antagonism is not discussed [105].

Acromegaly as consequence of pituitary acidophil adenoma results in excessive secretion of growth factor (GH) and also causes associated severe insulin resistance and diabetes mellitus [106]. The excess of GH will generate further synthesis of insulin growth factor 1 (IGH-1) which exerts anabolic effect and subsequent proliferation of connective tissue, cartilages, bones, and organs. Screening of IGH-1 provides valuable information for diagnosis of acromegaly in cats with overt insulin resistance, although both monitoring of GH and IGH-1 should be considered in addition with imaging diagnosis [107-109].

Hyperthyroidism generates excess of thyroxine and triiodothyronine, which increase the bodily demands of glucose. Thus, supplementary glucose is produced in liver via gluconeogenesis and Cori cycle. Furthermore, fasting period allows adipose tissue lipolysis which provide glycerol and fatty acids. Under these metabolic circumstances gluconeogenesis is initiated, glycerol resulted from lipolysis and amino acids resulted from proteolysis being used as basic resources. Hyperthyroid status is featured by decreased insulin-stimulated glycogen synthesis and increased anaerobic glycolysis. Lactate resulted from muscle anaerobic glycolysis and conversion to glucose into the liver maintains high levels of glycemia and facilitates preservation of adipose reserves [110].

Insulin antagonism was also described as being associated with excessive secretion of catecholamines in animals with pheocromocytomas. Catecholamines action as inhibitors of insulin release and generate mild to moderate glucose intolerance [111]. Diuretics (hydrochlorothiazide, furosemide) induce glucose intolerance by diminishing insulin-stimulated glucose transport into skeletal muscle and adipose tissue [112].

8. Diabetic ketoacidosis and non-ketotic hyperosmolar diabetes

Diabetic ketoacidosis features complicated diabetes mellitus in dog and cat, being one of the most severe complications. Concurrent diseases as pancreatitis, hypercorticosolism, tumoral diseases, infections, renal and heart failure or poor management of insulin therapy create a stressful status by enhancing circulating levels of insulin antagonists such as catecholamines, cortisol, glucagon and growth hormone. Bodily energetic demands are shifted to lipolysis, followed by an increase uptake of fatty acids into the liver. The absence of insulin and glucose into the cytoplasm will favor oxidation of fatty acids, β-hydroxibutiric and acetoacetic acids being released. Some of ketoacids are converted into acetone, volatilization through the lungs giving a specific ketone breath [113]. Clinically, the onset of ketoacidosis manifests as severe hyperglycemia, acidosis, ketonemia, ketonuria, hyperosmolarity, massive loss of magnesium, sodium, potassium, dehydration, and hypovolemic shock [114, 115].

Non-ketotic hyperosmolar diabetes is characterized by hypeglicemia, hyperosmolarity, osmotic diuresis and subsequent dehydration. Thus, deleterious effects on central nervous system activity are clinically expressed as ataxia, nystagmus, seizures, hyperthermia and coma [116].

9. Lesions of diabetes mellitus in dog and cats

Postmortem gross lesions are very little expressed in diabetic animals. Atrophy of skeletal muscle, dehydration and fatty liver are the principal findings. Usually, pancreas is normal, excepting the situation when postnecrotic scarring, chronic pancreatitis and tumors occur [3].

Juvenile onset of diabetes in dog is represented by lymphocytic insulitis in almost a half of total number of islets. Inflammatory infiltrate is represented chiefly by T-lymphocytes, disposed around and inside the islets [47]. The rest of Langerhans islets presented severe atrophy and massive loss of β-cells. In addition to islet inflammatory lesions, other cases are featured by cytoplasmic vacuoles in islets cell and ductal epithelium due to massive glycogen accumulation (fig.1). Lees damaged islets may present mitotic figures (fig 2). When insulitis do not occur, histological examination reveals only a lower number of pancreatic islets [49]. Amyloid deposition is characteristic for cat diabetes. The deposits are mainly extracellular, with particular concentration at the periphery of islets and around the capillaries and concurrent with depletion of islet cells (fig. 3) [79, 117].

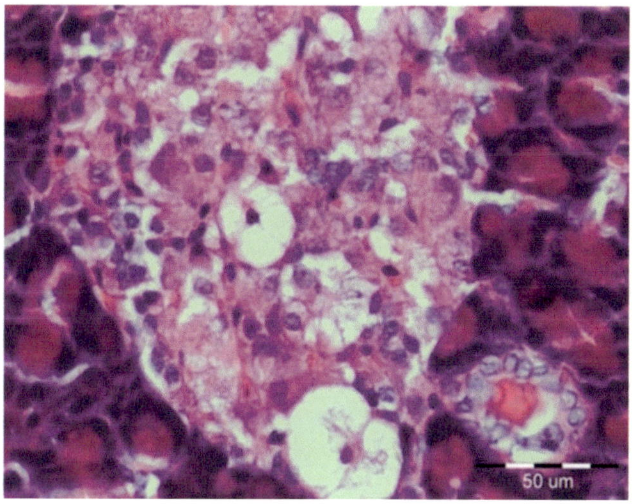

Figure 1. Cytoplasmic vacuoles in cells of Langerhans islets in a dog with diabetes mellitus

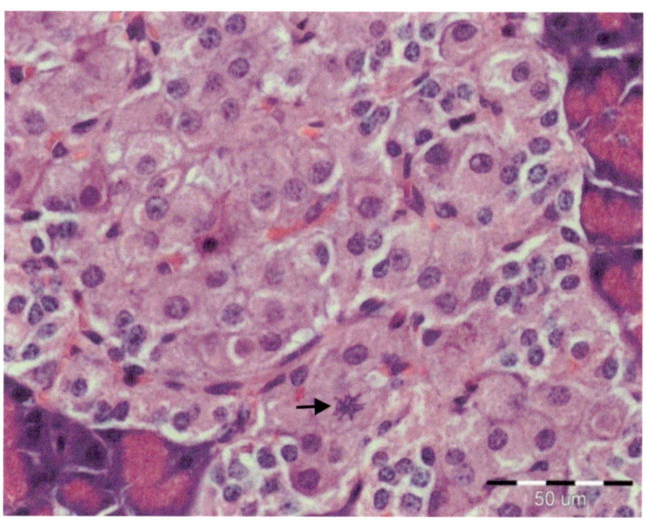

Figure 2. Mitotic figure (arrow) in a less damaged islets.

Hepatocytes and epithelium of bile ducts express also vacuolation of the cytoplasm due to lipid accumulation and glycogen, respectively. Renal epithelial cells show the same glycogen deposits, mainly in loops of Henle and distal convoluted tubules. Renal lipidosis is featured by vacuoles in proximal convoluted tubes and lipidic emboli in glomerular capillaries [3].

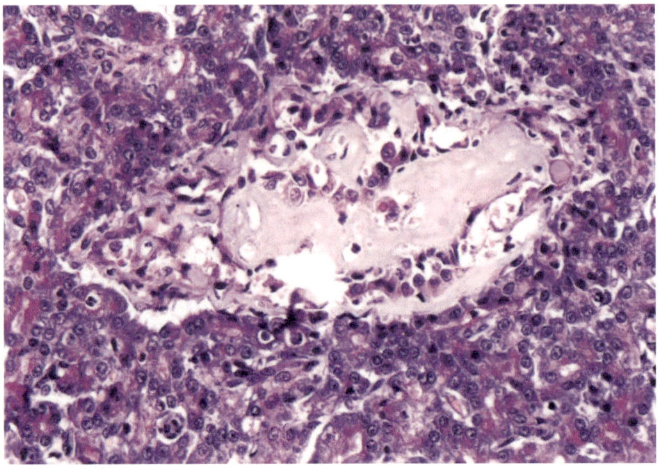

Figure 3. Islet amyloidosis, extracellular depositions and depletion of islet cells in cat diabetes mellitus. (Courtesy of M. Militaru)

The functional and structural disorders in other organs, chiefly in kidney and retina but also in other organs are attributable to altered vasomotor responsiveness, vasoactive mediators, plasma volume enhancement and tissue hypoxia, generating diabetic microangiopathy. Thus, increased vascular pressure and enhanced permeability in capillaries are followed by cell proliferation into the capillary walls and macromolecule transfer towards extravascular space respectively. Furthermore, these pathological effects are responsible for the thickening of basement membrane of the capillaries and vascular wall which induce compensatory dilation of less altered capillaries [118].

Focal or diffuse diabetic glomerulosclerosis is one of the morphological expressions of diabetic microangiopathy. It is commonly encountered in dog and cats and indicate a long evolution of the disease. Basal membrane of glomerular capillaries present thickening caused by hyaline deposits, being followed by subsequent sclerosis of the tufts. Similar sclerosis occurs in mesangium and also thickening of the basement membrane of Bowman capsule and convoluted tubules. Dysfunctional filtration are clinically expressed in cats as microalbuminuria and proteinuria [119].

Diabetic lesions of the eye are represented by diabetic retinopathy and cataracts. As renal complications, retinal involvement proves a long evolution disease. Dogs and cats express retinopathy as microaneurysms and varicous dilations of capillaries, degenerative processes which result in loss of endothelial cells and pericytes and further formation of acellular non-perfused capillaries. Neovascularization within the retina may occur [120, 121]. Cataract onset in dog and cats is a common event and represent the reason for which diabetes is suspected. The incidence is higher in dogs than cats [122], suggesting that lens capsule in diabetic dogs is more permeable to circulating glucose [118, 123].

The cats express frequently diabetic neuropathy, being clinically revealed by plantigrade position, hindlimb paresis and subsequent muscle atrophy [124]. The lesions are usually confined to pelvic sensitive and motor nerves, but thoracic limb involvement was also described in juvenile onset [125]. Axonal injuries (glycogen deposition, accumulation of membranous deposits or neurofilaments and loss of fibers) of both myelinated and unmyelinated fibers, degeneration of myeline sheath featured by discontinuity (rows of myelin balls and ovoids), and demyelination are frequently described in feline and canine diabetes [126]. Microvascular changes were noticed in feline diabetic neuropathy, those being consistent with endoneurial dilation of capillaries and thickening of basement membrane [127]. Remyelination may occur if the therapy management in glucose control is achieved and revealed by fibers with thin myelin sheaths [128].

Diabetic dog and cats are prone to secondary infections. Glucosuria creates good growth conditions for glucose and albumin fermenting bacteria (*E. coli, Clostridium sp, Proteus sp, Staphylococcus aureus, Aerobacter aerogenes*) [129] which creates gas accumulation in kidneys, ureters and urinary bladder. Urinary bladder wall has spongy consistency, with multiple cyst-like structures filled with gas, which confer floating ability when the tissue specimens are put into fixative solution. Hemorrhages and inflammatory cell infiltration are observed in lamina propria [130, 131].

Pulmonary lesions may occur in cats with diabetes mellitus. The lesions are diverse and require careful clinical assessment of the individuals. Furthermore, the onset of pulmonary lesions are linked to vascular disturbances (congestion, edema, smooth muscle hypertrophy), inflammatory (pneumonia, type II pneumocytes hyperplasia, fibrosis), degenerative (mineralization) and neoplasia [132].

Impaired pigmentation (vitiligo) and canine diabetic dermathopathy are rarely seen and may be expressed as erythema, erosions, ulcers and crusts which feature superficial necrolytic dermatitis. The lesions have bilateral disposal on muzzle, lips, periocular skin, pinae and extremities. The onset of the lesions is attributable to decreased levels of amino acids which are extensively used in hepatic gluconeogenesis [3].

10. Diabetes mellitus in wildlife

Spontaneous diabetes mellitus in humanoid and non-humanoid primates was described in captive animals and it is consistent with clinical and morphological features of type 2 diabetes mellitus [133-139]. Thus, previous results, comparative studies and creation of animal models emphasized many similarities with human non-insulin dependent diabetes mellitus (insulin resistance, long prediabetic status and impaired β-cell function). Furthermore, spontaneous amyloidosis is described in various species such as rhesus (*Macaca mulatta*), squirrel monkey (*Saimiri sciureus*), baboons (*Papio hamadryas*), *drills (Mandrillus leucophaeus, Mandrillus sphynx)* , macaques (*Macaca fascularis, Macaca cyclopis, Macaca nemestrina, Macaca nigra*), *Cercopithecus diana, Cercopithecus nictitans* , orangutan (*Pongo pygmaeus*) and chimpanzee (*Pan troglodytes*). Amyloid deposits appear not only in pancreas, but also in spleen, liver, kidney and adrenal gland. In this context islets amyloidosis was immunohistochemically positive for islet amyloid polypeptide (IAPP) and calcitonine gene-related peptide (CGRP) [138]. Histologically, the lesions present obvious resemblance with those described in cat: amyloid deposition around capillaries, with little or severe deleterious effect on islet cell density [134, 138, 140-142]. Complications of diabetes mellitus in primates are cardiomiopathy, myocardial fibrosis, nephropathy and venous thrombosis [143]. Secondary diabetes mellitus is described in non-humanoid monkeys with pituitary adenoma which creates condition for insulin antagonism [144].

Diabetes mellitus was described in wild captive rodents, one of the broader studies being conducted on golden mantled ground squirrel (*Spermophilus lateralis*). Grossly, the animals present cataract (multifocal subcapsular areas of opacity), retinal atrophy, and islet cell vacuolation in both α and β cells [145]. Other species of captive rodents such as tuco-tuco (*Ctenomys talarum*) [146] and plains viscachas (*Lagostomus maximus*) [147] may develop diabetes mellitus in both adults and offspring which have been diagnosed with cataract, hepatic lipidosis and significant high level of glucose and fructosamine. High energetic diet and lack of physical exercises seem to be the cause of the onset of diabetes. Wild bank vole (*Clethrionomys glareolus*) developed type 1 diabetes mellitus in adults and offspring after few months of captivity. The animals express typical markers for insulin dependent diabetes mellitus such as GAD65, IA-2 and insulin autoantibodies and vacuolation of pancreatic islets. A novel Picornavirus (Ljungan virus) was identified in affected islets [148, 149].

Secondary diabetes mellitus was also described in rock hyraxes (*Procavia capensis*) diagnosed with pancreatic islet fibrosis [150] and in California sea lion due to chronic pancreatitis [151].

Wild carnivores develop diabetes in captive or captive-born individuals such as jaguar [152] and african spotted leopard [153]. Thus, secondary diabetes occurred in a female of jaguar (*Panthera onca*) with prolonged administration of megestrol acetate for preventing pregnancy and subsequent metastatic uterine scirrhous adenocarcinomas [152].

A case of diabetes mellitus is described in a 50 years of age captive elephant. The bull had a medical history of necrotizing laminitis, poliarthritis and preputial edema treated with phenylbutazone, prednisolone, dexamethasone and diuretics (chlorothiazide). Pancreas presented atrophy and fibrosis of the islets. The authors mention that a previous infection with endotheliotropic elephant herpes virus should be considered as a potential cause of this case. Therapy protocol is also important. Although is not discussed, the usage of insulin antagonists in the therapy protocol may be envisaged [167].

Glucose metabolism in granivorous birds presents important differences comparing with mammals. Normal glycemia records higher values than other vertebrates with corresponding body weight, intracellular glycogen reserve is lower and plasma glucose concentration is not regulated via insulin intervention. Glucagon, insulin, somatostatin and avian pancreatic polypeptide are synthesized in three different types of islets [154]. The levels of glucagon in pancreas and plasma are higher than in mammals, this being essential for glucose metabolism. The absorption of glucose from gastrointestinal tract is performed by sodium-glucose co-transporters and glucose transport protein. These mechanisms are very efficient in kidneys, avian urine being glucose-free [155]. Finally, it is postulated that the onset of avian diabetes is probably a consequence of glucagon excess and less due to insulin deficiency. This has been supported by studies in ducks which have developed hypoglycemia after total pancreatectomy. Controversially, some experiments conducted in duck and goose proved the onset of diabetes after administration of anti-insulin serum or subtotal pancreatectomy respectively [154]. Furthermore, some cases of avian diabetes mellitus have been managed successfully by insulin therapy for a long time. Carnivorous birds have the same insulin-coordinated glucose metabolism as described in mammals [156].

Spontaneous diabetes mellitus in birds is rarely reported and it is consistent with type 1 diabetes mellitus. Small parrots such as nanday conure (*Nandayus nenday*) [157] or in chestnut-fronted macaw (*Ara severa*) [158] present diabetes clinically expressed as polyuria, polydipsia, hyperglycemia, hypoinsulinemia, glucosuria and ketonuria. Pancreatic islets were almost totally destructed with absent immunohistochemical reaction to insulin. Lymphoplasmocytic pancreatitis features the lesions of exocrine pancreas in almost all cases described [157]. A similar situation was described in African grey parrot (*Psittacus erithacus erithacus*), in which destructions produced by pancreas inflammation were concurrent with compensatory proliferation and hypertrophy of the islets cells [159]. Negative results were obtain for identification of concurrent bacteriological and viral infection in almost all reviewed cases. A cockatiel (*Nymphicus hollandicus*) diagnosed with type 1 diabetes mellitus present chronic pancreatitis and associated viral inclusions in acinar and ductal epithelial cells due to Psittacid herpesvirus infection which indicates the diagnosis of Pacheco's disease [160]. This condition is specific for Psittaciforme and it is featured by hepatic, renal and splenic coagulative necrosis, syncitial cells into respiratory epithelium, intestinal crypts, parathyroid, thymus and both intracytoplasmic and intranuclear inclusions [161, 162]. Although Psittacid viral infection in pancreas is rarely mentioned, the authors recommend differential diagnosis in avian pancreatitis with or without diabetes mellitus. It is noteworthy that diabetes mellitus was associated with excessive iron storage, this being a condition described in chestnut-fronted macaw (*Ara severa*), military macaw (Ara militaris) and also in humans [163]. This association is well documented in humans and rodent models of haemochromatosis, iron being preferentialy stored in β-cells and generating insulin deficiency [164]. Although pancreatic biopsies revealed no lesions attributable to iron storage in pancreatic islets, specific long term therapy succeeded to prolong survival of the birds more than 20 months [163].

Diabetes mellitus in raptors is little documented. Experimental pancreatectomy in a great horned owl was followed by hyperglicemia and subsequent death, proving that carnivorous birds develop a similar disease with humans [165]. Spontaneous diabetes mellitus was described in a female of red-tailed hock (*Buteo jamaicensis*). Kidneys, lungs and air sacs present different types of inflammation, as interstitial lymphocytic nephritis associated with cysts of proximal tubules and suppurative bronchopneumonia and aerosaculitis. Hepatic lipidosis was featured by isolated foci. Severe degeneration of pancreatic islets was confined to β-cells, characteristic glycogen granules being absent. Although bacteriological investigation did not identified any bacterial colonies, histological section detected cocci in kidneys and lungs. Postmortem examination of pituitary and adrenal glands did not identified tumoral lesions attributable, the etiology of the condition remaining unknown [166].

11. Conclusions

Spontaneous diabetes mellitus in animals includes all types of diabetes described in humans. Although rarely diagnosed, the horses express IDDM, NIDDM and secondary diabetes. Cattle and dogs present IDDM, while the cat is the animal prototype of spontaneous NIDDM featured by islet amyloidosis. Gestational, diestrus and persistent corpora luteal diabetes were described in dog. The onset of diabetes in wildlife is frequently correlated with captivity, diet changes, low physical exercises or concurrent lesions of the pancreas followed by endocrine insufficiency.

Diabetes mellitus in animals represent not only a generous field for research purpose due to numerous resemblances with human conditions, but also an important area in practice of veterinary medicine. The surveillance and treatment of diabetic animals include many issues to be considered, beginning with the diagnosis, continuing with causes which are responsible for the onset of diabetes and finishing with the setting of the most appropriate therapeutical protocol. Although the human diagnosis and classification of diabetes mellitus is not entirely applicable to animals, spontaneous onset of this disease represented the first steps in creating adequate animal models which became more refined to meet the various requirements of the research.

Author details

Emilia Ciobotaru
University of Agronomic Science and Veterinary Medicine, Faculty of Veterinary Medicine, Bucharest, Romania

12. References

[1] Nelson, R.W., *Canine Diabetes Mellitus*, in *Textbook of Veterinary Internal Medicine*, E.C.F. Stephen J Ettinger, Editor 2010, Saunders Elsevier: Canada. p. 1782-1796.
[2] Stogdale, L., *Definition of diabetes mellitus.* Cornell Vet, 1986. 76(2): p. 156-174.
[3] Charles, J., *Pancreas*, in *Jubb, Kennedy and Palmer's Pathology of Domestic Animals*, M.G. Maxie, Editor 2007, Elsevier Limited. p. 389-424.
[4] Rees, D.A. and J.C. Alcolado, *Animal models of diabetes mellitus.* Diabetic Medicine, 2004. 22: p. 395-370.
[5] *Diagnosis and classification of diabetes mellitus, American Diabetes Association*, 2004: Diabetes Care. p. S5-S10.
[6] Kronfeld, D.S., *Equine syndrome X, the metabolic disease, and equine grain-associated disorders: Nomenclature and dietetics.* Journal of Equine Veterinary Science, 2003. 23(12): p. 567-569.
[7] Johnson, P.J., et al., *Endocrinopathic laminitis in the horse.* Clin. Tech. Eq. Prac., 2004. 3(1): p. 45-56.
[8] Kronfeld, D.S., Treiber K.H., Hess T.M., Boston R.C., *Insulin resistance in the horse: Definition, detection and dietetics.* J Anim Sci, 2005. 83: p. E22-E31.

[9] Hoffman R. M., et al., *Obesity and diet affect glucose dynamics and insulin sensitivity in Thoroughbred geldings.* J Anim Sci, 2003. 81: p. 2333-2342.

[10] Wreiole, M., *The horse (Equs cabalus) as an animal reserch model for human diabetes,* 2011, Drexel University College of Medicine. p. 10.

[11] Jeffery, J.R., *Diabetes mellitus secondary to a chronic pancreatitis in pony.* J Am Vet Med Assoc., 1968. 153: p. 1168-1175.

[12] Baker, J.R. and R.H. E., *Diabetes mellitus in the horse: A case report and review of the literature.* Equine Vet J, 1974. 6: p. 7-11.

[13] Collobert C., et al., *Chronic pancreatitis associated with diabetes mellitus in a standardbred race horse: A case report.* Journal of Equine Veterinary Science, 1990. 10(1): p. 58-61.

[14] Giri, J.K., K.G. Magdesian, and P.M. Gaffney, *Insulin-dependent diabetes mellitus associated with presumed autoimmune polyendocrine syndrome in a mare.* Can Vet J, 2011. 52(5): p. 506-12.

[15] Johnson, P.J., et al., *Diabetes mellitus in a domesticated Spanish mustang.* J Am Vet Med Assoc, 2005. 226(4): p. 584-8, 542.

[16] Durham, A.E., et al., *Type 2 diabetes mellitus with pancreatic beta cell dysfunction in 3 horses confirmed with minimal model analysis.* Equine Vet J, 2009. 41(9): p. 924-9.

[17] Navas de Solis, C. and J.H. Foreman, *Transient diabetes mellitus in a neonatal Thoroughbred foal.* J Vet Emerg Crit Care (San Antonio), 2010. 20(6): p. 611-5.

[18] Gould, A.C., *Diabetes mellitus in cattle.* Vet Rec, 1981. 109(24): p. 539.

[19] Nafizi, S., T. Karimi, and Rowshan Ghasrodashti A., *Diabetes mellitus and fatty liver in a cow: case report.* Comp Clin Path, 2004. 13: p. 82-85.

[20] Kaneko, J.J. and E.A. Rhode, *Diabetes Mellitus in a Cow.* J Am Vet Med Assoc, 1964. 144: p. 367-73.

[21] Kitchen, D.L. and A.J. Roussel, Jr., *Type-I diabetes mellitus in a bull.* J Am Vet Med Assoc, 1990. 197(6): p. 761-3.

[22] Clark, Z., *Diabetes mellitus in a 6-month-old Charolais heifer calf.* Can Vet J, 2003. 44: p. 921-922.

[23] Taniyama, H., et al., *Spontaneous diabetes mellitus in young cattle: histologic, immunohistochemical, and electron microscopic studies of the islets of Langerhans.* Vet Pathol, 1993. 30(1): p. 46-54.

[24] Tajima, M., et al., *Possible causes of diabetes mellitus in cattle infected with bovine viral diarrhoea virus.* Zentralbl Veterinarmed B, 1999. 46(3): p. 207-15.

[25] Taniyama, H., et al., *Histopathological and immunohistochemical analysis of the endocrine and exocrine pancreas in twelve cattle with insulin-dependent diabetes mellitus (IDDM).* J Vet Med Sci, 1999. 61(7): p. 803-10.

[26] Taniyama, H., et al., *Immunohistochemical detection of the enzyme glutamic acid decarboxylase and hormones of the islets of Langerhans in spontaneous insulin-dependent diabetes mellitus in cattle.* Vet Pathol, 1999. 36(6): p. 628-31.

[27] von Herrath, M., C. Filippi, and K. Coppieters, *How viral infections enhance or prevent type 1 diabetes-from mouse to man.* J Med Virol, 2011. 83(9): p. 1672.

[28] Richter, W., et al., *Sequence homology of the diabetes-associated autoantigen glutamate decarboxylase with coxsackie B4-2C protein and heat shock protein 60 mediates no molecular mimicry of autoantibodies.* J Exp Med, 1994. 180(2): p. 721-6.

[29] Tracy, S., K.M. Drescher, and N.M. Chapman, *Enteroviruses and type 1 diabetes.* Diabetes Metab Res Rev, 2011. 27(8): p. 820-3.

[30] Lee, M.S., I. Chang, and S. Kim, *Death effectors of beta-cell apoptosis in type 1 diabetes.* Mol Genet Metab, 2004. 83(1-2): p. 82-92.

[31] Thomas, H.E., J.A. Trapani, and T.W. Kay, *The role of perforin and granzymes in diabetes.* Cell Death Differ, 2010. 17(4): p. 577-85.

[32] Pearl-Yafe, M., et al., *Pancreatic islets under attack: cellular and molecular effectors.* Curr Pharm Des, 2007. 13(7): p. 749-60.

[33] Almawi, W.Y., H. Tamim, and S.T. Azar, *Clinical review 103: T helper type 1 and 2 cytokines mediate the onset and progression of type I (insulin-dependent) diabetes.* J Clin Endocrinol Metab, 1999. 84(5): p. 1497-502.

[34] Falcone, M. and N. Sarvetnick, *The effect of local production of cytokines in the pathogenesis of insulin-dependent diabetes mellitus.* Clin Immunol, 1999. 90(1): p. 2-9.

[35] Harrison, L.C., et al., *MHC molecules and beta-cell destruction. Immune and nonimmune mechanisms.* Diabetes, 1989. 38(7): p. 815-8.

[36] Fall, T., *Characterisation of Diabetes Mellitus in Dogs*, in *Department of Clinical Sciences*2009, Swedish University of Agricultural Sciences: Uppsala. p. 70.

[37] Fall, T., et al., *Diabetes mellitus in a population of 180,000 insured dogs: incidence, survival, and breed distribution.* J Vet Intern Med, 2007. 21(6): p. 1209-16.

[38] Fall, T., et al., *Diabetes mellitus in elkhounds is associated with diestrus and pregnancy.* J Vet Intern Med, 2010. 24(6): p. 1322-8.

[39] Barbour, L.A., et al., *Human placental growth hormone causes severe insulin resistance in transgenic mice.* Am J Obstet Gynecol, 2002. 186(3): p. 512-7.

[40] Davison, L.J., M.E. Herrtage, and B. Catchpole, *Study of 253 dogs in the United Kingdom with diabetes mellitus.* Vet Rec, 2005. 156(15): p. 467-71.

[41] Kramer, J.W., et al., *Inheritance of diabetes mellitus in Keeshond dogs.* Am J Vet Res, 1988. 49(3): p. 428-31.

[42] Sai, P., et al., *Anti-beta-cell immunity in insulinopenic diabetic dogs.* Diabetes, 1984. 33(2): p. 135-40.

[43] Short, A.D., et al., *Analysis of candidate susceptibility genes in canine diabetes.* J Hered, 2007. 98(5): p. 518-25.

[44] Catchpole, B., et al., *Canine diabetes mellitus: can old dogs teach us new tricks?* Diabetologia, 2005. 48(10): p. 1948-56.

[45] Guptill, L., L. Glickman, and N. Glickman, *Time trends and risk factors for diabetes mellitus in dogs: analysis of veterinary medical data base records (1970-1999).* Vet J, 2003. 165(3): p. 240-7.

[46] Charles, J., *Pancreas*, in *Pathology of Domestic Animals*, M.G. Maxie, Editor 2007, Elsevier Limited. p. 389-424.

[47] Jouvion, G., et al., *Lymphocytic insulitis in a juvenile dog with diabetes mellitus.* Endocr Pathol, 2006. 17(3): p. 283-90.

[48] Neiger, R., V.B. Jaunin, and C.E. Boujon, *Exocrine pancreatic insufficiency combined with insulin-dependent diabetes mellitus in a juvenile German shepherd dog.* J Small Anim Pract, 1996. 37(7): p. 344-9.
[49] Kang, J.H., et al., *Juvenile diabetes mellitus accompanied by exocrine pancreatic insufficiency in a dog.* J Vet Med Sci, 2008. 70(12): p. 1337-40.
[50] Catchpole, B., et al., *Canine diabetes mellitus: from phenotype to genotype.* J Small Anim Pract, 2008. 49(1): p. 4-10.
[51] Hoenig, M. and D.L. Dawe, *A qualitative assay for beta cell antibodies. Preliminary results in dogs with diabetes mellitus.* Vet Immunol Immunopathol, 1992. 32(3-4): p. 195-203.
[52] Davison, L.J., et al., *Autoantibodies to GAD65 and IA-2 in canine diabetes mellitus.* Vet Immunol Immunopathol, 2008. 126(1-2): p. 83-90.
[53] Kramer, J.W., et al., *Inherited, early onset, insulin-requiring diabetes mellitus of Keeshond dogs.* Diabetes, 1980. 29(7): p. 558-65.
[54] Lund, E.M., et al., *Prevalence and risk factors for obesity in adult dogs from private US veterinary practices.* Intern J Appl Res Vet Med, 2006. 4(2): p. 177-186.
[55] Mattheeuws, D., et al., *Glucose tolerance and insulin response in obese dogs.* J. Amer. Anim. Hosp. Assoc., 1982. 20: p. 287-293.
[56] Mattheeuws, D., et al., *Diabetes mellitus in dogs: relationship of obesity to glucose tolerance and insulin response.* Am. J. Vet. Res., 1984. 45: p. 98-103.
[57] Kaiyala, K.J., et al., *Reduced beta-cell function contributes to impaired glucose tolerance in dogs made obese by high-fat feeding.* Am J Physiol, 1999. 277(4 Pt 1): p. E659-67.
[58] Fall, T., et al., *Gestational diabetes mellitus in 13 dogs.* J Vet Intern Med, 2008. 22(6): p. 1296-300.
[59] Norman, E.J., K.J. Wolsky, and G.A. MacKay, *Pregnancy-related diabetes mellitus in two dogs.* N Z Vet J, 2006. 54(6): p. 360-4.
[60] Sorenson, R.L. and T.C. Brelje, *Adaptation of islets of Langerhans to pregnancy: beta-cell growth, enhanced insulin secretion and the role of lactogenic hormones.* Horm Metab Res, 1997. 29(6): p. 301-7.
[61] Eigenmann, J.E. and A. Rijnberk, *Influence of medroxyprogesterone acetate (Provera) on plasma growth hormone levels and on carbohydrate metabolism. I. Studies in the ovariohysterectomized bitch.* Acta Endocrinol (Copenh), 1981. 98(4): p. 599-602.
[62] Nelson, L.W. and W.A. Kelly, *Progestogen-related gross and microscopic changes in female Beagles.* Vet Pathol, 1976. 13(2): p. 143-56.
[63] Hoenig, M., *Comparative aspects of diabetes mellitus in dogs and cats.* Mol Cell Endocrinol, 2002. 197(1-2): p. 221-9.
[64] Scott-Moncrieff, J.C., *Insulin resistance in cats.* Vet Clin North Am Small Anim Pract, 2010. 40(2): p. 241-57.
[65] Rand, J., *Current understanding of feline diabetes: part 1, pathogenesis.* J Feline Med Surg, 1999. 1(3): p. 143-53.
[66] Lutz, T.A. and J.S. Rand, *Pathogenesis of feline diabetes mellitus.* Vet Clin North Am Small Anim Pract, 1995. 25(3): p. 527-52.
[67] Reusch, C., *Feline Diabetes Mellitus,* in *Textbook of Veterinary Internal medicine,* S.J. Ettinger and E.C. Feldman, Editors. 2010, Saunders Elsevier: Canada. p. 1796-1816.

[68] Hoenig, M., C. Reusch, and M.E. Peterson, *Beta cell and insulin antibodies in treated and untreated diabetic cats.* Vet Immunol Immunopathol, 2000. 77(1-2): p. 93-102.

[69] Hall, D.G., et al., *Lymphocytic inflammation of pancreatic islets in a diabetic cat.* J Vet Diagn Invest, 1997. 9(1): p. 98-100.

[70] Panciera, D.L., et al., *Epizootiologic patterns of diabetes mellitus in cats: 333 cases (1980-1986).* J Am Vet Med Assoc, 1990. 197(11): p. 1504-8.

[71] McCann, T.M., et al., *Feline diabetes mellitus in the UK: the prevalence within an insured cat population and a questionnaire-based putative risk factor analysis.* J Feline Med Surg, 2007. 9(4): p. 289-99.

[72] Lederer, R., et al., *Frequency of feline diabetes mellitus and breed predisposition in domestic cats in Australia.* Vet J, 2009. 179(2): p. 254-8.

[73] Thoresen, S.I., et al., *Diabetes mellitus and bilateral cataracts in a kitten.* J Feline Med Surg, 2002. 4(2): p. 115-22.

[74] O'Brien, T.D., et al., *Immunohistochemical morphometry of pancreatic endocrine cells in diabetic, normoglycaemic glucose-intolerant and normal cats.* J Comp Pathol, 1986. 96(4): p. 357-69.

[75] Dohan, F.C. and F.D. Lukens, *Experimental diabetes mellitus produced by intraperitoneal injections of glucose.* Fed Proc, 1947. 6(1 Pt 2): p. 97.

[76] Robertson, R.P., et al., *Beta-cell glucose toxicity, lipotoxicity, and chronic oxidative stress in type 2 diabetes.* Diabetes, 2004. 53 Suppl 1: p. S119-24.

[77] Zini, E., et al., *Hyperglycaemia but not hyperlipidaemia causes beta cell dysfunction and beta cell loss in the domestic cat.* Diabetologia, 2009. 52(2): p. 336-46.

[78] Li, L.O., E.L. Klett, and R.A. Coleman, *Acyl-CoA synthesis, lipid metabolism and lipotoxicity.* Biochim Biophys Acta, 2010. 1801(3): p. 246-51.

[79] Hoenig, M., et al., *A feline model of experimentally induced islet amyloidosis.* Am J Pathol, 2000. 157(6): p. 2143-50.

[80] Johnson, K.H., et al., *Amyloid in the pancreatic islets of the cougar (Felis concolor) is derived from islet amyloid polypeptide (IAPP).* Comp Biochem Physiol B, 1991. 98(1): p. 115-9.

[81] Yano, B.L., D.W. Hayden, and K.H. Johnson, *Feline insular amyloid. Ultrastructural evidence for intracellular formation by nonendocrine cells.* Lab Invest, 1981. 45(2): p. 149-56.

[82] Woldemeskel, M., *A Concise Review of Amyloidosis in Animals*, 2012, Hindawi Publishing Corporation: Veterinary Medicine International. p. 11.

[83] Johnson, K.H., et al., *Feline insular amyloid: immunohistochemical and immunochemical evidence that the amyloid is insulin-related.* Vet Pathol, 1985. 22(5): p. 463-8.

[84] O'Brien, T.D., *Pathogenesis of feline diabetes mellitus.* Mol Cell Endocrinol, 2002. 197(1-2): p. 213-9.

[85] Verchere, C.B., et al., *Transgenic overproduction of islet amyloid polypeptide (amylin) is not sufficient for islet amyloid formation.* Horm Metab Res, 1997. 29(6): p. 311-6.

[86] Henson, M.S., et al., *Evaluation of plasma islet amyloid polypeptide and serum glucose and insulin concentrations in nondiabetic cats classified by body condition score and in cats with naturally occurring diabetes mellitus.* Am J Vet Res, 2011. 72(8): p. 1052-8.

[87] O'Brien, T.D., et al., *Islet amyloid polypeptide: a review of its biology and potential roles in the pathogenesis of diabetes mellitus.* Vet Pathol, 1993. 30(4): p. 317-32.

[88] Laflamme, D.P., *Obesity in dogs and cats: what is wrong with being fat?* J Anim Sci, 2011.

[89] Rand, J.S., et al., *Canine and feline diabetes mellitus: nature or nurture?* J Nutr, 2004. 134(8 Suppl): p. 2072S-2080S.

[90] Zoran, D.L., *Obesity in dogs and cats: a metabolic and endocrine disorder.* Vet Clin North Am Small Anim Pract, 2010. 40(2): p. 221-39.

[91] Rand, J.S. and G.J. Martin, *Management of feline diabetes mellitus.* Vet Clin North Am Small Anim Pract, 2001. 31(5): p. 881-913.

[92] Feldhahn, J.R., J.S. Rand, and G. Martin, *Insulin sensitivity in normal and diabetic cats.* J Feline Med Surg, 1999. 1(2): p. 107-15.

[93] Mori, A., et al., *Decreased gene expression of insulin signaling genes in insulin sensitive tissues of obese cats.* Vet Res Commun, 2009. 33(4): p. 315-29.

[94] Hess, R.S., et al., *Evaluation of risk factors for fatal acute pancreatitis in dogs.* J Am Vet Med Assoc, 1999. 214(1): p. 46-51.

[95] Cullen, J.M. and D.L. Brown, *Hepatobiliary system and exocrine pancreas*, in *Pathologic Basis of Veterinary Disease*, J.F. Zachary and M.D. McGavin, Editors. 2012, Elsevier. p. 405-457.

[96] Strombeck, D.R., E. Wheeldon, and D. Harrold, *Model of chronic pancreatitis in the dog.* Am J Vet Res, 1984. 45(1): p. 131-6.

[97] Watson, P.J., et al., *Characterization of chronic pancreatitis in English Cocker Spaniels.* J Vet Intern Med, 2011. 25(4): p. 797-804.

[98] Watson, P.J. and M.E. Herrtage, *Use of glucagon stimulation tests to assess beta-cell function in dogs with chronic pancreatitis.* J Nutr, 2004. 134(8 Suppl): p. 2081S-2083S.

[99] Watson, P.J., et al., *Observational study of 14 cases of chronic pancreatitis in dogs.* Vet Rec, 2010. 167(25): p. 968-76.

[100] Mizuno, T., et al., *Superficial necrolytic dermatitis associated with extrapancreatic glucagonoma in a dog.* Vet Dermatol, 2009. 20(1): p. 72-9.

[101] Lowe, A.D., et al., *A pilot study comparing the diabetogenic effects of dexamethasone and prednisolone in cats.* J Am Anim Hosp Assoc, 2009. 45(5): p. 215-24.

[102] Nelson, R.W., E.C. Feldman, and M.C. Smith, *Hyperadrenocorticism in cats: seven cases (1978-1987).* J Am Vet Med Assoc, 1988. 193(2): p. 245-50.

[103] Watson, P.J. and M.E. Herrtage, *Hyperadrenocorticism in six cats.* J Small Anim Pract, 1998. 39(4): p. 175-84.

[104] Meij, B.P., et al., *Melanotroph pituitary adenoma in a cat with diabetes mellitus.* Vet Pathol, 2005. 42(1): p. 92-7.

[105] Baker, J.R. and H.E. Ritchie, *Diabetes mellitus in the horse: a case report and review of the literature.* Equine Vet J, 1974. 6(1): p. 7-11.

[106] Niessen, S.J., et al., *Feline acromegaly: an underdiagnosed endocrinopathy?* J Vet Intern Med, 2007. 21(5): p. 899-905.

[107] Fracassi, F., et al., *Acromegaly due to a somatroph adenoma in a dog.* Domest Anim Endocrinol, 2007. 32(1): p. 43-54.

[108] Peterson, M.E., et al., *Acromegaly in 14 cats.* J Vet Intern Med, 1990. 4(4): p. 192-201.

[109] Fracassi, F., et al., *Pituitary macroadenoma in a cat with diabetes mellitus, hypercortisolism and neurological signs.* J Vet Med A Physiol Pathol Clin Med, 2007. 54(7): p. 359-63.

[110] Mitrou, P., et al., *Insulin resistance in hyperthyroidism: the role of IL6 and TNF alpha.* Eur J Endocrinol, 2010. 162(1): p. 121-6.
[111] Nestler, J.E. and M.A. McClanahan, *Diabetes and adrenal disease.* Baillieres Clin Endocrinol Metab, 1992. 6(4): p. 829-47.
[112] Dimitriadis, G., et al., *Furosemide decreases the sensitivity of glucose transport to insulin in skeletal muscle in vitro.* Eur J Endocrinol, 1998. 139(1): p. 118-22.
[113] Kerl, M.E., *Diabetic ketoacidosis: pathophysiology and clinical and laboratory presentation.* Compendium Small Animal/Exotics, 2001. 23(3): p. 220-229.
[114] De Causmaecker, V., Daminet S., and D. Paepe, *Diabetes ketoacidosis and diabetes ketosis in 54 dogs: a retrospective study.* Vlaams Diergeneeskundig Tijdschrift, 2009. 78: p. 327-337.
[115] Hume, D.Z., K.J. Drobatz, and R.S. Hess, *Outcome of dogs with diabetic ketoacidosis: 127 dogs (1993-2003).* J Vet Intern Med, 2006. 20(3): p. 547-55.
[116] Umpierez, G.E., M.B. Murphy, and A.E. Kitabchi, *Diabetic ketoacidosis and hyperglycemic hyperosmolar syndrome.* Diabetes Spectrum, 2002. 15(1): p. 28-38.
[117] Militaru, M., et al., *Meningiom psamomatos la o pisica diabetica.* Revista Romana de Medicina Veterinara, 2005. 3: p. 77-92.
[118] Fowler, M.J., *Microvascular and macrovascular complications of diabetes.* Clinical Diabetes, 2008. 26(2): p. 77-82.
[119] Al-Ghazlat, S.A., et al., *The prevalence of microalbuminuria and proteinuria in cats with diabetes mellitus.* Top Companion Anim Med, 2011. 26(3): p. 154-7.
[120] Feit-Leichman, R.A., et al., *Vascular damage in a mouse model of diabetic retinopathy: relation to neuronal and glial changes.* Invest Ophthalmol Vis Sci, 2005. 46(11): p. 4281-7.
[121] Joussen, A.M., et al., *A central role for inflammation in the pathogenesis of diabetic retinopathy.* FASEB J, 2004. 18(12): p. 1450-2.
[122] Salgado, D., C. Reusch, and B. Spiess, *Diabetic cataracts: different incidence between dogs and cats.* Schweiz Arch Tierheilkd, 2000. 142(6): p. 349-53.
[123] Engerman, R.L., *Pathogenesis of diabetic retinopathy.* Diabetes, 1989. 38(10): p. 1203-6.
[124] Kramek, B.A., et al., *Neuropathy associated with diabetes mellitus in the cat.* J Am Vet Med Assoc, 1984. 184(1): p. 42-5.
[125] Anderson, P.G., et al., *Polyneuropathy and hormone profiles in a chow puppy with hypoplasia of the islets of Langerhans.* Vet Pathol, 1986. 23(4): p. 528-31.
[126] Dahme, E., et al., *[Diabetic neuropathy in dogs and cats--a bioptic electron microscopic study].* Tierarztl Prax, 1989. 17(2): p. 177-88.
[127] Estrella, J.S., et al., *Endoneurial microvascular pathology in feline diabetic neuropathy.* Microvasc Res, 2008. 75(3): p. 403-10.
[128] Mizisin, A.P., et al., *Comparable myelinated nerve pathology in feline and human diabetes mellitus.* Acta Neuropathol, 2007. 113(4): p. 431-42.
[129] Thomas, A.A., et al., *Emphysematous cystitis: a review of 135 cases.* BJU Int, 2007. 100(1): p. 17-20.
[130] Oliveira, S.T.d., et al., *Emphysematous cystitis in a diabetic bitch: case report.* Medvep (Revista Científica de Medicina Veterinária. Pequenos Animais e Animais de Estimação), 2006. 4(13): p. 210-214.

[131] Matsuo, S., et al., *Emphysematous cystitis in a chemically-induced diabetic dog.* J Toxicol Pathol, 2009. 22(4): p. 289-92.

[132] Mexas, A.M., et al., *Pulmonary lesions in cats with diabetes mellitus.* J Vet Intern Med, 2006. 20(1): p. 47-51.

[133] Rosenblum, I.Y., T.A. Barbolt, and C.F. Howard, Jr., *Diabetes mellitus in the chimpanzee (Pan troglodytes).* J Med Primatol, 1981. 10(2-3): p. 93-101.

[134] Davis, K.J., et al., *Immunohistochemical analysis of spontaneous pancreatic islet amyloid deposits in nonhuman primates.* Vet Pathol, 1994. 31(4): p. 479-80.

[135] Koning, E.J.P.d., et al., *Diabetes mellitus in Macaca mullata monkeys is characterized by islet amyloidosis and reduction in beta-cell population.* Diabetologia, 1993. 36: p. 378-384.

[136] Howard, C.F., Jr. and J.L. Palotay, *Spontaneous diabetes mellitus in Macaca cyclopis and Mandrillus leucophaeus: case reports.* Lab Anim Sci, 1975. 25(2): p. 191-6.

[137] O'Brien, T.D., et al., *Islet amyloid and islet amyloid polypeptide in cynomolgus macaques (Macaca fascicularis): an animal model of human non-insulin-dependent diabetes mellitus.* Vet Pathol, 1996. 33(5): p. 479-85.

[138] Hubbard, G.B., et al., *Spontaneous pancreatic islet amyloidosis in 40 baboons.* J Med Primatol, 2002. 31(2): p. 84-90.

[139] Hubbard, G.B., et al., *Spontaneous amyloidosis in twelve chimpanzees, Pan troglodytes.* J Med Primatol, 2001. 30(5): p. 260-7.

[140] Pirarat, N., et al., *Immunohistochemical analysis of pancreatic amyloidosis in two captive diabetic mandrills,* in *The 11th International Symposium of the World Association of Veterinary Laboratory Diagnosticians and OIE Seminar of Biotechnology*2003. p. P28-P29.

[141] Wagner, J.D., et al., *Diabetes mellitus and islet amyloidosis in cynomolgus monkeys.* Lab Anim Sci, 1996. 46(1): p. 36-41.

[142] McClure, H.M. and F.W. Chandler, *A survey of pancreatic lesions in nonhuman primates.* Vet Pathol Suppl, 1982. 7: p. 193-209.

[143] Pirarat, N., et al., *Spontaneous diabetes mellitus in captive Mandrillus sphinx monkeys: a case report.* J Med Primatol, 2008. 37(3): p. 162-5.

[144] Remick, A.K., et al., *Histologic and immunohistochemical characterization of spontaneous pituitary adenomas in fourteen cynomolgus macaques (Macaca fascicularis).* Vet Pathol, 2006. 43(4): p. 484-93.

[145] Heidt, G.A., et al., *Spontaneous diabetes mellitus in a captive golden-mantled ground squirrel, Spermophilus lateralis (Say).* J Wildl Dis, 1984. 20(3): p. 253-5.

[146] Weir, B.J., *The development of diabetes in the tuco-tuco (Ctenomys talarum).* Proc R Soc Med, 1974. 67(9): p. 843-6.

[147] Gull, J., et al., *Occurrence of cataract and fatty liver in captive plains viscachas (Lagostomus maximus) in relation to diet.* J Zoo Wildl Med, 2009. 40(4): p. 652-8.

[148] Niklasson, B., et al., *Type 1 diabetes in Swedish bank voles (Clethrionomys glareolus): signs of disease in both colonized and wild cyclic populations at peak density.* Ann N Y Acad Sci, 2003. 1005: p. 170-5.

[149] Niklasson, B., et al., *Development of type 1 diabetes in wild bank voles associated with islet autoantibodies and the novel ljungan virus.* Int J Exp Diabesity Res, 2003. 4(1): p. 35-44.

[150] Gamble, K.C., et al., *Pancreatic islet fibrosis in rock hyraxes (Procavia capensis), Part 1: Case histories, clinical pathology, and epizootiology.* J Zoo Wildl Med, 2004. 35(3): p. 361-9.
[151] Meegan, J.M., et al., *Chronic pancreatitis with secondary diabetes mellitus treated by use of insulin in an adult California sea lion.* J Am Vet Med Assoc, 2008. 232(11): p. 1707-12.
[152] Kollias, G.V., Jr., M.B. Calderwood-Mays, and B.G. Short, *Diabetes mellitus and abdominal adenocarcinoma in a jaguar receiving megestrol acetate.* J Am Vet Med Assoc, 1984. 185(11): p. 1383-6.
[153] Prowten, A.W., *Case report: diabetes mellitus in an African spotted leopard,* 1975: American Association of Zoo Veterinarians. p. 215-217.
[154] Sitbon, G. and P. Mialhe, *[The endocrine pancreas of birds].* J Physiol (Paris), 1980. 76(1): p. 5-24.
[155] Braun, E.J. and K.L. Sweazea, *Glucose regulation in birds.* Comp Biochem Physiol B Biochem Mol Biol, 2008. 151(1): p. 1-9.
[156] Pollock, C., *Carbohydrate regulation in avian species.* Seminars in Avian and Exotic Pet Medicine, 2002. 11(2): p. 57-64.
[157] Desmarchelier, M. and I. Langlois, *Diabetes mellitus in a nanday conure (Nandayus nenday).* J Avian Med Surg, 2008. 22(3): p. 246-54.
[158] Pilny, A.A. and R. Luong, *Diabetes mellitus in a chestnut-fronted macaw (Ara severa).* J Avian Med Surg, 2005. 19(4): p. 297-302.
[159] Candeletta, S.C., et al., *Diabetes mellitus associated with chronic lymphocytic pancreatitis in an African grey parrot (Psittacus erithacus erithacus).* Journal of the Association of Avian Veterinarians, 1993. 7(1): p. 39-43.
[160] Phalen, D.N., M. Falcon, and E.K. Tomaszewski, *Endocrine pancreatic insufficiency secondary to chronic herpesvirus pancreatitis in a cockatiel (Nymphicus hollandicus).* J Avian Med Surg, 2007. 21(2): p. 140-145.
[161] Tsai, S.S., et al., *Herpesvirus infections in psittacine birds in Japan.* Avian Pathology, 1993. 22(1): p. 141-156.
[162] Gravendyck, M., et al., *Quantification of the herpesvirus content in various tissues and organs, and associated post mortem lesions of psittacine birds which died during an epornithic of pacheco's parrot disease (PPD).* Avian Pathology, 1998. 27(5): p. 478-489.
[163] Gancz, A.Y., et al., *Diabetes mellitus concurrent with hepatic haemosiderosis in two macaws (Ara severa, Ara militaris).* Avian Pathology, 2007. 36(7): p. 331-336.
[164] Iancu, T.C., R.J. Ward, and T.J. Peters, *Ultrastructural changes in the pancreas of carbonyl iron-fed rats.* J Pediatr Gastroenterol Nutr, 1990. 10(1): p. 95-101.
[165] Nelson, N., S. Elgart, and A.I. Mirsky, *Pancreatic diabetes in the owl.* Endocrinology, 1942. 31: p. 119-123.
[166] Wallner-Pendleton E. A., Rogers D., and A. Epple, *Diabetes mellitus in a red-tailed hawk (Buteo jamaicensis).* Avian Pathology, 1993. 22(3): p. 631-635.
[167] van der Kolk, J.H., et al., *Diabetes mellitus in a 50-year-old captive Asian elephant (Elaphas maximus) bull.* Vet Q, 2011. 31(2): p. 99-101.

Chapter 16

A New Behavioral Model (Health Belief Model Combined with Two Fear Models): Design, Evaluation and Path Analysis of the Role of Variables in Maintaining Behavior

Alireza Shahab Jahanlou, Masoud Lotfizade and Nader Alishan Karami

Additional information is available at the end of the chapter

http://dx.doi.org/10.5772/52966

1. Introduction

With the increased pace of industrialization and higher life expectancy in the present century, lifestyles across the world have changed significantly. Some of these changes include changes in the pattern of diseases and prevalence of chronic diseases, such as diabetes (Narayan et al., 2000). Diabetes is one of the most prevalent noninfectious diseases in the world that affects approximately 6% of the world population (Task Force on Community Preventive, 2002). The prevalence of this condition is at the epidemic level in locations where obesity and inactive lifestyles prevail (Campbell, 2001). Diabetes has several side effects, including retinopathy, renal diseases, neuropathy and critical metabolic disorders (Alavi et al., 2007) and is also recognized as an important and costly health problem both for the patients and for the healthcare systems. Diabetes may also cause irreparable harms such as lost life, amputation, blindness, kidney failure and lost working days which, together with their associated costs, can be avoided through blood sugar level monitoring (Clarke et al., 2002). Patient training is the best method for achieving this goal.

According to the World Health Organization, patient training is the best method to monitor blood sugar level in diabetic patients. WHO, however, reported that ordinary people, healthcare staff and policy makers are inadequately educated and knowledgeable about noninfectious diseases and their associated risk factors (Group, 1997). Diabetic patients as well need guidance to acquire new skills and change their lifestyles so that they can acquire the required attitude and functioning for the control of their blood sugar (Jahanlou et al., 2010). Diabetes management primarily depends on the behavior and self-care of the patient (Clarke et al., 2002). Studies show that there is a gap between what patients actually do and what they actually need to do to control their diabetes (Kamel et al., 1999). Patient training is shown to have a positive effect on enhancing the knowledge, attitude and performance of patients. Patient willingness and ability to learn depends on their needs and personal beliefs and the presented training can be effective only if the target audience is willing to learn (DeWalt et al., 2007).

2. An overview of behavior training models

Today various models are used to train diabetic patients and make a change in their behaviors so that through acquiring new skills and controlling their blood sugar level they can prevent or delay the side effects of diabetes (Sarkar et al., 2006). Common models and theories include *Health Belief Model, Social Behavior Model*. These training models and theories support the basic knowledge about the effective environmental and psychological mechanisms of the patients for acceptance and following of appropriate behaviors which may ameliorate the short-term and long-term effects of diabetes and provide instructions for researchers to develop appropriate training approaches. These instructions greatly enhance acceptance and following of appropriate behaviors (such as nutrition regiment) and eventually lead to the long-term control of blood sugar level in diabetic patients (Campbell, 2001). The authors attempt to develop a model to improve training intervention in diabetic patients and decrease related costs through existing training models or their combination. To create a new model, the developers need to be knowledgeable in the field.

In the present chapter, we introduce an extended training model based on *Health Belief Model* and two models of fear. We have chosen to combine these two models because previous studies have shown no distinction between perceived threat and fear. Health belief model is a behavior prediction model which involves no intervention. Nevertheless, most researchers after using this model and identifying its constructs, such as perceived threat or perceived barriers, attempt to develop an intervention for behavior change in patients. Most studies utilize perceived threat to design the intervention while failing to distinguish between perceived threat and fear arousal. Through making a distinction between perceived threat and fear arousal we attempt to develop a model to help design the appropriate intervention for behavior change in diabetic patients. Among various models of fear, we came to find those of Leventhal and Ruiter to be more suitable for our new model based on health belief. In the last section of this chapter, you will be introduced to how to measure the effect of model components on the behavior change using path analysis.

3. Health belief model

3.1. History

The Health Belief model was first proposed and developed by Godfery Hochbaum, Stephan Kegels and Irwin Rosenstock. This model was initially developed as a structural style for the expression and prediction of health and preventive behaviors (Campbell, 2001). The model underwent modifications in 1977 by Baker et al. and more in 1982 by -Pender (Figure 1).

The different constructs of the model include perceived benefits, perceived barriers, perceived susceptibility and perceived seriousness to be later joined by self-efficacy and guidance for practice.

The early studies using this model included preventive programs for oral and dental diseases, polio and timely identification of uterus cancer (Glanz et al., 1997).

The ground for utilizing this model in the study was denial of health problems by ordinary people and explaining the behavior in individuals who acquitted themselves of any health problems. Further studies concentrated on a wider range of areas, including the study of short-term and long-term health behaviors (including sexual behaviors and AIDS) (Campbell, 2001). PubMed has indexed approximately 1100 academic papers on health belief model to date.

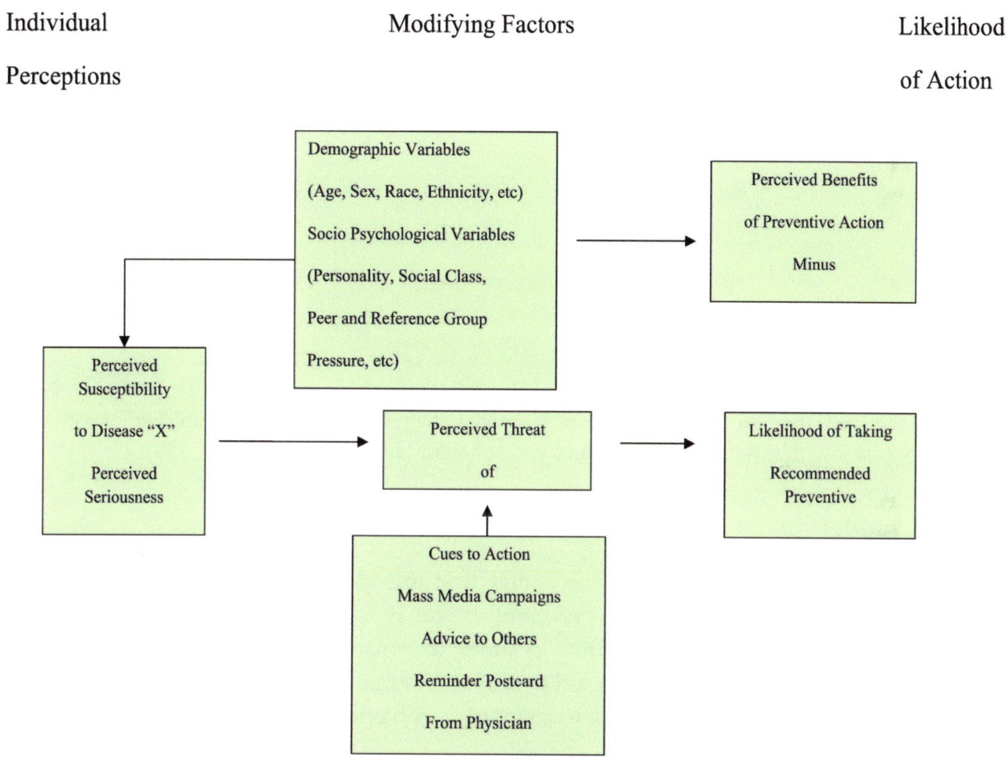

Figure 1. The Health Belief Model (Becker Mh: The Health Belief Model and sick role behavior. In Becker Mh (Ed): The Health Belief Model and Personal Health Behavior, P 89 .Thorrofare, New Jersey, Charles B Slack, (1974) *Fear Drive Model*

This model was first introduced by Leventhal et al in 1983 (Figure 2). This model is based on the assumption that knowledge and understanding are not adequate for creating behavior change in health matters and a feeling of fear is required and essential. Fear is a stimulating factor that causes change in health behaviors or early practices. This model includes several stages. At first, the individual receives a signal of fear, as in the form of pain or a defective stimulus, which is then followed by an emotional reaction (usually fear). Then the individual experiences a disturbing point in the fear (usually anxiety). This stimulus functions as a change in the individual's lifestyle routine.

Fear Drive model suggests that fear can be utilized as a behavior change agent. In addition, levels of fear are associated with change of behavior. For instance, after learning about the death of their aerobic fellows, overweight middle aged individuals decided to quit this exercise, which shows a change of behavior due to fear (Leventhal et al., 1983).(Figure 2).

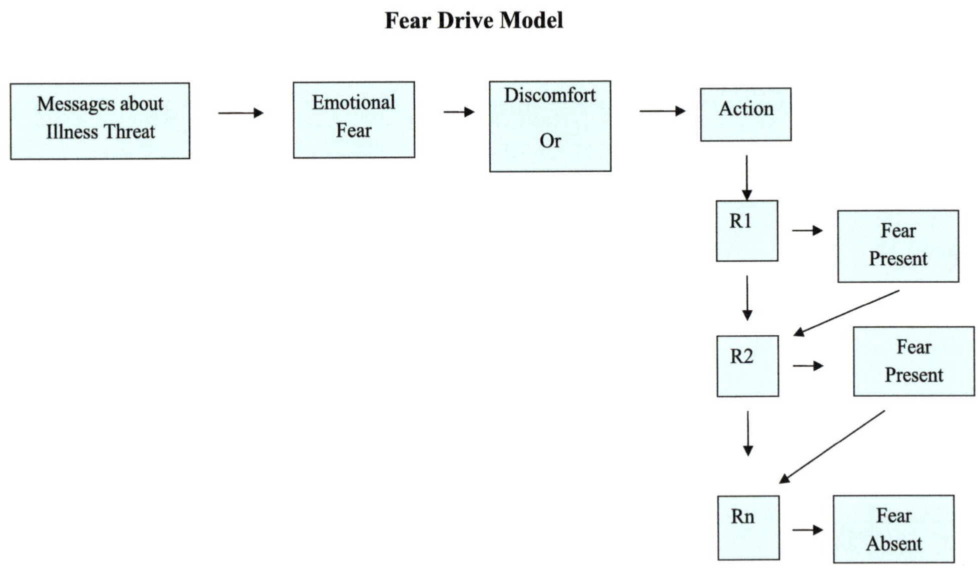

Figure 2. The Fear Drive Model. (Leventhal H, Safer M, Panagis D: The impact of communications on the self – regulation of health beliefs, decisions, and behavior Health Educ Q 10(1):7, 1983

3.2. Fear model

Inspired by earlier studies on fear, Rob Ruiter first introduced this model in 2001. In this model, the effect of fear arousal on perceived threat is identified. Fear arousal causes an individual to look for new information in order to control his fear. Eventually, through analysis of previous and new information the individual reaches an understanding that endows him with the adequate energy to change his behavior (Ruiter et al., 2001). (Figure 3).

3.3. How did the model evolve?

Previous studies on health belief model show that researchers' concentration on one construct and their attempt to combine perceived threat with perceived barriers and perceived benefits into a health motto leads to different expressions of the signal. This model in fact is a prediction model for behavior and includes no construct to receive intervention for. However, researchers consider a construct with the highest effect on the target population and design an intervention accordingly. For instance, Terry et al. showed that an individual would accept a health behavior if felt threatened by a disease.

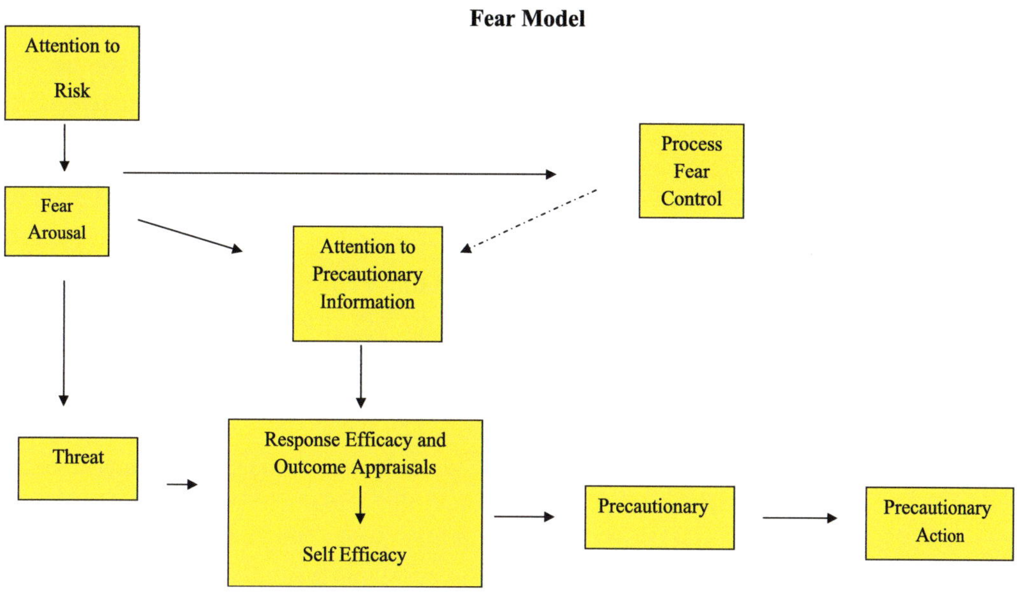

Figure 3. Ruiter RAC, Abraham C, Kok G. Scary warnings and rational precautions: a review of the psychology of fear appeals. Psychol Health 2001;16:613.

A study by Latoya et al. involved Spanish female patients with breast cancer and cervical cancer. Cancer monitoring barriers in Spanish women included a fear of cancer, deterministic judgments on cancer and a culture of self-consciousness. Perceived benefits had the lowest variance among the constructs of the model.

The study showed that cancer monitoring barriers occurred due to a fear of cancer and not the perceived threat by cancer. Of course, the researchers had used the model only as a predictor for the failure to monitor breast and cervical cancer. Latoya found a relationship between perceived benefits and acceptance of treatment program in diabetic patients (Austin et al., 2002). Bond found perceived benefits have a relationship with acceptance of treatment program by diabetic patients (Bond et al., 1992).

However, Ganz et al. and Harris et al. declared perceived barriers and perceived threat as having the strongest and weakest, respectively, predictors. In general, studies using the health belief model for diabetic patients show that priority is given foremost to perceived benefits and next to perceived susceptibility and perceived barriers, in that order, for adopting different behaviors. Perceived seriousness has been shown to have a mediocre effect (Jahanlou et al., 2008).

The foregoing models cannot adequately capture the distinction between affective (emotional) reactions, such as fear arousal, and cognitive reactions such as perceived threat against the impact of fear. In addition, there is yet to be a clear method in using the threat factor in control or induction of fear. There is a hazy intermediate state between fear arousal and perceived threat. The distinction between fear arousal as an emotional state and perceived threat as a cognitive state which is a reaction to fear arousal is not observable and existing models fail to support them (Leventhal et al., 1983).

Most studies based on the fear model show that another difference lies in subject learning which varies according to human conditions and states of the individual. Of course, the results are rather mixed (Witte, 1992) which could be attributed to the differences in measurement scales.

In this section we present the results of studies conducted on fear over the past 60 years to find the differences in these studies.

Janis and Feshback found tremendous changes in attitudes and behaviors associated to oral health in a group of high school students exposed to highly fearful messages. However, these results were not replicated in other experiments (Leventhal et al., 1983). In their study on weight loss, Wilson, Kincey, Ley and Bradshaw found that initiating and maintaining these behaviors over time was challenging. However, Clive et al. did not find any significant relationship between fear arousal and weight loss (Ishizaki et al., 2004). Lanyon et al. examined various fear measurement scales and found that paper-and-pencil self-report may reveal fear behavior in real situations (Lanyon and Manosevitz, 1966). Roland et al. showed that self-report has the highest sensitivity to the fear construct among various similar measurement scales. The most common way for fear arousal is through showing horror films which has a constant effect on measuring fear through paper-and-pencil self-reporting. These data support the validity of self-reporting fear and increase our confidence in fear arousal in various studies (Rogers and Mewborn, 1976). Beck and Davis in their study of smokers and non-smokers showed that attitude change in smokers is higher than in non-smokers and that greater fear leads to greater change in attitude (Montazeri and McEwen, 1997).

In a study on 220 female volunteers, Skilbeck et al. examined the effect of fear arousal, fear situation and exposure to fear on adopting a diet regiment in female participants with 10% overweight. They found that mild fear arousal had a better effect on the participants and that individuals exposed to a single fear-inducing message appear better than those receiving multiple fear-inducing messages (Bond et al., 1992). In a similar research, Sutton et al. studied two smoker groups in which one group was exposed to a film on the harmful effects of smoking and the other group watching a health-related film. The results showed that the film group received an instant effect which was followed by a rapid change of behavior in individuals. Likewise, Montazari (1997) found that smoking individuals preferred fear-inducing anti-tobacco advertisements (Koszegi, 2003). Tatsuro et al. studied individuals referring to ambulatory treatment division of a hospital where a SARS patient had been hospitalized. The results showed a 20% drop in visiting rate for individuals who observed the patient (Witte, 1992).

Werrij conducted a study on the effect of threat information in 2003. He found a significant relationship between threat information and fear and risk control. An individual holding the thought about breast cancer can be regarded as using a fear control measure which eventually decreases the feeling of fear in the patient. In addition, threat information can create an incentive for the patient to perform monthly breast cancer self-assessment. Werrij showed that threat information can moderate and balance individual's belief on their ability to fight the perceived threat. Although threat information may have a positive relationship with fear control, it shows lower effect compared to risk control. Werrij proposed that individuals need to be convinced without resort to threat information to adapt with health promotion behaviors (Ruiter et al., 2003).

The years from 1980 through 1990 mark the peak time when mass media campaigns inducing fear to change behavior were used, such as using the devil or tombstone images in anti-AIDS campaigns. The effectiveness of these advertisements is doubtful and even a review of interventions used in the related studies show that fear arousal and perceived threat were not clearly distinguished in those studies (Witte, 1992).

Hirschorn asserted that controlling the feelings rising from fear is a pivotal factor in social and health care. These feelings include a set of emotional states that are directed towards different behaviors. Thamson believed those individuals' reactions to fear depended on their understanding of fear arousal while Zagone believed that individual experiences of various fearful situations underlie the main reason for reaction to fear in different situations.

The foregoing studies show that even research on fear has failed to make a clear distinction between fear and perceived threat. Threat is in fact an external stimulus that develops from a message or an environment for the individual even if the individual knows it. If an individual comes to the understanding that he is subject to a threat we say the individual has perceived the threat (Campbell, 2001); but perception of the threat does not necessarily lead to fear. However, fear is an inner emotional reaction which includes both psychological and physiological components (Andersen and Guerrero, 1998). In other words, it is a reaction in a person following an experience or feeling of fearful and horrific content, situation or state(Campbell, 2001) , *(Jahanlou et al., 2008).*

Thus some studies purportedly on the fear of presented messages are in fact studies on perceived threats for the patient. For instance, in Montazari's study, health information on smoking was a perceived threat while the training film on lung cancer produced a type of fear arousal. Ruiter emphatically noted that on some occasions the border between fear arousal and perceived threat is not that clear (Ruiter et al., 2003).

In light of the foregoing discussion, we can see in Figure 4 that in the extended health model and the combined two fear models, the fear arousal box is positioned in the model in a way that has an effect both on perceived threat and on attention to precautionary information.

In order to apply the fear arousal model on patients, we needed different types of patient information. Therefore, we used 11 standardized questionnaires to collect various types of data on patient variables.

The preliminary results of our study showed that diabetic patients have very low information about threat perception of the disease. Fear assessment of these patients of the disease and its side effects (measured by a standard fear assessment scale) showed that patients had very low fear of the side effects of this disease. Next, we planned for fear arousal in these patients through presentation of frightening photos of diabetic feet (Figure 8) accompanied by related health information.

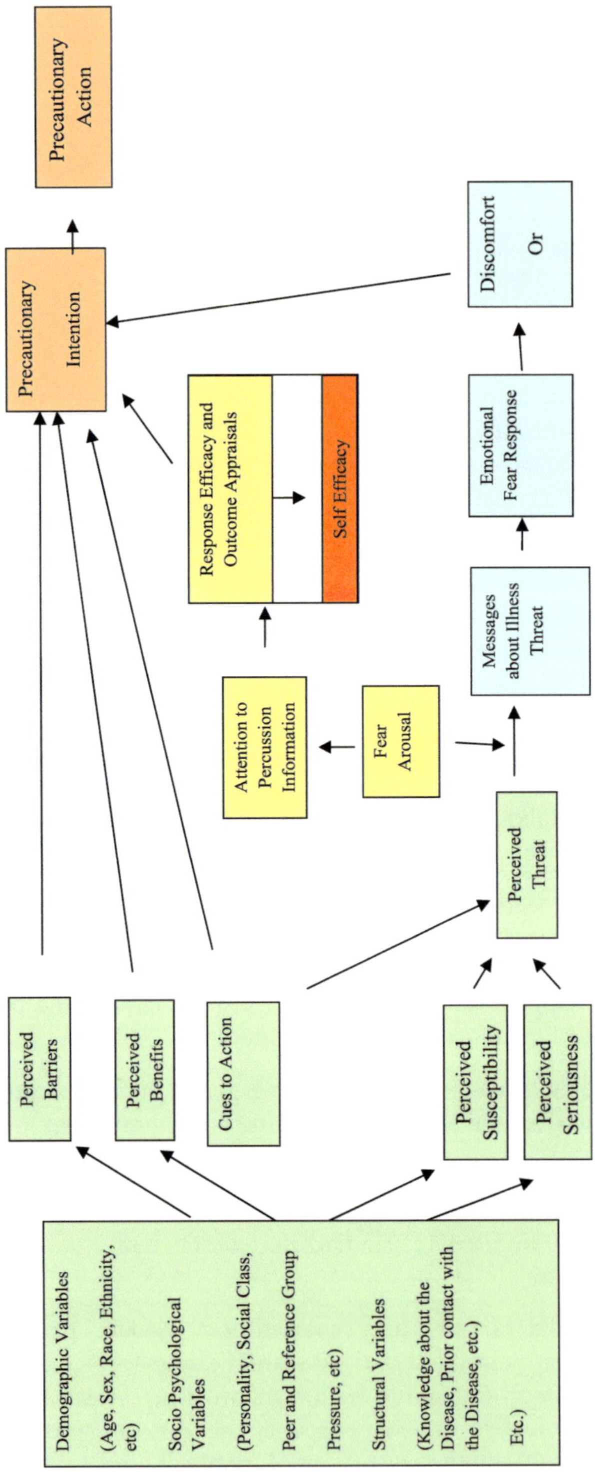

Figure 4. Expanded Health Belief Model Combined with Fear Drive Model & Fear Model

As Figure 2 represents, in this situation patients enter Leventhal's Fear Drive model and express en emotional response to fear, which develops into discomfort and tension in patients. Eventually, through the Leventhal's model patients are directed to precautionary action.

In addition, fear arousal in patients sensitized them to precautionary information, which is the same path predicted in Leventhal's model. Thus patients are placed in both Leventhal's and Ruiter's fear models. In other words, the emotional response of fear in patients leads them to response efficacy and outcome appraisal. The results show that self-efficacy in patient's increases and leads to precaution alongside discomfort or tension. These factors are eventually tantamount to precautionary action in patient.

Intended fear level in patients was set at moderate to be comparable with other studies. Fear inducement method and message type selection were inspired by previous studies using video and specific advertisements.

The results showed that 100% of diabetic patients who underwent this training model showed a significant behavior change in blood sugar control six months after the intervention. On average, patients cut down on two pills. In addition, 30% of Type II diabetes stopped using insulin and resorted only to diet and exercise to control their blood sugar. The mean number of pills in the intervention group was 3.78 at the outset, which decreased to 1.86 in six months after the intervention, which was a significant change. However, the medication in the control group increased in three months mainly due to failure to control their blood sugar. The mean level of HbA1c hemoglobin at the outset was 8.8 which decreased to 6.23 in six months with a concomitant decrease in their medication from an average number of 3.78 pills to 1.85 (mean: 1.93 pills). Moreover, insulin treatment was ceased in 30% of experimental patients. The initial average HbA1c hemoglobin in the control group was 8.2 which decreased to 7.81, which was not statistically significant though. However, the medication level in the control group significantly decreased six months after the intervention. In the intervention group, the average insulin dosage decreased from 63 units to 27.5 units within six months of the treatment, which is a significant change. However, no significant similar change was observed in the control group.(Graph1-2)

The foregoing results suggest that the new combined model intervention, consisting of three models, had a positive effect on behavior change in diabetic patients within six months of the intervention. In addition, using a stepwise multiple regression analysis we could obtain a formula to predict the effect of various variables on behavior change.

3.4. Resultant variables in the final model and their weights

After the intervention based on fear arousal , we selected 9 variables includes Health Belief Model's dimensions , knowledge and attitude, Outcome Appraisals, Response Efficacy, self-efficacy, intention, behavior maintenance, duration of affection, and satisfaction from treatment were selected to be assessed by Path Analysis method. In terms of theoretical aspects, Precautionary Intention and behavior maintenance, and in terms of practical aspects, the rate of HbAc1 were used. Five different data entry methods for the Path Analysis have been discussed in the next pages. In this part, it is intended to find the maximum association between the constructs by including or excluding a variable. Numbers on the fletchers demonstrate the Beta value, and all the associations are significant (Figure 5-9)

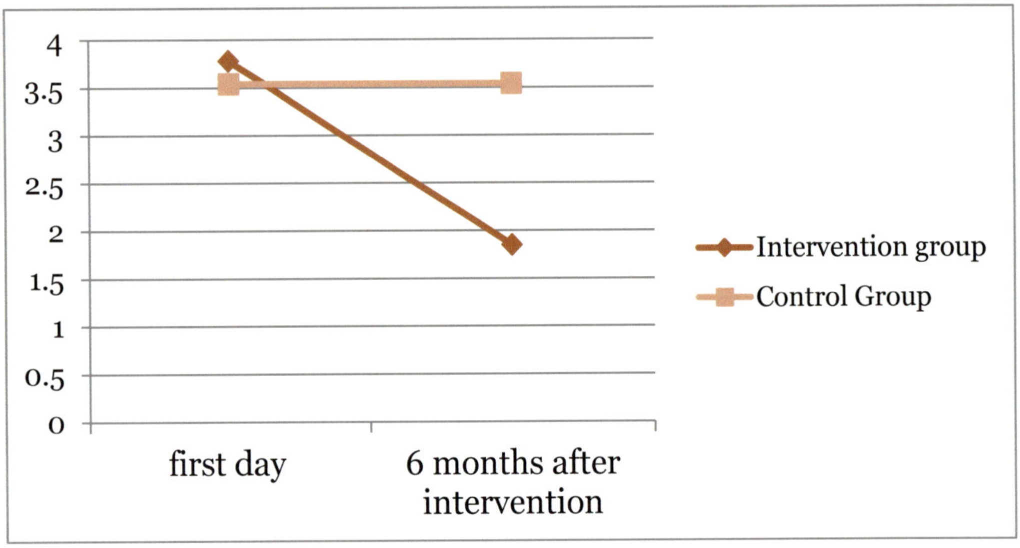

Graph 1. Mean of Metformin pills consumption by 2 groups of patients in the first day of survey and 6 months after intervention

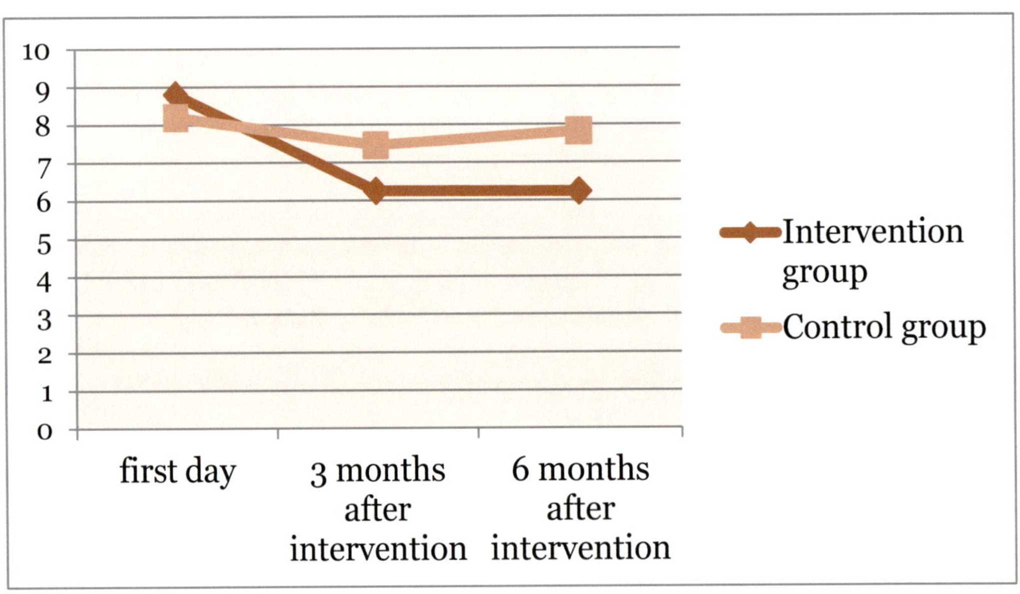

Graph 2. Mean Hba1c in 3 times: First day of the survey, 3 months after intervention, and 6 months after intervention

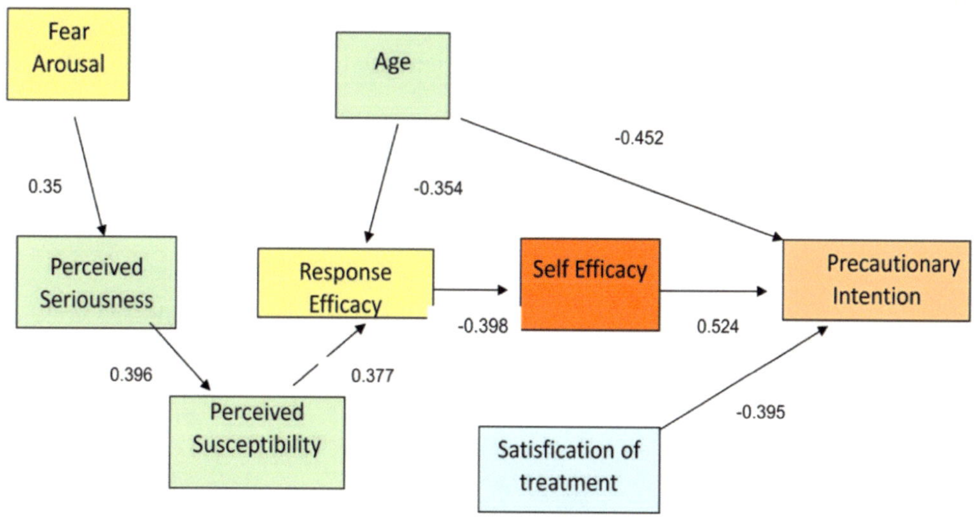

Figure 5. Path analysis for precautionary Intention based on: age, duration of diabetes, perceived benefits, perceived barriers, perceived seriousness, perceived susceptibility, response efficacy, self efficacy, satisfaction of treatment after itervention and fear arousal

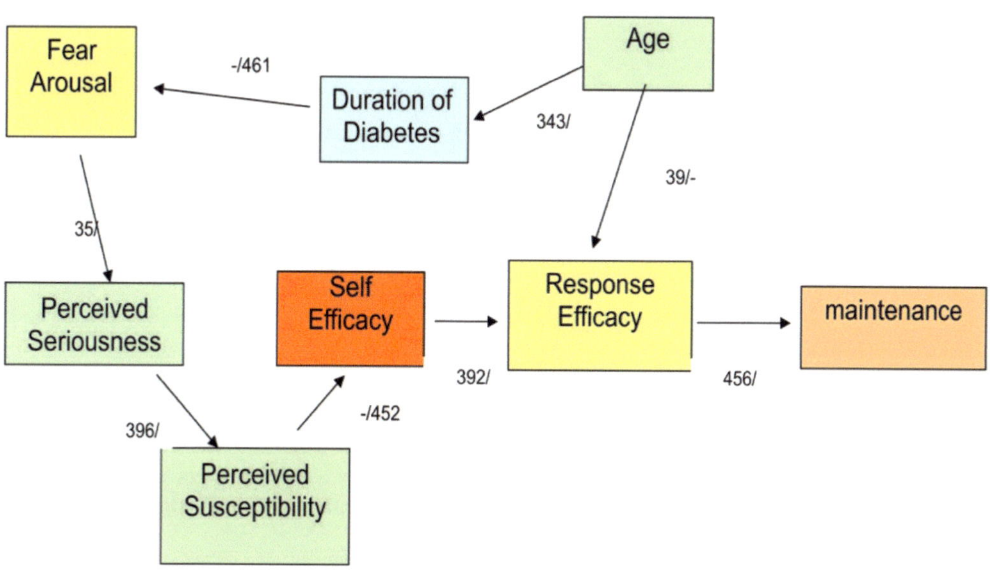

Figure 6. Path analysis for Behavioral Maintenance based on: age, duration of diabetes, perceived benefits, perceived barriers, perceived seriousness, perceived susceptibility, response efficacy, self efficacy, satisfaction of treatment after intervention and fear arousal

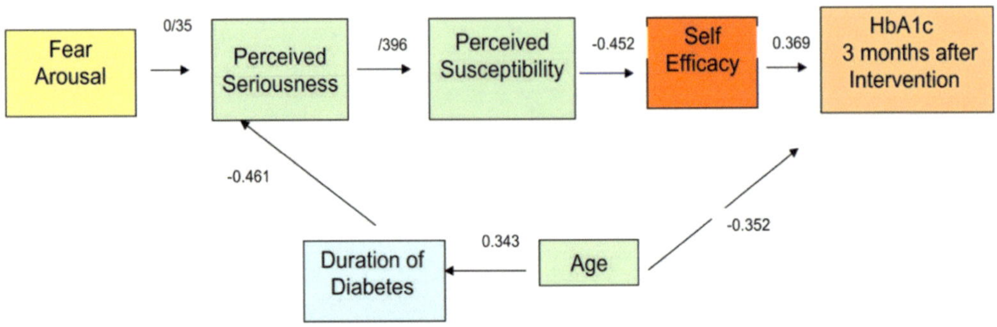

Figure 7. Path analysis for Behavioral Maintenance based on HbA1c 3 months after intervention: variables including age, duration of diabetes, perceived benefits, perceived barriers, perceived seriousness, perceived susceptibility, self efficacy, satisfaction of treatment , Knowledge, fear arousal after intervention and fear arousal

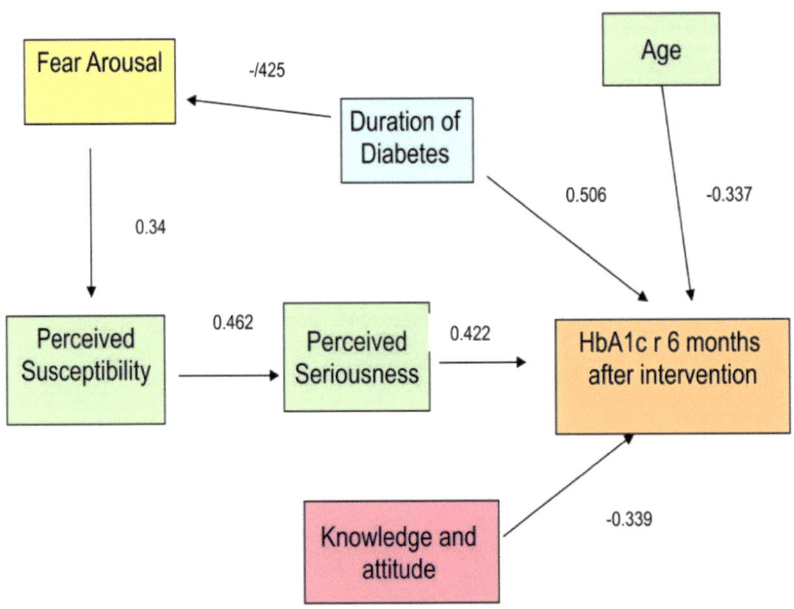

Figure 8. Path analysis for Behavioral Maintenance based on HbA1c 6 months after intervention: include 10 variables age, duration of diabetes, perceived benefits, perceived barriers, perceived seriousness, perceived susceptibility, self efficacy, satisfaction of treatment , Knowledge, fear arousal after intervention and fear arousal

After the completion of the research, which took one year, we used a path analysis to specify the role of 13 variables in maintaining behavior(Figure 9). The variables included patient age, duration of diabetes, treatment satisfaction, perceived benefits after intervention, perceived barriers after intervention, perceived susceptibility after intervention, , self-efficacy, and knowledge after intervention, fear arousal, response efficacy, and intention. In the following section, we discuss each of the foregoing variables in the final model and specify their values on the basis of the model.

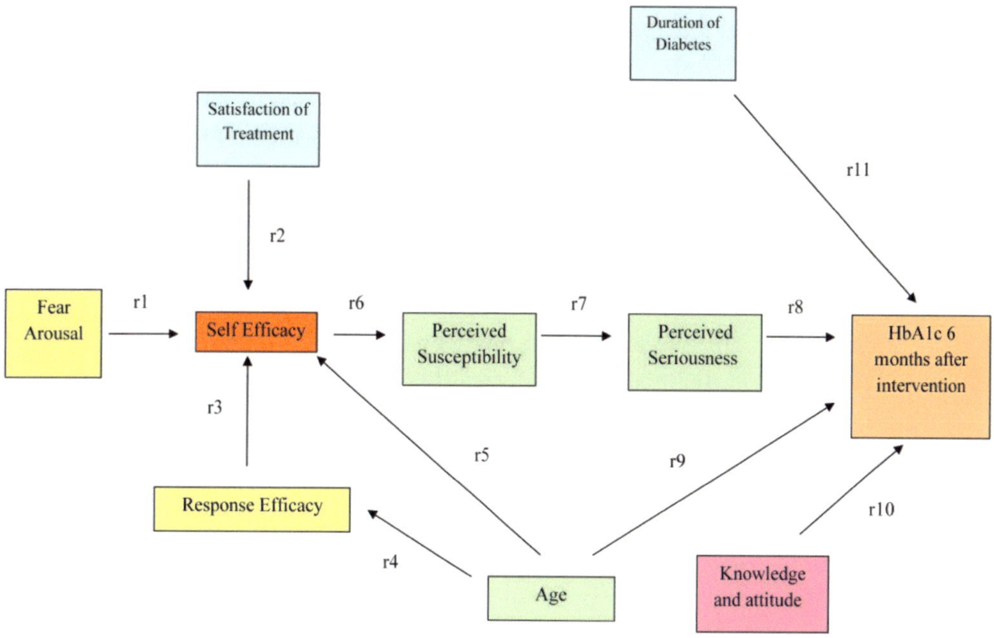

Figure 9. Path analysis for Behavioral Maintenance based on Hba1c 6 months after intervention: include 13 variables (age, duration of diabetes, perceived benefits, perceived barriers, perceived seriousness, perceived susceptibility, self efficacy, satisfaction of treatment , Knowledge, fear arousal , intention, behavioral maintenance, response efficacy after intervention and fear arousal)

According to the results of the path analysis and the initial model which was based on theoretical studies, we can observe that the principal form of the model consists of nine variables on behavior maintenance within six months of the study.

1. *Fear arousal*: This variable had a negative and direct effect on self-efficacy. We label this variable x1 and attach a value of e1 to it. This is an independent variable which is not affected by any other variable. The value of this variable is x1 = e1.
2. *Treatment satisfaction*: This variable had a positive and direct effect on self-efficacy. We label this variable x2 and assign a value of e2 to it. This is an independent variable which is not affected by any other variable. The value of this variable is x2 = e2.
3. *Response efficacy*: This variable, which is affected by age, had a positive and direct effect on self-efficacy. We label this variable x3 and attach a value of e3 to it. The value of this variable is x3 = e3+ [r4*X5].
4. *Self-efficacy*: This variable is affected by treatment satisfaction, fear arousal, age and response efficacy. We label this variable x4 and attach a value of e4 to it. The value of this variable is X4=e4+{[r1*X1]+[r2*X2]+[r3*X3]+[r5*X5}
5. *Age*: This variable, which was produced in the final model [Figure 5 in path analysis], had direct effect on self-efficacy, negative and direct effect on response efficacy and negative and direct effect on blood sugar control. We name this variable x 5 and give it

a value of e5. This is an independent variable which is not affected by any other variable. The value of this variable is x5 = e5.

6. *Perceived susceptibility*: This variable had a positive and direct effect on perceived seriousness. We label this variable x6 and assign a value of e6 to it. The value of this variable is x6 = e6+ [r6*X4].
7. *Perceived seriousness*: This variable had negative and direct effect on blood sugar control within six months of the treatment. We label this variable x7 and give it a value of e7. The value of this variable is x7 = e7+ [r7*X6].
8. *Knowledge*: This variable had positive and direct effect on blood sugar control within six months of the treatment. We label this variable x8 and give it a value of e8. This is an independent variable which is not affected by any other variable. The value of this variable is x8=e8.
9. *Duration of disease*: This variable had positive and direct effect on blood sugar control within six months of the treatment. We label this variable x9 and give it a value of e9. This is an independent variable which is not affected by any other variable. The value of this variable is x9=e9.
10. *Behavior maintenance*: This variable was affected by disease length, knowledge, patient age and perceived seriousness. We call this variable x10 and compute it as below:

$$X10= [[r9* X5] + [r8* X7] + [r10*X8] + [r11*X9]]$$

We also learn that fear arousing messages had a significant effect on behavior change, especially when they are accompanied by effective solutions, recommendations and methods (Witte et al., 2001).

4. Conclusion

With regard to the topics discussed earlier we showed that the fear box, which acts bilaterally, actually play the role of a relational bridge between the 3 models. In fact, the differentiation between fear and threat was clarified in this way in the new model. After examining the new model in practice (our study) and considering the previous studies, we can conclude that an average level fear can pave the ground for the patients to make the best decision for glycemic control.

In our study, we did not arouse a high level fear in our cases because 1)its effect disappears in the long run and/or 2) it may disappoint the hopes of patients for treatment.

Recommendations

Researchers are recommended to use the model for other chronic disorders too. Before intervention, the researcher should carefully evaluate their patients by the use of standardized questionnaires like WHOQOL, self-efficacy, self-care, self-management and etc. They should plan for fear arousal and be well prepared for proper response to patients' reactions seeking for precautionary information. After fear arousal it is better to provide the patients with the educational material he/she needs for controlling the aroused fear.

The researchers are also recommended to arrange the 2nd visit one week after fear arousal to fully meet the patient's information needs. Because during this week, the patients may receive inappropriate information which need to be corrected.

Author details

Alireza Shahab Jahanlou *
Health Education Unit, Cardiovascular Research Center,
Hormozgan University of Medical Sciences, Iran

Masoud Lotfizade
Public Healt Department, Shahre Kord University of Medical Sciences, Iran

Nader Alishan Karami
Healt Information Management Department, Hormozgan University of Medical Sciences, Iran

5. References

Alavi, N. M., Ghofranipour, F., Ahmadi, F. & Emami, A. 2007. Developing a culturally valid and reliable quality of life questionnaire for diabetes mellitus. *Eastern Mediterranean Health Journal,* 13.

Andersen, P. A. & Guerrero, L. K. 1998. *Handbook of communication and emotion : research, theory, applications, and contexts,* San Diego, Academic Press.

Austin, L. T., Ahmad, F., Mcnally, M. J. & Stewart, D. E. 2002. Breast and cervical cancer screening in Hispanic women: A literature review using the health belief model. *Womens Health Issues,* 12.

Bond, G. G., Aiken, L. S. & Somerville, S. C. 1992. The health belief model and adolescents with insulin-dependent diabetes mellitus. *Health psychology : official journal of the Division of Health Psychology, American Psychological Association,* 11.

Campbell, C. 2001. *Health Education Behavior Models and Theories-- A Review of the Literature - Part I* [Online]. Mississippi State University. Available: URL: http://msucares.com/health/health/appa1.htm [Accessed 2nd September 2012].

Clarke, J., Crawford, A. & Nash, D. B. 2002. Evaluation of a comprehensive diabetes disease management program: progress in the struggle for sustained behavior change. *Disease Management,* 5, 10.

Dewalt, D. A., Boone, R. S. & Pignone, M. P. 2007. Literacy and its relationship with self-efficacy, trust, and participation in medical decision making. *American Journal of Health Behavior,* 31.

Glanz, K., Lewis, F. M. & Rimer, B. K. 1997. *Health behavior and health education : theory, research, and practice,* San Francisco, Jossey-Bass.

Group, W. 1997. *Whoqol: measuring quality of life* [Online]. World Health Organization. [Accessed 2nd September 2012].

---

* Corresponding Author

Ishizaki, T., Imanaka, Y., Hirose, M., Hayashida, K., Kizu, M., Inoue, A. & Sugie, S. 2004. Estimation of the impact of providing outpatients with information about SARS infection control on their intention of outpatient visit. *Health Policy,* 69.

Jahanlou, A. S., Ghofranipour, F., Sobhani, A., Kimmiagar, M. & Vafaei, M. 2008. Evaluating curvilinear hypothesis in quality of life and glycemic control in diabetic patients. *Arak University of Medical Sciences Journal,* 11, 27-34.

Jahanlou, A. S., Sobhani, A. & Alishan, N. 2010. A comparison of two standard quality of life questionnaires for evaluation of the relationship between personality characteristics and glycemic control in diabetic patients. *Arak University of Medical Sciences Journal,* 13, 28-34.

Kamel, N. M., Badawy, Y. A., El-Zeiny, N. A. & Merdan, I. A. 1999. Sociodemographic determinants of management behaviour of diabetic patients. Part I. Behaviour of patients in relation to management of their disease. *Eastern Mediterranean health journal = La revue de sante de la Mediterranee orientale = al-Majallah al-ṣiḥḥiyah li-sharq al-mutawassiṭ,* 5.

Koszegi, B. 2003. Health anxiety and patient behavior. *Journal of Health Economics,* 22.

Lanyon, R. I. & Manosevitz, M. 1966. Validity of self-reported fear. *Behaviour research and therapy,* 4.

Leventhal, H., Safer, M. A. & Panagis, D. M. 1983. The impact of communications on the self-regulation of health beliefs, decisions, and behavior. *Health education quarterly,* 10.

Montazeri, A. & Mcewen, J. 1997. Effective communication: Perception of two anti-smoking advertisements. *Patient Education and Counseling,* 30.

Narayan, K. M. V., Gregg, E. W., Fagot-Campagna, A., Engelgau, M. M. & Vinicor, F. 2000. Diabetes - a common, growing, serious, costly, and potentially preventable public health problem. *Diabetes Research and Clinical Practice,* 50.

Rogers, R. W. & Mewborn, C. R. 1976. Fear appeals and attitude change: effects of a threat's noxiousness, probability of occurrence, and the efficacy of coping responses. *Journal of personality and social psychology,* 34.

Ruiter, R. A. C., Abraham, C. & Kok, G. 2001. Scary warnings and rational precautions: A review of the psychology of fear appeals. *Psychology & Health,* 16.

Ruiter, R. A. C., Verplanken, B., Kok, G. & Werrij, M. Q. 2003. The role of coping appraisal in reactions to fear appeals: Do we need threat information? *Journal of Health Psychology,* 8.

Sarkar, U., Fisher, L. & Schillinger, D. 2006. Is self-efficacy associated with diabetes self-management across race/ethnicity and health literacy? *Diabetes Care,* 29.

Task Force On Community Preventive, S. 2002. Recommendations for healthcare system and self-management education interventions to reduce morbidity and mortality from diabetes. *American journal of preventive medicine,* 22.

Witte, K. 1992. Putting the fear back into fear appeals: The extended parallel process model. *Communication Monographs,* 59, 329-349.

Witte, K., Meyer, G. & Martell, D. 2001. *Effective health risk messages : a step-by-step guide,* Thousand Oaks, Sage Publications.

Chapter 17

Development of Improved Animal Models for the Study of Diabetes

Emilia Ciobotaru

Additional information is available at the end of the chapter

http://dx.doi.org/10.5772/49985

1. Introduction

Medical research based on animal model is rightly considered a "necessary evil", being a "modus vivendi" in all research activities for more than 2,000 years. It is admitted that the major breakthroughs in medicine such as blood circulation, respiration physiology, the hormonal system used for research purpose different species of animals. In the last 150 years animals used in medical experiments brought huge benefits to humanity by providing crucial responses to the most intriguing questions about prevention and treatment of some devastating diseases. Furthermore, diseases as cancer, AIDS, malaria, tuberculosis, influenza, Alzheimer's disease and diabetes mellitus were approached by creating specific animal models with respect to pathogenesis, genetic insights and treatment. Despite to all these achievements, over the years a lot of people or organizations were and still are reluctant to animal research because this brings intolerable suffer and pain. All of those mentioned emphasized that animal models are not the only scientific methods to achieve important and reliable results. Consecutively, it was constantly sustained that animal research should be abandoned at once and further efforts should be invested in creating alternative methods. For preventing barbarity against animals which was rightly condemned in the past, new concepts were necessary to be enforced. Thus, "animal rights" (animals are granted to live a life free from abuse and exploitation which also includes prevention of use an animal for scientific research) and "animal welfare" (for the animals used in research this implies assessment of breeding, transport, housing, nutrition, disease prevention and treatment, handling and, where necessary, euthanasia) were two of the most invoked [1].

Laboratory animal welfare was first defined in *The Principles of Humane Experimental Technique* written by William Russell and Rex Burch. The essence of this work refers to the *three Rs (3Rs)*:

- *refinement:* decrease in the incidence of the severity of inhumane procedures applied to those animals used for research purpose;
- *reduction*: reduction in the number of animals used to obtain information of given amount and precision;
- *replacement*: the substitution of conscious living animals with insentient materials.

Nevertheless, the 3Rs were the subject of dispute between animal research supporters and those who are against animal experimentation. Animal welfare was consistently improved by implementing of the 3Rs, but some important issues were created in some area of medical research. For instance, validation of the alternative methods which replaces the animals, reliable results based on statistical analysis when a smaller number of animals are used or refinement of the methods for induce less pain and suffering (e.g. administration of analgesics after surgical procedures) were the most debated in the last forty years. The scientific world is still preoccupied by further implementing of the 3Rs [2, 3]. In USA, National Institute of Health stopped financing almost all new projects which use chimpanzees as the closest human's related animal model [4]. This species become nonessential due to alternative research tools and methods, this being one of the last benefits of Russell's and Burch's 3Rs.

2. Experimentally induced hyperglycemia

Hyperglycemia is one of the most important signs of diabetes mellitus, both surgical removal of the pancreas and administration of β-cell toxins being equally used. The first method has been used for the first time in a canine model designed by Oskar Minkowski and Josef von Mering. Partial or total surgical removal of the pancreas was followed by the most "popular" clinical sign of diabetes: glucosuria, body weight loss despite voracious appetite and intake of nourishing food, polyuria, polydipsia and ketonuria [5, 6]. This experiment was followed by another historical breakthrough accomplished by Frederick Banting and Charles Best. These two scientists performed a ligation of pancreas ducts to induce atrophy of exocrine acinar component and thereby to obtain a less contaminated extract of pancreatic islets. This extract succeeded to determine a substantial prolongation of life in dogs with pancreatectomy and also to save the life of a diabetic boy [7].

It is well known that the beginnings of the research in diabetes aimed as animal model the dogs and the rabbits. Later, the scientists preferred to conduct experiments in smaller animals, these being easier to manipulate and involve smaller expenses. Thus, rats and mice were subjected for pancreatectomy. This surgical procedure is challenging because of the particular anatomy of the pancreas and pancreatic ducts in this species. The rat pancreas is spread on a large anatomic area, being divided in three parts (biliary, duodenal and gastrosplenic portions). The duct system is quite polymorphic and represented by numerous independent pancreatic ducts which drain secretion from each corresponding part. The results of pancreatectomy in rat were not always followed by the rapid onset of the diabetes and do not reflect entirely the diabetes in humans, these being speculated by those who consider that larger species are more appropriate for diabetes study [8, 9].

Toxins as streptozotocin [10], alloxan [11], vacor [12], dithizone [13], and 8-hydroxyquinolone [14] were used as non surgical methods. Each toxins aim to induce various destruction of β-cells and produce diabetes and subsequent complications.

Both surgical removal of the pancreas and toxin induced diabetes are valuable methods used for studying the consequence of hyperglycemia and the onset of diabetes complications such as diabetic microangiopathy and macroangiopathy, retinopathy, neuropathy, and cardiomiopathy. Cardiomiopathy, as a complication of streptozotocin induced diabetes was revealed by gravimetric assessments and morphometry. Diabetic rats present hypertrophy of left ventricle, revealed by increased values of ventricular ratio, comparing with control group. Same groups exhibited significant increasing of heart weight/body weight ratio and liver weight/body weight ratio, comparing with control group [15]. Considering that cardiac hypertrophy is the result of potential interstitial fibrosis, thickening of arteriolar media, endothelial cells and basement membrane changes, morphometry of arteriolar media of heart arterioles and cellular density of media were assessed. Arteriolar media/diameter of arteriolar lumen was significantly bigger in rats with streptozotocin induced diabetes, this being the result of fibrosis in arteriolar media [16].

Islet cell transplantation and its consequence is one of the current research targets, being conducted on either surgical removal of the pancreas and toxin induced diabetes. Successful transplantation was achieved for the first time in 1966 in patients with diabetic nephropathy subjected for simultaneous pancreas and kidney transplantation [17]. Despite to consistent benefits of this therapeutic management, the lack of donors, the acquired chronic immunosupression, postoperative complications and graft rejection have to be considered. Thus, islet transplantation era began with two experiments in rodents previously rendered diabetic by the methods described above [17-19]. The methods of transplantation became more refined correlated with and requested by all the shortcomings resulted by immunosupression and graft rejection. Therefore, pancreatic islets graft may be transplanted as alginate or alginate-polylysine immunoisolated microcapsules [20-22], which are implanted in various anatomic sites (subcutaneously, into the splenic parenchyma, under renal capsule, into the peritoneum, into the portal vein for further colonization in the liver) [17-19, 23]. Unfortunately, the lifetime of transplanted islets is shortened by the deleterious immune reaction of the host. Without microcapsule protection and immunosuppressive treatment, islets transplanted into the liver are immediately surrounded by thrombi placed into the vessels of the surrounding tissue. Allogeneic islets from liver and spleen present lymphocytic infiltrations in 2 days after transplantation and are destroyed rapidly by the host [24].

Diabetic rodents are frequently used in research concerning pharmaceutical compounds aimed to lower the level of glycemia in diabetic persons. New formulas are previously tested on diabetic rodents in order to estimate efficacy, and potential toxic effect on the patients.

3. Experimentally induced glycosuria

Phlorizin is an organic compound, member of chalcone class, extracted for the first time from the bark of the apple tree. The compound was also isolated from roots bark, shoots, leaves and fruits, proving that phlorizin is usually ingested by humans. It was observed that ingestion of more than 1g of phlorizin is followed by glycosuria. Knowing that diabetes mellitus expresses urinary symptoms such as glucosuria and polyuria, an important correlation has been made between these symptoms and the effect of phlorizin. Chronic administration in dog was followed by glucosuria, polyuria and weight loss, creating this way an obvious resemblance between human spontaneous diabetes mellitus and phlorizin effect [25]. Diabetic rats treated with phlorizin express values of glycemia almost equal with normal parameter. This model was used to clarify the implication of hyperglycemia in the progression of islet lesions. The results proved that chronic hyperglycemia might have no effect of islets histopathological changes [26].

4. Chemically induced insulin dependent diabetes mellitus – animal models

Considering that insulin dependent diabetes mellitus (IDDM) features the immune-mediated destruction of β-cells and subsequent insulinopaenia, animal models which reproduce damage of pancreatic islets have been created. For this purpose, streptozotocin and alloxan induced diabetes mellitus were considered the handiest manners to create this condition, although naturally, β-cells become dysfunctional after a long period without evident clinical signs. Streptozotocin and alloxan are diabetogenic chemicals, both being framed in the group of glucose analogues. The onset of β-cells destruction is induced via different mechanisms. Alloxan was the first used as a toxic agent against β-cells, its ability being to generate both reactive oxygen species (ROS) and inhibition of glucose mediated insulin secretion through glucokinase blockage. During the destructive process, β-cells express reversible transformation of cytoplasmic organelles (cytoplasmic vacuolization, dilation of rough endoplasmic reticulum, reduced Golgi apparatus, scattered insulin content secretory granules and swollen mitochondria) finalizing with irreversible damaging of DNA (TUNEL positive staining of β-cells nuclei) [11]. Streptozotocin has antibiotic and chemotherapeutic properties, being isolated from *Streptomyces achromogenes*. The main action of streptozotocin is focused on β-cells DNA via alkylation process. Finally, DNA methylation results into the fragmentation and ultimately generates cell death [11, 14, 27]. Streptozotocin diabetes mellitus can be induced via a single large dose or multiple low doses administration. It is possible that the first option to induce diabetes because of direct toxic effect of streptozotocin, while, low doses repeatedly administrated may exert blockage of insulin secretion [14].

Other diabetogenic compounds were used in experimental models such as dithizone [28]. Administration of this chelator in rabbit has a particular effect expressed as initial hyperglycemia after 2 hours, followed by normoglycemia in 8 hours and finalized by permanent hyperglycemia due to degranulation of β-cells [29].

5. Spontaneous IDDM based on animal models

The non-obese diabetic (NOD) mouse (table 1) is a spontaneous IDDM animal model. This was spontaneously obtained in one of two sublines derived from CTS mice (Immune Deficiency of Cataract Shionogi). The diabetic line was established after six generations of breeding [30]. About 20% of males and 80% of females develop type 1 diabetes mellitus around 30 weeks of age in particular environment (the incidence of diabetes is higher in colonies maintained in relatively germ-free conditions). The lesions of Langerhans islets are expressed as insulitis, the onset of insulinopaenia being recorded in 12-week-old females. Polyuria, polydipsia, hyperglycemia, glucosuria and hypercholesterolemia are the main clinical signs [30, 31]. Daily administration of insulin improves consistently the body weight and life span, although the mice can survive for weeks without insulin supplement. It is noteworthy that the low level of insulin in NOD mice is correlated with increase secretion of glucagon in treatead and non-treated with insulin individuals. Thus, is concluded that insulin deficiency and glucagon hypersecretion might have an important role in the development and clinical progress of diabetes in NOD mice [32]. Pinealectomy in newborn mice is followed by a more rapid onset of diabetes in female and supplementary melatonin administration protects the animals. The results are somehow intriguing, knowing that melatonin induces increase of insulin autoantibodies [33]. NOD mice are prone to develop autoimmune inflammations, especially those with anti-diabetogenic MHC haplotype and programmed death cell deficiency (sialadenitis of submandibular gland, thyroiditis, gastritis, vasculitis of renal arteries, neuritis) [34-36]. The most important studies which have been run on NOD mice targeted gene implication, MHC genes class II having an important role. Also, knowing that NOD mouse develop cell immune mediated diabetes, many of the experiments aim to picture the immunological status which is responsible for the onset of diabetes [37, 38]. It is important to bear in mind that diabetes in NOD mice is not only the result of cell mediated immunity but also of humoral factors as GAD and IgM [39].

Akita mouse ($Ins2^{Akita}$) was obtained from a spontaneous point mutation in a female of C57BL/6 line. This mutation disrupts normal synthesis of insulin via incapacity to produce and secrete mature insulin. Clinical signs of diabetes are clearly expressed in male, comparing with female. Heterozygous mutant mice present hyperglycemia, hypoinsulinemia, polydipsia and polyuria. The mice are lean and do not present insulitis. Pancreatic islets exhibit decreased density of β-cells and decreased density of secretory granules in the existing β-cells, increase amount of endoplasmic reticulum and swollen mitochondria [40]. Progressive diabetic retinopathy begins around 12 weeks of age after the onset of hyperglycemia and is consistent with increased vascular permeability, morphological abnormalities of astrocytes and microglia, apoptosis and thinning of inner layer of the retina [41]. Heterozygous $Ins2^{Akita}$ are suited for allogeneic and xenogeneic islet transplantation, because it provides a biological status free of unwanted toxic effect of streptozotocin and alloxan and without β-cell autoimmunity [42].

BB (bio breeding) rat also known as BBDP (bio-breeding diabetes prone) rat is an inbred laboratory rodent which spontaneously develops IDDM. The animals between 2 and 4 months of age develop spontaneous hyperglycemia, different degrees of mononuclear infiltration of the pancreatic islets or total loss of β-cells, insulinopaenia and ketogenesis [43-45]. The overt diabetes can be reversed in 36% of diabetic rats when BB/Worchester (BB/W) are treated with rabbit anitiserum to rat lymphocytes. These results highlight that diabetes mellitus in BB rats is a cell-mediated autoimmune disease [46]. Destruction of β-cells is performed

Rodents	**Mouse**	Non-obese diabetic (NOD) mouse Akita mouse
	Rat	BB/BBDP Long Evans Tokushima Lean (LETL) Komeda Diabetes Prone (KDP)
	Rabbit	New Zealand White Rabbit
	Hamster	Chinese hamster (*Cricetulus griseus*)
Dog		Keeshond dog

Table 1. Animal models for insulin dependent diabetes mellitus

by a cohort of immune cells such as T and B-lymphocytes, macrophages and natural killer cells [38, 47]. The BB/Worchester diabetic rats may develop lymphocytic thyroiditis in individuals between 8 and 10 months of age [48]. The onset of diabetes in BB rats is attributable to many genes, the most important being those which trigger the age of the onset of diabetes, diabetes susceptibility, severity of islet infiltration with inflammatory cells and islet atrophy [49].

As an overview of either differences or resemblances between NOD mouse, BB rats and human IDDM data are presented in table 2 [50].

Characteristics	**Human**	**NOD mice**	**BB rats**
Genetic predisposition (MHC class II)	yes	yes	yes
Genetic control	polygenic	polygenic	polygenic
Haemopoietic stem cell transfer	yes	yes [50]	yes [50]
Lymphocytic insulitis (with T-lymphocytes)	yes	yes	yes
Lymphocytic infiltrates in other organs	sometimes	yes	yes
Humoral reactivity to β-cells	yes	yes [39]	no
Diabetic ketoacidosis (without treatment)	yes	mild	yes
Detection of retroviral antigens expressed in beta cells	no	yes [51]	no
Sex predisposition	no	yes	no

Table 2. Comparative overview in human, NOD mouse and BB IDDM

Long Evans Tokushima Lean (LETL). An outbred colony of Long-Evans rats developed spontaneously remarkable signs attributable to diabetes (polyuria, polyphagia, and polydipsia). This line has been maintained since 1983 in Tokushima Research Institute (Otsuka Pharmaceutical, Yokushima, Japan) and generated another line (Long Evans Tokushima Lean - LETL). LETL rats present no sex predilection concerning the onset of the disease or severity, sudden onset of the diabetes expressed as hyperglycemia, polyuria, polydipsia and weight loss, lymphocytic insulitis at 120-220 days of age followed by the destruction of β-cells, normal levels of T-lymphocytes, lymphocytic infiltration of salivary and lacrimal glands [52, 53].

Komeda Diabetes Prone (KDP) rat is a substrain of LETL, all the individuals presenting moderate to mild insulitis around 220 days of age. The onset of diabetes is 70% at 120 days and 82% within 220 days. This strain present a major IDDM susceptibility gene named

Iddm/kdp1 placed on chromosome 11. Homozigous alleles at this locus are strongly linked with the capacity to develop moderate or severe insulitis [54-56]

New Zealand White Rabbit developed spontaneous diabetes mellitus for the first time in a female in 1969. By inbreeding this female and her offspring, a diabetic line was obtained. The overt diabetes was diagnosed in 19% of animals aged between 1 and 3 years. The diabetic animals present fasting hyperglycemia, hypoinsulinemia and absent ketoacidosis [57]. The lesions of β-cells are expressed as cytoplasmic hypergranulation, this being different comparing with previous animal models featured by insulitis, islet atrophy, degranulation of β-cells. It was postulated that the lesion is the consequence of a secretion defect. In addition, diabetic rabbits present mineral deposits in kidney, particularly in basement membrane of the tubules and Bowman capsules and into the lining cells of proximal convoluted tubules [58, 59].

Certain lines of *Keeshond dog* may develop inherited IDDM expressed as overt diabetes around 2-6 months of age. The dogs have low level of insulin as a consequence of β-cells aplasia. In addition, glucagon secretion is also depressed. The dogs can survive 2-4 months without insulin supplement. Concurrent lesions such as cataracts, skin infections and poor bodily growth are observed. The incidence of diabetes is higher in females. The fertility in diabetic individuals is very low, non-diabetic dogs being used to obtain diabetic offspring. An autosomal recessive disorder is consistent with the onset of diabetes. Keeshond dogs are suitable for studying long term complications of diabetes [60, 61].

Chinese hamster (Cricetulus griseus) has become the subject of research in diabetes mellitus as an animal model since 1959 [62]. The incidence of diabetes in Chinese hamster sublines is more than 85%. At the time of birth, the pups are prediabetic. The overt diabetes range from mild to severe and it is characterized by polyphagia, hyperglycemia, severe polyuria, glucosuria and elevated gluconeogenesis. β-cells present degranulation and hydropic degeneration [63-65]. Other morphologic changes occur in kidneys (glomerulosclerosis), brain (vascular lesions expressed as duplication and thickening of the basement membrane, degeneration in either dendrites or axons, focal demyelination and synaptic degeneration) [66], exocrine pancreas (pancreatic adenoma and adenocarcinoma) [67], teeth (periodontal disease) [68], and macroangiopathy of the thoracic aorta [69]. Genetic defects are responsible for the onset of diabetes, four autosomal recessive genes being involved [70]. Chinese hamster with IDDM have an impaired humoral antibody response similar to that developed in human diabetes, which makes it suitable for research concerning the consequence of diabetes mellitus induced by impaired immune response [71], as well as for diabetic nephropathy [72].

6. Animal models of non-insulin dependent diabetes mellitus (NIDDM)

NIDDM is generated by the failure of β-cells to adapt to a more challenging conditions created by insulin resistance, this being induced by over-nutrition and lack of physical exercises. Mechanisms as oxidative stress, islet amyloidosis, glucotoxicity and lipotoxicity were associated with inappropriate secretory behavior of β-cells. Autoimmune attack and islet inflammation considered previously as a hallmark for IDDM, is now associated with

NIDDM. This concept is sustained by the fact that all mentioned mechanisms may initiate inflammation or are initiated by the inflammation. One of the reasons is that human pancreatic islets release IL-1β as response to glucotoxicity. The inflamation is somehow blocked in the initial stages for allowing β-cell regeneration. The more necrosis and apoptosis become obvious, the more infiltration with inflammatory cells (e.g. macrophages) are seen in pancreatic islets [73, 74].

Creation of animal models of NIDDM needs to meet the heterogeneous background which features human condition. Roughly, the animals have to express insulin resistance, impaired insulin secretion in the condition of fasting or post-challenge hyperglycemia. On the other hand the existent animal models present as dominant at least one characteristic: some animals are insulin resistant, other express mainly glucose intolerance as a part of obesity, others express NIDDM because of a particular sensitivity to dietary components. The animal models used for research in NIDDM present an important diversity, although mice and rats are constantly preferred (table 2).

Rodents	Mouse	Obese	ob/ob mouse db/db mouse KK mouse NZO mouse NONcNZO10 mouse NSY mouse TH mouse TSOD mouse M16 mouse CBA/ca mouse	Gene mutation
		Diet induced	C57/BL 6J mouse	Diet-gene interaction
	Rat	Obese	ZDF rat Wistar fatty rat OLETF rat SHR/NIH-cp	Gene mutation
		Non-obese	GK rat Torii rat	Gene mutation
		Diet induced	Cohen diabetic rat Israeli sand rat Nile rat	Diet-gene interaction
Pig [75]		-	Yucatan minipig Göttingen minipigs Sinclair minipigs Yorkshire and Yorkshire crossed strains Chinese Guizhou minipig Ossabaw minipigs Familial hypercholesterolemic pigs Low-birth-weight pigs	Cardiovascular complications
Cat [76]		-	Shorthaired males	Islet amyloidosis
Monkey [77]		-	Non human primates	Islet amyloidosis

Table 3. Animal models for NIDDM

Ob/Ob mouse was created in Jackson Laboratories in 1949 and resulted from mutation on both obese (ob) genes [78]. The main characteristic of this mutant is the uncontrolled appetite which results rapidly in the onset of obesity and NIDDM around 11 weeks of age. Polyphagia in ob/ob mouse is generated by ob genes mutations which also encode leptine. This hormone is synthesized by adipose tissue and has an important role in appetite downregulation and regulation of body weight. Leptin is absent in obese mice, the treatment with this monomer lowers consistently the food intake and body weight and also improve up to normal the plasma levels of glucose and insulin [79]. Persistent mild hyperglycemia is linked with 60% enlargement of pancreatic islets and subsequent hyperinsulinemia comparing with lean mice. Interestingly, β-cell from obese mice secretes insulin at a lower threshold of glucose that lean mice [80]. High level of plasma insulin may result from metabolic alteration of β-cells that leads to insulin overproduction or is the consequence of the heterogeneity in glucose sensitivity of these cells. Increased concentration of glucose is followed by recruitment of new β-cells with increased glucose sensitivity [81]. Infertility is a current feature in obese mouse, this being supported by fatty degeneration of the ovaries, follicular atresia, damaged mitochondria and apoptosis of the ovocytes [82]. Many studies have been run in ob/ob mice such as amelioration of insulin resistance [83], hypoglycemic effects of some polysaccharids [84, 85] and complication of NIDDM as diabetic cardiomiopathy [86] and peripheral neuropathy [87].

Db/db mouse is a diabetic mutant mouse created in Dunn Nutritional Laboratory, Cambridge, United Kingdom in 1966. Particularly, this mutant expresses a mutation on db gene which encodes the leptin receptor [88]. Thus, leptin signaling in the hypothalamus is absent leading to persistent high levels of both insulin and leptin. The mouse becomes obese around 4-6 weeks of age and develops progressively high levels of plasma insulin and glucose. All characteristic clinical signs are recorded: polyuria, polydipsia, polyphagia, proteinuria, and glucosuria. One of the most intriguing aspects is that the mice of some strains maintain hyperinsulinemia despite severe depletion of β-cells. This can be attributed to stem cells differentiation from pancreatic ducts. Body weight and insulin levels begin to decrease in association with β-cell degeneration when the mouse reaches 5-6 months of age. The cause of death remains unclear, although the mice present ketonuria, hematuria and gastrointestinal hemorrhages in terminal stage [89]. Db/db mouse has a long history in comparative research to human diabetes. Thus, human dietary habits were reproduced in db/db mouse. High lipid and cholesterol reach diet induce dyslipidemia and create similarities with the patients with type 2 diabetes mellitus [90]. Furthermore, diabetic nephropathy in db/db mice is consistent with some features encountered in human diabetic nephropathy such as renal hypertrophy, glomeruli enlargement, albuminuria, and mesangial matrix expansion [91].

KK mouse history began in 1957, this line being derived from numerous strains of Japanese native mice. Later, after many inbreeding procedures, Nakamura obtained KK mouse strain, which was a polygenic model, spontaneously diabetic and named after the region where the strain was founded (Kasukabe in Saitama prefecture) [92]. The KK mice become obese once with the onset of adulthood and develop insulin resistance, subsequent hyperinsulinemia and β-cell hyperplasia. Particularly, KK mice present a chemical diabetic stage preceded by prediabetes stage accompanied by renal, neurological and retinal complications [93]. The severity of diabetes is strongly correlated with environmental factors such as diet, food intake and social isolation of the animals, the chemical diabetic state being replaced with overt diabetes [94, 95]. Diabetes and obesity in KK mouse has a moderate expression. Introduction of A^y allele creates a new line (KK- A^y) which present enhanced pathophysiological characteristics especially for glucose intolerance [96].

New Zealand obese (NZO) mouse is a polygenic animal model which is prone to express obesity, insulin resistance, glucose intolerance and also autoimmunity featured by perturbation of splenic lymphocyte function and IgM antibodies to insulin receptor. These characteristics are concomitant with poor breeding performance due to ovarian degeneration [97] and diabetic nephropathy expressed as glomerular proliferation, mesangial deposits, mild thickening of basement membrane, glomerular eosinophilic nodules and glomerulosclerosis [98-100]. There are research which concluded that the obesity develops independently to dietary content, the onset of diabetes being recorded earlier in mice fed with carbohydrates and fat reach diet [101]. Other studies emphasized that obesity in NZO individuals is the results of hyperphagia and low energy expenditure due to insufficient physical activity [102].

NONcNZO10 mouse is a recombinant congenic new strain of NIDDM developed by introgressing 5 genomic intervals containg NZO/H1Lt (NZO) diabetogenic quantitative trait loci onto non-obese non-diabetic (NON/Lt or NON) genetic background [103]. Particularly, these mice do not express polyphagia, morbid obesity, poor fertility and variable frequency of hyperglycemia as their parental NZO males do. NONcNZO10 males are normophagic, moderately obese and exhibit normal fertility. NONcNZO10 males become hyperglycemic in 12-20 weeks of age and present atrophy of pancreatic islets and hepatic lipidosis. The resemblance between NONcNZO10 mice and human obesity/diabetes syndrome in higher than ob/ob and db/db mice because of lack of hyperphagia, normal levels of leptin and leptin signaling, normal thermoregulation and lack of hypercorticism [104].

Nagoya-Shibata-Yasuda (NSY) mouse is a spontaneous model of NIDDM, having the same ancestor with NOD mouse (Jcl ICR line). Surprisingly, three major loci contributing to susceptibility to NIDDM in the NSY mouse presented overlapping with the region where susceptibility genes for IDDM have been mapped in NOD mouse. It was postulated that some responsible genes for the onset of diabetes come from the same ancestor genes which express IDDM phenotype in NOD mice and NIDDM in NSY mice [105]. Age and sex related onset of diabetes is the most prominent characteristic for NSY mice. Males develop diabetes at 48 weeks of age as mild obesity and mild hyperinsulinemia. The impaired insulin secretion via glucose challenge is observed after 24 weeks of age. There were no morphological changes in pancreatic islets in NSY mice at any age, these findings suggesting that defective secretion of β-cells may be one of the causes in NIDDM in the NSY mouse. Fasting hyperinsulinemia may contribute to the pathogenesis of diabetes in NSY mouse, insulin sensitivity being under genetic control of *Nidd2nsy* and *Nidd3nsy* genes. Genetic analysis of NSY identified a specific gene mutation of *Tcf2* responsible for encoding hepatocyte nuclear factor 1β (HNF-1β) and implicated in MODY pathogenesis [106, 107]. Spontaneous amyloidosis was reported in old individuals, deposits being remarked mainly in kidneys, but also in the different segments of digestive system, lung, heart and adrenal glands [108]. NSY mice as well as ob/ob mice prove recently to be the source of creating of new animal models for simultaneous development and research of Allzheimer's disease and NIDDM [109].

TallyHo (TH) mouse is a relatively new NIDDM animal model, reported for the first time in 2001. The mice present obesity, hyperinsulinemia, hyperlipidemia and male-limited hyperglycemia, insulin resistance and glucose intolerance. It has been postulated that female diabetes resistance is the consequence of estrogens which enhance hepatic insulin sensitivity [110]. The genome wide scan proves polygenic involvement and also additional gene-gene interactions to express hyperglycemic phenotype [111]. Comparing with ob/ob and db/db mice, which present severe obesity attributable to leptin synthesis and leptin receptor deficiencies respectively, TH has normal levels of this hormone and also intact leptin signaling. Carbohydrates and fat reach diet enhance the levels of leptin and also the other specific features of NIDDM [112]. The treatment with leptin results in decreased glucose-stimulated insulin secretion, which demonstrate that letin plays an important role in initiation of glucose intolerance in TH mice [113]. Both males and females develop early moderate hyperplasia and hypertrophy of pancreatic islets, but only the males continue these lesions with β-cell degranulation, discrete vacuolization, different degrees of islet atrophy and fibrosis [114]. Vascular dysfunction occurs in TH mice, expressed mainly in aorta, carotid arteries and cerebral arterioles as a consequence of PGH2/TxA2 receptor activation and cytochrome p450 products and oxidative stress and elevated activity of Rho kinase, respectively [115, 116].

Tsumura Suzuki obese diabetic (TSOD) mouse resulted from inbreeding procedure of ddY strain. The diabetic line includes only moderate obese males with polyphagia, polydipsia, glucosuria, hyperglycemia, hyperinsulinemia, and hyperlipidemia. Pancreatic islets exhibit hypertrophy and hyperplasia, without any signs of insulitis or islet fibrosis [117]. Diabetic nephropathy is consistent with thickened basement membrane of the glomeruli and increased mesangial area. Peripheral neuropathy involves both sensitive and motor nerves and expresses high resemblance with human counterpart. The most prominent lesions of the nerve are decreased density of nervous fibers due to endoneurial fibrosis, degeneration of myelin sheath, intralamellar edema and remyelination, total destruction of lamellar structure associated with macrophage invasion around and into the myelin sheath [118]. Insulin resistance in TSOD mouse is probably induced, at least partially, by a decreased GLUT 4 translocation by insulin in skeletal muscles and adipose tissue [119].

M16 mouse is a new obese animal model created in Institute of Cancer Research, London, UK. Both male and female express early onset of a moderate obesity due to hyperphagia and have high levels of insulin, leptin and cholesterol. The diabetic phenotype of M16 permits research of obesity/diabetes syndrome with early onset as it recorded in human population as a current tendency [120].

CBA/Ca mouse diabetes is recorded only in 10-20% of males. The incidence can be enhanced by inbreeding. Hyperphagia, obesity, hyperglycemia, glucose intolerance, hyperinsulinemia, hypertriglyceridemia occur around 12-16 week of age. Pancreatic islets are hypertrophied, with increased insulin content that persist up to 48 weeks of age. The islet degeneration as a prove of β-cell exhaustion does not appear in this mouse [121, 122].

Zucker diabetic fatty rats (ZDF rats) resulted from inbred as well as outbred lines of rats, which maintain hyperglycemia and glucose intolerance featuring NIDDM. The scientist Lois M. Zucker and Theodore F. Zucher created in 1961 a line of rats which express a gene responsible for the onset of obesity (fatty gene/fa). Usually these rats are not hyperglycemic and present leptine-receptor deficiency, although both male and female express some parameters attributable to insulin resistance. The original colony began spontaneously to present hyperglycemia and glucose intolerance in some bucks and does. These individuals were the founders of the Zucker diabetic fatty rats. ZDF rats develop hyperglycemia with concomitant β-cell death. Compensatory proliferation is maintained as long as plasma glucose levels remain moderate [123-125]. Subsequent exhaustion of β-cells is followed by an increased rate of apoptosis [126]. Lipotoxicity is also considered as a potential cause of β-cell population reduction. Thus, elevated lipogenesis prior to, or in association with hyperglycemia results in excessive accumulation of fatty acid into the β-cell cytoplasm [127]. ZDF rats are frequently used in comparative studies with non-diabetic fatty rats and lean ZDF.

Besides the ZDF rats, other strains have been created, all receiving fa-gene from Zucker rats. *Wistar fatty rats* (fa/fa) resulted from mating of Zucker with Wistar-Kyoto individuals. The rats from this line are obese, and present hyperlypidemia, hyperinsulinemia and insulin resistance. Wistar fatty rats are prone to develop hypertrophy of pancreatic islets and degranulation of β-cells. The symptoms of diabetes have been observed only in males [125].

Otsuka Long-Evans Tokushima fatty (OLETF) rat resulted from an outbred colony of Long-Evans rats which spontaneously develop polyuria, polydipsia and mild obesity. The onset of hyperglycemia occurs in male and relatively late comparing with other lines (after 18 weeks of age). Particularly, OLETF rats present a specific diabetogenic gene associated with X-chromosome Implication of testosterone is considered to have an important influence in the onset of diabetes in male. This feature is sustained also by the administration of estrogen in castrated males which suppress or delay diabetes. The lesions of pancreatic islets begin with discrete lymphocytic infiltration, followed by the second stage expressed as islet hyperplasia with or without fibrosis in or around the islets and final stage represented by islet atrophy [128, 129]. OLETF are prone to develop diabetic nephropathy, some features of this complication comparable with human diabetes being recorded (diffuse glomerulosclerosis, thickening of basement membrane, PAS-positive deposits in the mesangium or capillaries). Mesangial lesions might express some nodular aspect similar but not identical with specific Kiemmelstiel-Wilson lesions [130].

Spontaneously Hypertensive rat/National Institute of Health-cp (SHR/NIH-cp) was created in Bethesda Maryland USA and associates obesity, NIDDM and hypertension. This rat presents a homozygous genotype for corpulent gene (cp/cp). The males are early hyperphagic and become obese and express hyperglycemia, impaired glucose tolerance, hyperinsulinemia, insulin resistance, high plasma levels of cholesterol and triglycerides, hyperleptinemia and mild essential hypertension [131].

JCR/LA-cp rat (James C. Russel/LA-cp rat) was reported in 1984 as a homozygous genotype for cp gene which develops hyperphagia, obesity, insulin resistance, hyperinsulinemia, glucose intolerance, hyperlipidemia and leptin receptor deficiency. Obese males also manifest cardiovascular lesions such as atherosclerosis and myocardial lesions. Hyperinsulinemia is caused by β-cell hyperplasia followed by islet hypertrophy and fibrosis [132]. Pharmacological researches use this animal model to determine the effectiveness of anti-obesity compounds and also to evaluate long-term benefit to prevent atherosclerosis [133-135]

Goto Kikazaki rat (*GK*) is one of the polygenic non-obese models of NIDDM which exhibit high resemblances with human condition, especially on hormonal, metabolic and vascular disorders. The line was founded in Japan (Tohoku University in 1975) based on selective repeated inbreeding of non-diabetic Wistar-Kyoto rats with minor glucose intolerance. Diabetes became overt and stable after 30 generations. Despite minor differences between subcolonies of GK, common characteristics were noticed such as decreased β-cell mass, moderate and stable hyperglycemia in adults, hepatic and peripheric insulin resistance and polyuria. Defective function and morphology of pancreatic islets was recorded since embryonic and fetal period featured by reduction of β-cell mass and insulin levels [136-138]. The complications of diabetes in GK rats refer to nephropathy (significant enhancement of kidney weight, glomerular volume, basement membrane thickness, mesangial fraction and total mesangial volume) [139], peripheral neuropathy [140, 141], diabetic osteopathy (trabecular osteopaenia) [142] and diabetic retinopathy (reduction of retinal blood flow, pericytes ghosts, acellular capillaries, increased production of vascular endothelial growth factor) [143, 144].

Spontaneously Diabetic Torii (SDT) rat has been developed from Sprague-Dawley rats in 1997 in Research Laboratories of Torii Pharmaceutical, Ohnodai, Chiba, Japan. This rat is particularly characterized by non-obese, sex related onset of NIDDM with insulin hyposecretion and severe diabetic retinopathy. The males develop glucosuria around 20 weeks of age. All males are diabetic by 40 weeks, while only 33% of female rats present diabetes even by 65 weeks of age. Glucose intolerance is noticed in 16-week-old individuals and continues with the onset of hyperglycemia, hypoinsulinemia, long-term survival without insulin treatment and hypertriglyceridemia. Fibrosis of pancreatic islets and ocular lesions such as hypermature cataract, hemorrhages in anterior chamber, tractional retinal detachment and subsequent retinal fibrovascular proliferation are the most important histopathological findings in SDT rats [145, 146]. The attempt to clarify the genetic basis of diabetes in SDT rats succeeded to identify seven quantitative trait loci which affect the levels of plasma glucose and one for body weight. One of them (*Dmsdt1*) have particular involvement in islet inflammation and fibrosis. It was suspected that this gene might also have implication in retinal lesions [147].

Cohen diabetic rat (CD) is a particular experimental model for study in NIDDM, which make it distinctive comparing with the other models presented. Diet-induced diabetes correlated with a genetic sensitivity is truly considered the most prominent feature of this rat, although it is still unclear which of the dietary components are responsible for the onset of the diabetes. It was observed that CD rats become overtly diabetic when their diet has a high-sucrose low copper content. In addition with diet profile, a sex predilection can be observed: male record a lower growth rate and more severe glucose intolerance than female. CD rats fed with diabetogenic diet do not express obesity or hyperlipidemia [148]. Other studies concluded that high-casein low copper diet is responsible for the onset of the diabetes. This result is based on genetic analysis, a gene (*Ica1*) being associated with diabetes and bovine casein. Routine histopathological investigation reveals intact pancreas islets and replacement of exocrine acini with adipose tissue. Degeneration of exocrine pancreas remains intact when diabetogenic diet is replaced with a regular one [149]. CD rats develop early hyperinsulinemia and insulin resistance, followed by the exhaustion of β-cells and hypoinsulinemia. The most common complications are diabetic retinopathy and nephropathy [150, 151].

The Israeli sand rat (Psammomys obesus) is a terrestrial mammal, being mostly found in the desert area of North Africa and Middle East. The sand rat is another experimental model for diet induced NIDDM. The high resemblance with human condition derives from distribution of adipose tissue into the subcutaneous and visceral compartments. This animal readily becomes obese when the diet from the natural habitat is replaced with usual laboratory rat chow. It was suspected but not proved yet that some components from the natural diet might have hypoglycemic effect. Thus, the juice from *Atriplex halimus* (saltbush which has low energy, high water and electrolyte content and represents the basis of the food intake), as well as water extract and dialysate induce a significant decrease of glucose in diabetic sand rat [152]. The development of obesity is accompanied by hyperglycemia, hyperinsulinemia, decreased insulin sensitivity in adipose tissue and liver, and glucosuria, [153, 154]. Comparing with normoglycemic individuals, pancreatic β-cell volume begin to decrease in the obese and diabetic sand rats, as well as GLUT 2 glucose transporter on the cellular membrane and glucokinase in the cytoplasm of β-cells [155, 156]. Progressive loss of β-cells due to cell death is accompanied by hypoinsulinemia and persistent hyperglycemia, generating an irreversible diabetic state in sand rat. Proinflammatory cytokines such as IL-1β are not involved in producing deleterious effect on β-cells [157]. However, initiation of inflammation in sand rat NIDDM seems to be induced by other pathogenic pathways. For instance, a gene named Tanis (the Hebrew word for fasting) and expressed as hepatic receptor for serum amyloid A (SAA) is regulated by glucose and become dysfunctional when diabetes occur. Knowing that SAA and other acute-phase protein received special attention because their implication in cardiovascular disease, Tanis gene may provide answers for questions about the link between diabetes, inflammation and cardiovascular disease [158].

Nile rat (Arvicanthis niloticus) is a recently reported diet-induced model which expresses the features of both Metabolic Syndrome and NIDDM. Nile rats fed with current lab diet present characteristic signs as excessive abdominal adipose tissue, hyperglycemia, hyperinsulinemia, impaired peripheral insulin sensitivity, dyslipidemia (high level of cholesterol and triglycerides), microalbuminuria, and hypertension. Sex predilection was observed in males, which present segregation in two groups: early-onset diabetes and late-onset diabetes. Dietary modulation (high-fat diet) induce the early onset, as well as more accumulation of body fat [159].

7. Transgenic and knockout models used for research in diabetes mellitus

The specific techniques of molecular biology had a valuable contribution for the study of diabetes mellitus. As it was mentioned before, diabetes mellitus involves a considerable heterogeneity given by the multifactorial genetic and environmental conditions. Thus, interpretation of the results in a particular experiment is challenged by this complicated background. For this particular reason, the scientists have felt the need to create transgenic animal model which provide good conditions for studying the effect or implication of a specific gene and corresponding product according to physiological and environmental conditions. The most important outcomes of the transgenic animals are knowledge about gene regulation and development, pathogenesis of diabetes and new approaches in the therapy of this disease.

Transgenic animals, particularly mice, result from two basic techniques of genetic engineering. The first aims to transfer a gene (a new genetic material presented as a foreign DNA construct containing a regulatory region and a coding region for a protein), into the pronucleus of a fertilized ovocyte. After the gene inoculation, the modified ovocytes are transferred in the uterus of a foster mother for further development. After the birth, the pups are genetically scanned to verify whether the new genetic material was incorporated into the host genome. The animals which manifest the transgene are bred and the pups are also analyzed for the same DNA construct. Positive offspring of the second generation are further bred to establish a transgenic line for studying a particular transgenic phenotype. This revolutionary technique has both advantages and disadvantages. The major advantage is that the method enables to obtain transgenic animals with minimal cost and in a short time. The disadvantages are generated by the hazardous integration of the DNA construct in the genome of the host. The locus of integration, as well as the number of copies is unpredictable. Transgene phenotype expression is limited to use for studying a specific protein or RNA. Therefore, this protein will be overexpressed in the transgenic animal. If the target of experimentation is to reduce the expression of a protein, a RNA antisense transgene is used. It is noteworthy that this technique is also disadvantageous because of unpredictable complications and misinterpretation of the results [160].

The second method used for obtaining genetically engineered mice is focused on deleting a specific endogenous gene or gene fragment (knockout) and replacing with an exogenous DNA which present homologous sequences with the endogenous DNA fragment (homologous recombination). The engineered DNA fragment (a vector which is designed to produce a disruption in the target gene) is inoculated in an embryonic stem cell culture. The positive targeted cells are inoculated in a mouse embryo, which will be finally transferred into the uterus of a foster mother. If the experiment is successful, this embryonic stem cells will participate to generate germ cells and finally organs, all having the new recombinant gene [161].

Double transgenic mice can be obtained by maiting. Thus, the offspring of transgenic mice expressing the hemagglutinin of influenza virus under the insulin promoter and transgenic mice expressing T-lymphocytes with receptor for immunodominant epitope of the same virus present typical features for IDDM. The mice are hyperglycemic, hypoinsulinemic, present lymphocytic insulitis, glucosuria and poor bodily growth, features which are consistent with IDDM. The mortality is up to 90% at 3 months of age [162]. This line (TCR-HA Ins-HA) has consistent improvement glucose levels when treated with potato buds lectin [163, 164].

8. Conclusions

The experimentation in diabetes mellitus has known a long history, as well as a continuous and diverse development. Banting and Best as discoverers of insulin and Minkowski as the scientist who create the first experimental model of diabetes mellitus are truly recognized as the pioneers of the research in this area. Although the diversity of animal models created in the last fifty years is somehow overwhelming, their classification and usefulness follows the pathogenesis, corresponding lesions and subsequent complications recorded in human diabetes mellitus. The scientific literature describes many animal models of IDDM, NIDDM and secondary diabetes, although mice and rats are constantly used regardless the purpose of the research. It is easily noticed that the most famous research centers and laboratories developed their own experimental models and also provided genetic material for the creation of other colonies. Considering that hyperglycemia and glucosuria are two of the most important clinical signs of diabetes, some basic substances which induce these signs are described. Thus, Streptozotocin, Alloxan, Vacor, 8-hydroxyquinolone, Dithizone are usually used in experimentation which reproduce hyperglycemia, while phlorizin is recognized as a vegetal component which is responsible for glucosuria. The animal models of spontaneous diabetes mellitus are consistently represented by rodents, although other species as dog, cat, pig and primates are recommended. The research in NIDDM is sustained by experimental models divided in three major categories: obese, non-obese and diet-induced models. Molecular biology techniques have an important contribution in creation of transgenic animals for research the depth of the pathogenesis of diabetes mellitus.

Author details

Emilia Ciobotaru
University of Agronomic Science and Veterinary Medicine Bucharest Romania

9. References

[1] *The ethics of research involving animals*, 2005, Nuffield Council on Bioethics: http://www.nuffieldbioethics.org/animal-research.
[2] Flecknell, P., *Replacement, reduction and refinement.* ALTEX, 2002. 19(2): p. 73-8.
[3] Sechzer, J.A., *Historical issues concerning animal experimentation in the United States.* Soc Sci Med F, 1981. 15(1): p. 13-7.
[4] Nolen, R.S. *NIH suspends new chimp research grants. Agency adopts strict conditions set out in IOM report*. JAVMA News, 2012.

[5] Jörgens, V., *Oskar Minkowski (1858-1931). An outstanding master of diabetes research.* Hormones, 2006. 5(4): p. 310-311.

[6] Minkowski, O., *Perspectives in diabetes. Historical development of the theory of pancreatic diabetes (introduction and translation by Rachmiel Levine).* Diabetes, 1989. 38: p. 1-6.

[7] Simoni, R.D., R.L. Hill, and M. Vaughan, *The discovery of insulin: the work of Frederick Banting and Charles Best.* J Biol Chem, 2002. 277(26): p. 31-32.

[8] Scow, R.O., *"Total" pancreatectomy in the rat: operation, effects, and postoperative care.* Endocrinology, 1957. 60(3): p. 359-367.

[9] Kara, M.E., *The anatomical study on the rat pancreas and its ducts with emphasis on the surgical approach.* Ann Anat, 2005. 187(2): p. 105-12.

[10] Junod, A., et al., *Diabetogenic action of streptozotocin: relationship of dose to metabolic response.* J Clin Invest, 1969. 48(11): p. 2129-39.

[11] Lenzen, S., *The mechanisms of alloxan- and streptozotocin-induced diabetes.* Diabetologia, 2008. 51(2): p. 216-26.

[12] Esposti, M.D., A. Ngo, and M.A. Myers, *Inhibition of mitochondrial complex I may account for IDDM induced by intoxication with the rodenticide Vacor.* Diabetes, 1996. 45(11): p. 1531-4.

[13] Lazaris, J.A. and Z.E. Bavelsky, *Dithisone diabetes in rabbits and its prevention by sulfhydryl and imidazole containing compounds.* Endocrinol Exp, 1984. 18(3): p. 157-67.

[14] Rees, D.A. and J.C. Alcolado, *Animal models od diabetes mellitus.* Diabetic Medicine, 2005. 22: p. 359-370.

[15] Ciobotaru, E., et al., *Gravimetric and morphometric assessments in Wistar rats with experimental diabetes mellitus type 1 and cardiac failure.* Acta Veterinaria Beograd, 2008. 58(5-6): p. 583-592.

[16] Ciobotaru, E., et al., *Morphological chages of myocardial arterioles in rats with experimentally induced diabetes mellitus and cardiac failure (unpublished)*, 2012.

[17] Jamiolkowski, R.M., et al., *Islet transplantation in type I diabetes mellitus.* Yale J Biol Med, 2012. 85(1): p. 37-43.

[18] Reckard, C.R. and C.F. Barker, *Transplantation of isolated pancreatic islets across strong and weak histocompatibility barriers.* Transplant Proc, 1973. 5(1): p. 761-3.

[19] Ballinger, W.F. and P.E. Lacy, *Transplantation of intact pancreatic islets in rats.* Surgery, 1972. 72(2): p. 175-86.

[20] Kulseng, B., T. Espevik, and G. Skjak-Braek, *Treatment of diabetes mellitus with transplantation of immunoprotected pancreatic islet tissue.* Tidsskr Nor Laegeforen, 1999. 119(28): p. 4219-23.

[21] Kulseng, B., et al., *Transplantation of alginate microcapsules: generation of antibodies against alginates and encapsulated porcine islet-like cell clusters.* Transplantation, 1999. 67(7): p. 978-84.

[22] Rabanel, J.M., et al., *Progress technology in microencapsulation methods for cell therapy.* Biotechnol Prog, 2009. 25(4): p. 946-63.

[23] Fiedor, P.S., S.F. Oluwole, and M.A. Hardy, *Localization of endocrine pancreatic islets.* World J Surg, 1996. 20(8): p. 1016-22; discussion 1022-3.

[24] Franklin, W.A., J.A. Schulak, and C.R. Reckard, *The fate of transplanted pancreatic islets in the rat.* Am J Pathol, 1979. 94(1): p. 85-95.

[25] Ehrenkranz, J.R.L., et al., *Phlorizin: a review.* Diabetes-Metabolism Research and Reviews, 2005. 21(1): p. 31-38.

[26] Janssen, S.W., et al., *Phlorizin treatment prevents the decrease in plasma insulin levels but not the progressive histopathological changes in the pancreatic islets during aging of Zucker diabetic fatty rats.* J Endocrinol Invest, 2003. 26(6): p. 508-15.
[27] Bono, V.H., Jr., *Review of mechanism of action studies of the nitrosoureas.* Cancer Treat Rep, 1976. 60(6): p. 699-702.
[28] Meiramov, G.G. and N.I. Trukhanov, *[The ultrastructure of pancreatic beta cells in dithizone diabetes and its prevention by sodium diethyldithiocarbamate].* Probl Endokrinol (Mosk), 1975. 21(6): p. 92-5.
[29] Goldberg, E.D., V.A. Eshchenko, and V.D. Bovt, *The diabetogenic and acidotropic effects of chelators.* Exp Pathol, 1991. 42(1): p. 59-64.
[30] Makino, S., et al., *Breeding of a non-obese, diabetic strain of mice.* Jikken Dobutsu, 1980. 29(1): p. 1-13.
[31] Kikutani, H. and S. Makino, *The murine autoimmune diabetes model: NOD and related strains.* Adv Immunol, 1992. 51: p. 285-322.
[32] Ohneda, A., et al., *Insulin and glucagon in spontaneously diabetic non-obese mice.* Diabetologia, 1984. 27(4): p. 460-3.
[33] Conti, A. and G.J. Maestroni, *Role of the pineal gland and melatonin in the development of autoimmune diabetes in non-obese diabetic mice.* J Pineal Res, 1996. 20(3): p. 164-72.
[34] Jiang, F., et al., *Identification of QTLs that modify peripheral neuropathy in NOD.H2b-Pdcd1-/- mice.* Int Immunol, 2009. 21(5): p. 499-509.
[35] Cihakova, D., et al., *Animal models for autoimmune myocarditis and autoimmune thyroiditis.* Methods Mol Med, 2004. 102: p. 175-93.
[36] Rose, N.R., R. Bonita, and C.L. Burek, *Iodine: an environmental trigger of thyroiditis.* Autoimmun Rev, 2002. 1(1-2): p. 97-103.
[37] Bonifacio, E., et al., *International Workshop on Lessons From Animal Models for Human Type 1 Diabetes: identification of insulin but not glutamic acid decarboxylase or IA-2 as specific autoantigens of humoral autoimmunity in nonobese diabetic mice.* Diabetes, 2001. 50(11): p. 2451-8.
[38] Yoon, J.W. and H.S. Jun, *Cellular and molecular pathogenic mechanisms of insulin-dependent diabetes mellitus.* Ann N Y Acad Sci, 2001. 928: p. 200-11.
[39] Shieh, D.C., et al., *Insulin-dependent diabetes in the NOD mouse model. I. Detection and characterization of autoantibody bound to the surface of pancreatic beta cells prior to development of the insulitis lesion in prediabetic NOD mice.* Autoimmunity, 1993. 15(2): p. 123-35.
[40] Izumi, T., et al., *Dominant negative pathogenesis by mutant proinsulin in the Akita diabetic mouse.* Diabetes, 2003. 52(2): p. 409-16.
[41] Barber, A.J., et al., *The Ins2Akita mouse as a model of early retinal complications in diabetes.* Invest Ophthalmol Vis Sci, 2005. 46(6): p. 2210-8.
[42] Mathews, C.E., S.H. Langley, and E.H. Leiter, *New mouse model to study islet transplantation in insulin-dependent diabetes mellitus.* Transplantation, 2002. 73(8): p. 1333-6.
[43] Marliss, E.B., A.F. Nakhooda, and P. Poussier, *Clinical forms and natural history of the diabetic syndrome and insulin and glucagon secretion in the BB rat.* Metabolism, 1983. 32(7 Suppl 1): p. 11-7.
[44] Rossini, A.A., et al., *Spontaneous diabetes in the gnotobiotic BB/W rat.* Diabetes, 1979. 28(11): p. 1031-2.

[45] Lam-Tse, W.K., A. Lernmark, and H.A. Drexhage, *Animal models of endocrine/organ-specific autoimmune diseases: do they really help us to understand human autoimmunity?* Springer Semin Immunopathol, 2002. 24(3): p. 297-321.

[46] Like, A.A., et al., *Spontaneous diabetes mellitus: reversal and prevention in the BB/W rat with antiserum to rat lymphocytes.* Science, 1979. 206(4425): p. 1421-3.

[47] Bone, A.J., et al., *Insulitis and mechanisms of disease resistance: studies in an animal model of insulin dependent diabetes mellitus.* J Mol Med (Berl), 1999. 77(1): p. 57-61.

[48] Sternthal, E., et al., *Lymphocytic thyroiditis and diabetes in the BB/W rat. A new model of autoimmune endocrinopathy.* Diabetes, 1981. 30(12): p. 1058-61.

[49] Wallis, R.H., et al., *Type 1 diabetes in the BB rat: a polygenic disease.* Diabetes, 2009. 58(4): p. 1007-17.

[50] Leiter, E.H. and M. von Herrath, *Animal models have little to teach us about type 1 diabetes: 2. In opposition to this proposal.* Diabetologia, 2004. 47(10): p. 1657-60.

[51] Tsumura, H., et al., *Detection of endogenous retrovirus antigens in NOD mouse pancreatic beta-cells.* Lab Anim, 1998. 32(1): p. 86-94.

[52] Komeda, K., et al., *Establishment of two substrains, diabetes-prone and non-diabetic, from Long-Evans Tokushima Lean (LETL) rats.* Endocr J, 1998. 45(6): p. 737-44.

[53] Kawano, K., et al., *New inbred strain of Long-Evans Tokushima lean rats with IDDM without lymphopenia.* Diabetes, 1991. 40(11): p. 1375-81.

[54] Yokoi, N., et al., *A non-MHC locus essential for autoimmune type I diabetes in the Komeda Diabetes-Prone rat.* J Clin Invest, 1997. 100(8): p. 2015-21.

[55] Yokoi, N., et al., *Establishment and characterization of the Komeda diabetes-prone rat as a segregating inbred strain.* Exp Anim, 2003. 52(4): p. 295-301.

[56] Yokoi, N., *Identification of a major gene responsible for type 1 diabetes in the Komeda diabetes-prone rat.* Exp Anim, 2005. 54(2): p. 111-5.

[57] Conaway, H.H., et al., *Spontaneous diabetes mellitus in the New Zealand white rabbit: physiologic characteristics.* Metabolism, 1981. 30(1): p. 50-6.

[58] Roth, S.I., et al., *Spontaneous diabetes mellitus in the New Zealand white rabbit: preliminary morphologic characterization.* Lab Invest, 1980. 42(5): p. 571-9.

[59] Roth, S.I. and H.H. Conaway, *Animal model of human disease. Spontaneous diabetes mellitus in the New Zealand white rabbit.* Am J Pathol, 1982. 109(3): p. 359-63.

[60] Kramer, J.W., et al., *Inherited, early onset, insulin-requiring diabetes mellitus of Keeshond dogs.* Diabetes, 1980. 29(7): p. 558-65.

[61] Kramer, J.W., *Animal model of human disease: Inherited early-onset, insulin-requiring diabetes mellitus in keeshond dogs.* Am J Pathol, 1981. 105(2): p. 194-6.

[62] Meier, H. and G.A. Yerganian, *Spontaneous hereditary diabetes mellitus in Chinese hamster (Cricetulus griseus). 1. Pathological findings.* Proc Soc Exp Biol Med, 1959. 100(4): p. 810-5.

[63] Gerritsen, G.C., *The Chinese hamster as a model for the study of diabetes mellitus.* Diabetes, 1982. 31(Suppl 1 Pt 2): p. 14-23.

[64] Green, M.N., G. Yerganian, and H.J. Gagnon, *Prediction of spontaneous hereditary diabetes mellitus in Chinese hamsters by means of elevated alpha-2 serum levels.* Nature, 1963. 197: p. 396.

[65] Gerritsen, G.C. and W.E. Dulin, *Characterization of diabetes in the Chinese hamster.* Diabetologia, 1967. 3(2): p. 74-84.

[66] Luse, S.A., *The ultrastructure of the brain in the diabetic Chinese hamster with special reference to synaptic abnormalities.* Electroencephalogr Clin Neurophysiol, 1970. 29(4): p. 410.
[67] Poel, W.E. and G. Yerganian, *Adenocarcinoma of the pancreas in diabetes-prone Chinese hamsters.* Am J Med, 1961. 31: p. 861-3.
[68] Cohen, M.M., G. Shklar, and G. Yerganian, *Periodontal pathology in a strain of Chinese hamster, Cricetulus griseus, with hereditary diabetes mellitus.* Am J Med, 1961. 31: p. 864-7.
[69] McCombs, H.L., et al., *Morphologic changes in the aorta of the diabetic Chinese hamster.* Diabetologia, 1974. 10 Suppl: p. 601-6.
[70] Gerritsen, G.C., et al., *Epidemiology of Chinese hamsters and preliminary evidence for genetic heterogeneity of diabetes.* Diabetologia, 1974. 10 Suppl: p. 581-8.
[71] Fletcher-McGruder, B.L. and G.C. Gerritsen, *Deficient humoral antibody response of the spontaneously diabetic Chinese hamster.* Proc Soc Exp Biol Med, 1984. 175(1): p. 74-8.
[72] Diani, A.R., et al., *Systematic evaluation of microangiopathy in diabetic Chinese hamsters. I. Morphometric analysis of minimal glomerular basement membrane thickness in 11- to 15- and 19- to 23-month-old Chinese hamsters.* Microvasc Res, 1986. 31(3): p. 306-16.
[73] Donath, M.Y., et al., *Islet inflammation impairs the pancreatic beta-cell in type 2 diabetes.* Physiology (Bethesda), 2009. 24: p. 325-31.
[74] Donath, M.Y., et al., *Islet inflammation in type 2 diabetes: from metabolic stress to therapy.* Diabetes Care, 2008. 31 Suppl 2: p. S161-4.
[75] Bellinger, D.A., E.P. Merricks, and T.C. Nichols, *Swine models of type 2 diabetes mellitus: insulin resistance, glucose tolerance, and cardiovascular complications.* ILAR J, 2006. 47(3): p. 243-58.
[76] Hoenig, M., et al., *A feline model of experimentally induced islet amyloidosis.* Am J Pathol, 2000. 157(6): p. 2143-50.
[77] Wagner, J.E., et al., *Old world nonhuman primate models of type 2 diabetes mellitus.* ILAR J, 2006. 47(3): p. 259-71.
[78] Ingalls, A.M., M.M. Dickie, and G.D. Snell, *Obese, a new mutation in the house mouse.* J Hered, 1950. 41(12): p. 317-8.
[79] McGarry, J.D., *Appetite control: Does leptin lighten the problem of obesity?* Curr Biol, 1995. 5(12): p. 1342-4.
[80] Tassava, T.M., T. Okuda, and D.R. Romsos, *Insulin secretion from ob/ob mouse pancreatic islets: effects of neurotransmitters.* Am J Physiol, 1992. 262(3 Pt 1): p. E338-43.
[81] Chen, N.G., T.M. Tassava, and D.R. Romsos, *Threshold for glucose-stimulated insulin secretion in pancreatic islets of genetically obese (ob/ob) mice is abnormally low.* J Nutr, 1993. 123(9): p. 1567-74.
[82] Serke, H., et al., *Leptin-deficient (ob/ob) mouse ovaries show fatty degeneration, enhanced apoptosis and decreased expression of steroidogenic acute regulatory enzyme.* Int J Obes (Lond), 2011.
[83] Takeshita, S., et al., *Amelioration of insulin resistance in diabetic ob/ob mice by a new type of orally active insulin-mimetic vanadyl complex: bis(1-oxy-2-pyridinethiolato)oxovanadium(IV) with VO(S(2)O(2)) coordination mode.* J Inorg Biochem, 2001. 85(2-3): p. 179-86.
[84] Xu, J., et al., *Hypoglycemic effects of MDG-1, a polysaccharide derived from Ophiopogon japonicas, in the ob/ob mouse model of type 2 diabetes mellitus.* Int J Biol Macromol, 2011. 49(4): p. 657-62.

[85] Kim, S.W., et al., *Proteomic analysis in ob/ob mice before and after hypoglycemic polysaccharide treatments.* J Microbiol Biotechnol, 2009. 19(10): p. 1109-21.

[86] Mazumder, P.K., et al., *Impaired cardiac efficiency and increased fatty acid oxidation in insulin-resistant ob/ob mouse hearts.* Diabetes, 2004. 53(9): p. 2366-74.

[87] Drel, V.R., et al., *The leptin-deficient (ob/ob) mouse: a new animal model of peripheral neuropathy of type 2 diabetes and obesity.* Diabetes, 2006. 55(12): p. 3335-43.

[88] Chen, H., et al., *Evidence that the diabetes gene encodes the leptin receptor: identification of a mutation in the leptin receptor gene in db/db mice.* Cell, 1996. 84(3): p. 491-5.

[89] Hummel, K.P., M.M. Dickie, and D.L. Coleman, *Diabetes, a new mutation in the mouse.* Science, 1966. 153(3740): p. 1127-8.

[90] Kobayashi, K., et al., *The db/db mouse, a model for diabetic dyslipidemia: molecular characterization and effects of Western diet feeding.* Metabolism, 2000. 49(1): p. 22-31.

[91] Sharma, K., P. McCue, and S.R. Dunn, *Diabetic kidney disease in the db/db mouse.* Am J Physiol Renal Physiol, 2003. 284(6): p. F1138-44.

[92] Taketomi, S., *KK and KKA y Mice*, in *Animal models of diabetes, Second Edition*, E. Shafrir, Editor 2007, CRC Press Taylor & Francis Group: USA. p. 335-348.

[93] Reddi, A.S. and R.A. Camerini-Davalos, *Hereditary diabetes in the KK mouse: an overview.* Adv Exp Med Biol, 1988. 246: p. 7-15.

[94] Nonogaki, K., K. Nozue, and Y. Oka, *Social isolation affects the development of obesity and type 2 diabetes in mice.* Endocrinology, 2007. 148(10): p. 4658-66.

[95] Ikeda, H., *KK mouse.* Diabetes Res Clin Pract, 1994. 24 Suppl: p. S313-6.

[96] Suto, J., et al., *Genetic analysis of non-insulin-dependent diabetes mellitus in KK and KK-Ay mice.* Eur J Endocrinol, 1998. 139(6): p. 654-61.

[97] Radavelli-Bagatini, S., et al., *The New Zealand obese mouse model of obesity insulin resistance and poor breeding performance: evaluation of ovarian structure and function.* J Endocrinol, 2011. 209(3): p. 307-15.

[98] Melez, K.A., et al., *Diabetes is associated with autoimmunity in the New Zealand obese (NZO) mouse.* Diabetes, 1980. 29(10): p. 835-40.

[99] Breyer, M.D., et al., *Mouse models of diabetic nephropathy.* J Am Soc Nephrol, 2005. 16(1): p. 27-45.

[100] Melez, K.A., et al., *Immune abnormalities in the diabetic New Zealand obese (NZO) mouse: insulin treatment partially suppresses splenic hyperactivity measured by flow cytometric analysis.* Clin Immunol Immunopathol, 1985. 36(1): p. 110-9.

[101] Mirhashemi, F., et al., *Diet dependence of diabetes in the New Zealand Obese (NZO) mouse: total fat, but not fat quality or sucrose accelerates and aggravates diabetes.* Exp Clin Endocrinol Diabetes, 2011. 119(3): p. 167-71.

[102] Jurgens, H.S., et al., *Hyperphagia, lower body temperature, and reduced running wheel activity precede development of morbid obesity in New Zealand obese mice.* Physiol Genomics, 2006. 25(2): p. 234-41.

[103] Haskell, B.D., et al., *The diabetes-prone NZO/HlLt strain. I. Immunophenotypic comparison to the related NZB/BlNJ and NZW/LacJ strains.* Lab Invest, 2002. 82(7): p. 833-42.

[104] Pan, H.J., et al., *Pharmacogenetic analysis of rosiglitazone-induced hepatosteatosis in new mouse models of type 2 diabetes.* Diabetes, 2005. 54(6): p. 1854-62.

[105] Ikegami, H., T. Fujisawa, and T. Ogihara, *Mouse models of type 1 and type 2 diabetes derived from the same closed colony: genetic susceptibility shared between two types of diabetes.* ILAR J, 2004. 45(3): p. 268-77.

[106] Ueda, H., et al., *Genetic analysis of late-onset type 2 diabetes in a mouse model of human complex trait.* Diabetes, 1999. 48(5): p. 1168-74.

[107] Ueda, H., et al., *The NSY mouse: a new animal model of spontaneous NIDDM with moderate obesity.* Diabetologia, 1995. 38(5): p. 503-8.

[108] Shimizu, K., et al., *Spontaneous amyloidosis in senile NSY mice.* Acta Pathol Jpn, 1993. 43(5): p. 215-21.

[109] Han, W. and C. Li, *Linking type 2 diabetes and Alzheimer's disease.* Proc Natl Acad Sci U S A, 2010. 107(15): p. 6557-8.

[110] Buck, D.W., 2nd and T.A. Mustoe, *Reply: TallyHo Diabetic Phenotype Limited to Male Mice: Female Mice Provide Obese, Nondiabetic Mouse Model.* Plast Reconstr Surg, 2012. 129(4): p. 727e-8e.

[111] Kim, J.H., et al., *Genetic analysis of a new mouse model for non-insulin-dependent diabetes.* Genomics, 2001. 74(3): p. 273-86.

[112] Kim, J.H., et al., *Type 2 diabetes mouse model TallyHo carries an obesity gene on chromosome 6 that exaggerates dietary obesity.* Physiol Genomics, 2005. 22(2): p. 171-81.

[113] Sung, Y.Y., et al., *Glucose intolerance in young TallyHo mice is induced by leptin-mediated inhibition of insulin secretion.* Biochem Biophys Res Commun, 2005. 338(4): p. 1779-87.

[114] Kim, J.H., et al., *Phenotypic characterization of polygenic type 2 diabetes in TALLYHO/JngJ mice.* J Endocrinol, 2006. 191(2): p. 437-46.

[115] Didion, S.P., C.M. Lynch, and F.M. Faraci, *Cerebral vascular dysfunction in TallyHo mice: a new model of Type II diabetes.* Am J Physiol Heart Circ Physiol, 2007. 292(3): p. H1579-83.

[116] Cheng, Z.J., et al., *Vascular dysfunction in type 2 diabetic TallyHo mice: role for an increase in the contribution of PGH2/TxA2 receptor activation and cytochrome p450 products.* Can J Physiol Pharmacol, 2007. 85(3-4): p. 404-12.

[117] Suzuki, W., et al., *A new mouse model of spontaneous diabetes derived from ddY strain.* Exp Anim, 1999. 48(3): p. 181-9.

[118] Iizuka, S., et al., *Diabetic complications in a new animal model (TSOD mouse) of spontaneous NIDDM with obesity.* Exp Anim, 2005. 54(1): p. 71-83.

[119] Miura, T., et al., *Impairment of insulin-stimulated GLUT4 translocation in skeletal muscle and adipose tissue in the Tsumura Suzuki obese diabetic mouse: a new genetic animal model of type 2 diabetes.* Eur J Endocrinol, 2001. 145(6): p. 785-90.

[120] Allan, M.F., E.J. Eisen, and D. Pomp, *The M16 mouse: an outbred animal model of early onset polygenic obesity and diabesity.* Obes Res, 2004. 12(9): p. 1397-407.

[121] Connelly, D.M. and P.V. Taberner, *Characterization of the spontaneous diabetes obesity syndrome in mature male CBA/Ca mice.* Pharmacol Biochem Behav, 1989. 34(2): p. 255-9.

[122] Figueroa, C.D. and P.V. Taberner, *Pancreatic islet hypertrophy in spontaneous maturity onset obese-diabetic CBA/Ca mice.* Int J Biochem, 1994. 26(10-11): p. 1299-303.

[123] Finegood, D.T., et al., *Beta-cell mass dynamics in Zucker diabetic fatty rats. Rosiglitazone prevents the rise in net cell death.* Diabetes, 2001. 50(5): p. 1021-9.

[124] Unger, R.H., *How obesity causes diabetes in Zucker diabetic fatty rats.* Trends Endocrinol Metab, 1997. 8(7): p. 276-82.

[125] Wind, D.S. *Type 2 diabetes, obesity, and bumblefoot: a possible correlation?* 2003 [cited 2012 24.04.].

[126] Pick, A., et al., *Role of apoptosis in failure of beta-cell mass compensation for insulin resistance and beta-cell defects in the male Zucker diabetic fatty rat.* Diabetes, 1998. 47(3): p. 358-64.

[127] Finegood, D.T. and B.G. Topp, *beta-cell deterioration - prospects for reversal or prevention.* Diabetes Obes Metab, 2001. 3 Suppl 1: p. 20-27.

[128] Kawano, K., et al., *Spontaneously diabetic rat "OLETF" as a model of NIDDM in humans,* in *Lessons from animal diabetes VI,* E. Shafrir, Editor 1996, Birkhausser Boston: USA. p. 225-236.

[129] Kawano, K., et al., *OLETF (Otsuka Long-Evans Tokushima Fatty) rat: a new NIDDM rat strain.* Diabetes Res Clin Pract, 1994. 24 Suppl: p. S317-20.

[130] Kawano, K., et al., *Examination of the pathogenesis of diabetic nephropathy in OLETF rats.* J Vet Med Sci, 1999. 61(11): p. 1219-28.

[131] Velasque, M.T., S.J. Bhathena, and C.T. Hansen, *Leptin and its relation to obesity and insulin in the SHR/N-corpulent rat, a model of type II diabetes mellitus.* Int J Exp Diabetes Res, 2001. 2(3): p. 217-23.

[132] Russell, J.C., et al., *Insulin resistance and impaired glucose tolerance in the atherosclerosis-prone LA/N corpulent rat.* Arteriosclerosis, 1987. 7(6): p. 620-6.

[133] Brindley, D.N., et al., *Sustained decreases in weight and serum insulin, glucose, triacylglycerol and cholesterol in JCR:LA-corpulent rats treated with D-fenfluramine.* Br J Pharmacol, 1992. 105(3): p. 679-85.

[134] Brindley, D.N. and J.C. Russell, *Metabolic abnormalities linked to obesity: effects of dexfenfluramine in the corpulent rat.* Metabolism, 1995. 44(2 Suppl 2): p. 23-7.

[135] Russell, J.C., et al., *Cardioprotective effect of probucol in the atherosclerosis-prone JCR:LA-cp rat.* Eur J Pharmacol, 1998. 350(2-3): p. 203-10.

[136] Gauguier, D., et al., *Chromosomal mapping of genetic loci associated with non-insulin dependent diabetes in the GK rat.* Nat Genet, 1996. 12(1): p. 38-43.

[137] Galli, J., et al., *Pathophysiological and genetic characterization of the major diabetes locus in GK rats.* Diabetes, 1999. 48(12): p. 2463-70.

[138] Zhou, H., et al., *Network screening of Goto-Kakizaki rat liver microarray data during diabetic progression.* BMC Syst Biol, 2011. 5(Suppl 1): p. S1-S16.

[139] Schrijvers, B.F., et al., *Long-term renal changes in the Goto-Kakizaki rat, a model of lean type 2 diabetes.* Nephrol Dial Transplant, 2004. 19(5): p. 1092-7.

[140] Wada, R., et al., *Effects of long-term treatment with alpha-glucosidase inhibitor on the peripheral nerve function and structure in Goto-Kakizaki rats: a genetic model for type 2 diabetes.* Diabetes Metab Res Rev, 1999. 15(5): p. 332-7.

[141] Murakawa, Y., et al., *Impaired glucose tolerance and insulinopenia in the GK-rat causes peripheral neuropathy.* Diabetes Metab Res Rev, 2002. 18(6): p. 473-83.

[142] Ahmad, T., et al., *Skeletal changes in type-2 diabetic Goto-Kakizaki rats.* J Endocrinol, 2003. 178(1): p. 111-6.

[143] Sone, H., et al., *Ocular vascular endothelial growth factor levels in diabetic rats are elevated before observable retinal proliferative changes.* Diabetologia, 1997. 40(6): p. 726-30.

[144] Yatoh, S., et al., *Antioxidants and an inhibitor of advanced glycation ameliorate death of retinal microvascular cells in diabetic retinopathy.* Diabetes Metab Res Rev, 2006. 22(1): p. 38-45.

[145] Shinohara, M., et al., *A new spontaneously diabetic non-obese Torii rat strain with severe ocular complications.* Int J Exp Diabetes Res, 2000. 1(2): p. 89-100.

[146] Sasase, T., *Pathophysiological characteristics of diabetic ocular complications in spontaneously diabetic torii rat.* J Ophthalmol, 2010. 2010: p. 615641.

[147] Yokoi, N., M. Fuse, and S. Seino, *Genetics of the spontaneously diabetic Torii rat.* The Open Diabetes Journal, 2011. 4: p. 21-25.

[148] Weksler-Zangen, S., et al., *The newly inbred cohen diabetic rat: a nonobese normolipidemic genetic model of diet-induced type 2 diabetes expressing sex differences.* Diabetes, 2001. 50(11): p. 2521-9.

[149] Yagil, C., et al., *Metabolic and genomic dissection of diabetes in the Cohen rat.* Physiol Genomics, 2007. 29(2): p. 181-92.

[150] Hammes, H.P., et al., *Islet transplantation inhibits diabetic retinopathy in the sucrose-fed diabetic Cohen rat.* Invest Ophthalmol Vis Sci, 1993. 34(6): p. 2092-6.

[151] Yagil, C., et al., *Nonproteinuric diabetes-associated nephropathy in the Cohen rat model of type 2 diabetes.* Diabetes, 2005. 54(5): p. 1487-96.

[152] Aharonson, Z., J. Shani, and F.G. Sulman, *Hypoglycaemic effect of the salt bush (Atriplex halimus)--a feeding source of the sand rat (Psammomys Obesus).* Diabetologia, 1969. 5(6): p. 379-83.

[153] Frenkel, G., P.F. Kraicer, and J. Shani, *Diabetes in the sand-rat: diabetogenesis, responses to mannoheptulose and atriplex ash.* Diabetologia, 1972. 8(5): p. 313-8.

[154] De Fronzo, R., E. Miki, and J. Steinke, *Diabetic syndrome in sand rat.* Diabetologia, 1967. 3(2): p. 140-142.

[155] Donev, S., et al., *Immunohistochemical investigations of the endocrine pancreas in normoglycemic sand rats (Psammomys obesus).* Acta Diabetol Lat, 1989. 26(4): p. 309-13.

[156] Jorns, A., et al., *Gradual loss of pancreatic beta-cell insulin, glucokinase and GLUT2 glucose transporter immunoreactivities during the time course of nutritionally induced type-2 diabetes in Psammomys obesus (sand rat).* Virchows Arch, 2002. 440(1): p. 63-9.

[157] Jorns, A., et al., *Beta cell death in hyperglycaemic Psammomys obesus is not cytokine-mediated.* Diabetologia, 2006. 49(11): p. 2704-12.

[158] Walder, K., et al., *Tanis: a link between type 2 diabetes and inflammation?* Diabetes, 2002. 51(6): p. 1859-66.

[159] Chaabo, F., et al., *Nutritional correlates and dynamics of diabetes in the Nile rat (Arvicanthis niloticus): a novel model for diet-induced type 2 diabetes and the metabolic syndrome.* Nutr Metab (Lond), 2010. 7: p. 29.

[160] Livingston, J.N., *Genetically engineered mice in drug development.* J Intern Med, 1999. 245(6): p. 627-35.

[161] Bronson, S.K. and O. Smithies, *Altering mice by homologous recombination using embryonic stem cells.* J Biol Chem, 1994. 269(44): p. 27155-8.

[162] Radu, D.L., et al., *Double transgenic mice with type 1 diabetes mellitus develop somatic, metabolic and vascular disorders.* J Cell Mol Med, 2004. 8(3): p. 349-58.

[163] Ciobotaru, E., et al., *Histological aspects in TCR-HA Ins-HA double transgenic mice treated with potato buds lectin*, in *24th Meeting of European Society of Veterinary Pathology*2006: Edinburgh. p. 135.

[164] Pop, A., et al., *Potato buds lectin reduces hyperglicemia in TCR-HA, INS-HA duble transgenic mice.* Buletin USAMV Cluj Napoca, 2005. 62: p. 259-261.